Insect Pests of Vegetable, Spice and Ornamental Crops

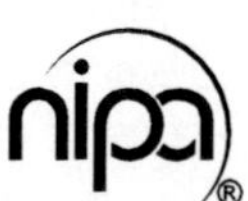

NIPA® GENX ELECTRONIC RESOURCES & SOLUTIONS P. LTD.
New Delhi-110 034

About the Authors

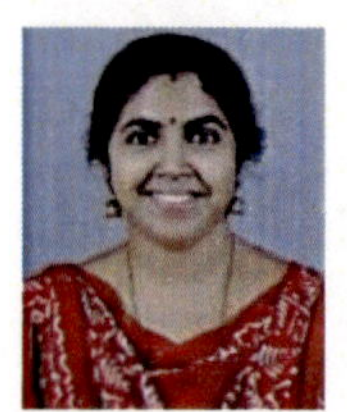

Dr. Deepthy K.B completed graduation, post-graduation, and Ph.D, from Kerala Agricultural University. She has published 20 peer-reviewed research articles, 11 symposium proceedings 4 book chapters, and 8 popular articles. She has successfully completed 8 external-aided projects as Principal Investigator (PI) and 3 as Co-Principal Investigator (Co-PI). She has guided 6 postgraduate students and 1 Ph.D. scholar to the successful completion of their research work. At present, she is nurturing the academic growth of 4 postgraduate and 2 Ph.D. students.

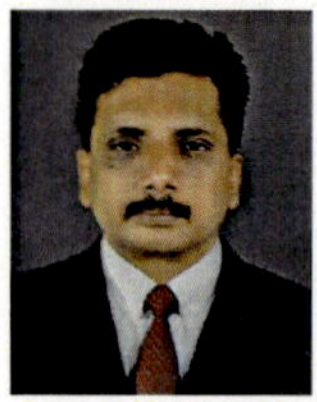

Dr. Pradeepkumar T. took PhD in Horticulture from IARI New Delhi and undergone overseas training at University of Wisconsin, USA. He is holding the charge of Vice Chancellor Kerala University of Fisheries and Ocean Studies, Kochin, Kerala and working as Professor and Head, Department of Vegetable Science, Kerala Agricultural University. Dr Pradeepkumar. T has experience of more than 30 years in horticultural research, teaching and extension as state and national level expert. He has developed 8 hybrids of different crops like water melon (Seedless types), salad cucumber (Parthenocarpic type), bitter gourd and ridge gourd. He was the editor of Journal of Tropical Agricul- ture for six years and reviewer of springer and elseiver publications. He is the recipient of Krishi vijnan award for the best agricultural scientist instituted by Govt. of Kerala and Harbhajan Singh Award by ISVS. He has published 9 2 research papers, 12 books, 18 book chapters and 45 popular article . He is fellow of , Indian Society of Vegetable Science (ISVS), Indian Academy of Horticultural Science (IAHS) and Indian Society for Spices (ISS).

Insect Pests of Vegetable Spice and Ornamental Crops

Deepthy K.B.
Pradeep Kumar T.

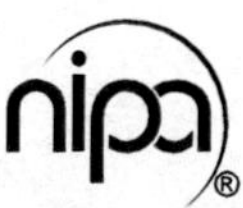

NIPA® GENX ELECTRONIC RESOURCES & SOLUTIONS P. LTD.
New Delhi-110 034

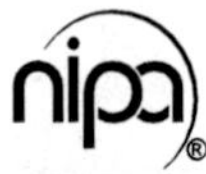

NIPA® GENX ELECTRONIC RESOURCES & SOLUTIONS P. LTD.

101,103, Vikas Surya Plaza, CU Block
L.S.C. Market, Pitam Pura, New Delhi-110 034
Ph : +91-11-43860225, Mob.: +91 9717133558, 9540816132
E-mail: newindiapublishingagency@gmail.com
Website: www.nipaersources.com

Print ISBN: 978-93-58871-67-8
ebook ISBN: 978-93-58872-54-5

Composed and Designed by NIPA®.

Preface

Pests are one of the most enduring and constantly changing issues in the agricultural industry, threatening the health, yield, and quality of crops, leading to significant economic losses for farmers, gardeners, and horticulturists alike. Despite being a normal component of the ecosystem, pests have a significant and frequently disastrous effect on vegetables, spices and ornamental plants.

Because of their short growing season, high yield, nutritional value, economic feasibility, and capacity to produce both on- and off-farm income, vegetables are crucial components of Indian agriculture and nutritional security. Vegetables are generally low in calories yet high in nutrients, including vitamins, minerals, and fibres. They also contain natural compounds known as antioxidants, which help protect our cells from damage. In 2023–2024, India exported approximately \$708 million worth of processed vegetables and over \$1.345 billion worth of raw vegetables. Insect pests pose a major threat to the production and productivity of vegetable crops.

Spices and condiments are a significant category of horticultural products and have long been considered essential in the culinary arts for adding flavor to meals. Some have colourant, preservative, antioxidant, antibacterial, and antibiotic qualities, while others are utilised in the pharmaceutical, cosmetic, and fragrance industries, among other sectors. They play a crucial role in the national economies of India contributing an export earnings of US\$ 4.46 billion during 2023-24. Major reason for the low productivity of spices in India is the incidence of pests and diseases.

Recently, India has become a prominent player in international ornamental business with an export earning of Rs. 575 crores in 2020-21 and Rs.777.4 crores during 2021-22, an increase of 34%. Major bottle neck in the production of ornamental crops is the presence of pests leading to a huge yield loss.

This book is a comprehensive guide aimed at addressing the challenges posed pests by providing a detailed and practical understanding of the insect pests and mites that affect vegetables, spices, and ornamental plants. This book mainly focusses on identification, biology, behaviour, and management techniques and serves as an essential resource for anybody dedicated to protecting crops and advancing sustainable agricultural practices, including students, farmers, researchers and agricultural extension officials.

In order to ensure the long-term survival of our crops and landscapes, this book highlights the significance of a comprehensive approach that strikes a balance between ecological health and efficient pest control by providing insights into integrated pest management (IPM).

We hope this book serves as a valuable resource and a guide toward healthier, more resilient plants in the gardens, fields, and greenhouses of tomorrow.

Authors

Contents

Pests of Vegetables

1

Pests of Amaranthus

Amaranthus is an important leafy vegetable and is grown all over the Indian subcontinent. *Amaranthus tricolor* Linn and *A. blittum* Linn. are the common varieties cultivated. These herbaceous annuals are a rich source of proteins, vitamins A and C, and iron. The foliage is a good source of calcium, iron, and vitamins A, B, and C. In contrast, grains are good sources of important amino acids, particularly lysine, and are rich in dietary fibre, calcium, and minerals such as iron, magnesium, phosphorus, copper, and manganese. It enhances the body's immune system and antioxidant status while lowering blood pressure and cholesterol. Fresh leaves and tender stems are used as vegetables. Production of amaranthus is affected by the incidence of pests. Cultivated amaranth is currently infested by a total of 92 different insect pests. (Rajeshkanna *et al*., 2017) among which the leaf webbers and amaranthus stem weevil are the most important pests.

Sl. No.	Common name	Scientific name	Family and Order	Site of oviposition	Site of pupation
			Webbers		
1	Leaf webber	*Hymenia/Spoladea recurvalis*	Crambidae, Lepidoptera	Leaves	Leaf webs
2	Leaf webber	*Psara / Herpetogramma basalis*	Crambidae, Lepidoptera	Leaves	Leaf webs
3	Leaf webber	*Eretmocera impactella*	Scythrididae, Lepidoptera	Leaves	Leaf webs
			Borers		
4	Amaranthus weevil	*Hypolixus truncatulus*	Curculionidae, Coleoptera	Stems, branches, petioles or mid ribs	Ground level or at the axil of a branch
			Defoliators		
5	Semilooper	*Plusia / Argyrogramma signata*	Noctuidae, Lepidoptera	Leaves	Within folded leaves/plant / soil
6	Hairy caterpillar	*Spilosoma / Diacrisia obliqua*	Erebidae, Lepidoptera	Leaves	Soil

Leaf Webber : *Hymenia/Spoladea recurvalis Fabricius*

Family : Crambidae

Order : Lepidoptera

Biology: Black moth with dark brown wings bearing white wavy markings on wings. Eggs are laid singly on leaves. Egg period 3 to 4 days. Larval duration will be completed within a period of 2 weeks. Pupation occurs among the leaf webbings and pupal duration lasts for 10 days. Several larvae can be seen inside each leaf web.

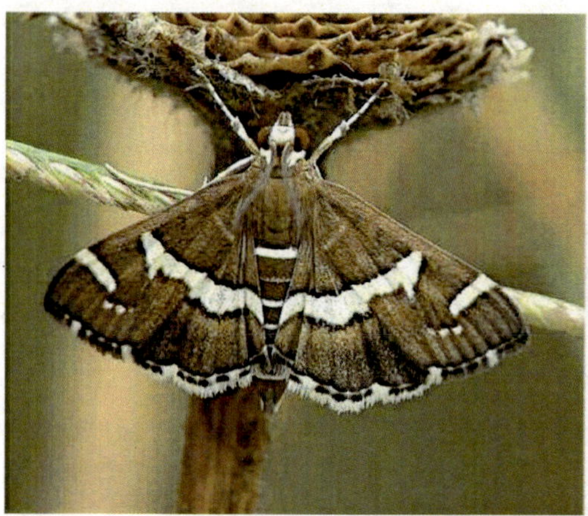

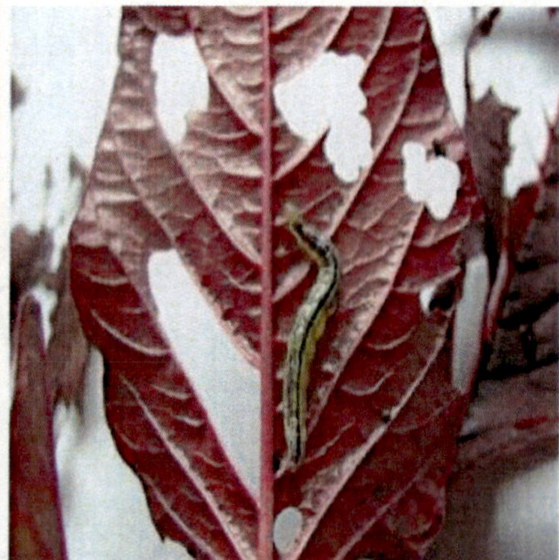

Adult and larvae of *Spoladea recurvalis* showing damage symptoms

Leaf Webber : *Psara / Herpetogramma basalis* Walker

Family : Crambidae

Order : Lepidoptera

The moth has yellow wings with faint black dots. The caterpillars are greenish in colour with five larval instars and are voracious feeders. Larvae usually web the leaves together and feed from within. Pupae can also be seen inside the webbings.

Nature of damage

Larvae cause damage to the plant by webbing the leaves and feeding from within the webbings. They skeletonise the leaves completely.

Symptoms

- Webbing of leaves and skeletonisation

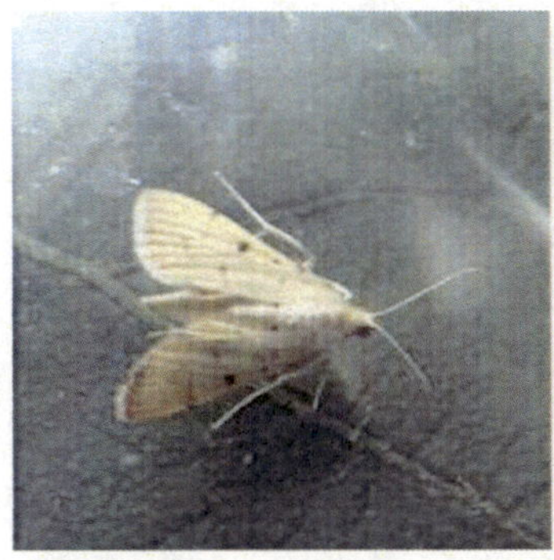
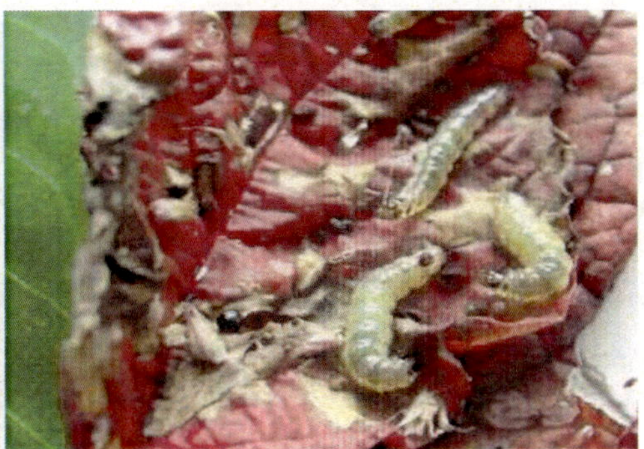

Adult and larvae of *Herpetogramma basalis* showing damage symptoms

Leaf Webber : *Eretmocera impactella* Walker

Family : Scythrididae

Order : Lepidoptera

Larvae roll the leaves and web the adjacent leaves together forming a web and feed by scraping chlorophyll. Several larvae and pupae can be seen inside the leaf webs.

Management of leaf webbers

- Collect and destroy the caterpillars
- As far as possible, avoid use of insecticides
- In severe cases, spray malathion 50EC @ 2 ml/l

Amaranthus Weevil : *Hypolixus truncatulus* F.

Order : Coleoptera

Family : Curculionidae

Distribution and status: Specific major pest. Widely distributed in India and neighbouring countries. It attacks both wild and cultivated crops and leafy vegetables with large leaves.

Biology: Medium sized ashy-grey weevil with white dots on the elytra. Eggs are laid singly in holes made in stems, branches, petioles or mid ribs. A single female lays about 30 eggs and incubation period is 2 to 4 days during Summer and 10-12 days during Winter (Srivastava and Butani, 2009). Grub tunnels within the stem and branches feeding on the internal tissues. Grub period lasts for 12 -24 days depending upon the prevailing weather conditions. It pupates in a cell at the ground level or the axil of a branch. The adult, upon emergence, remains within the stem for 5-6 days and then cuts the epidermal membrane before emerging. Weevils cause damage by feeding on leaves.

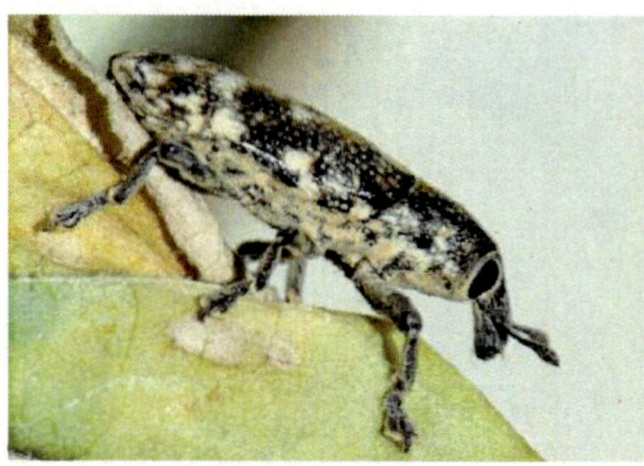

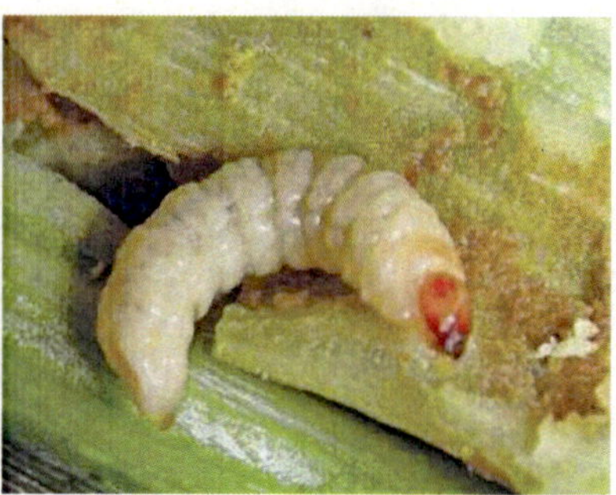

Adult and grub of *Hypolixus truncatulus*

Nature of damage

- Both adults and grubs cause damage
- Grubs bore into the stems feed on pith region causing irregular zigzag tunnels and finally girdle the stems
- The adult cause damage by feeding on leaves and tender stems

Symptoms of damage

- Inside the stem, tunneling by stout creamy white grubs can be seen with frass
- Irregular zigzag tunnels filled with excreta
- In severe cases, plants show yellowing of leaves and wilting
- A single plant may contain 17-18 grubs causing it to rapture and break off
- In affected plants, gall like swellings can be observed on the stem which is scarred with longitudinal white markings

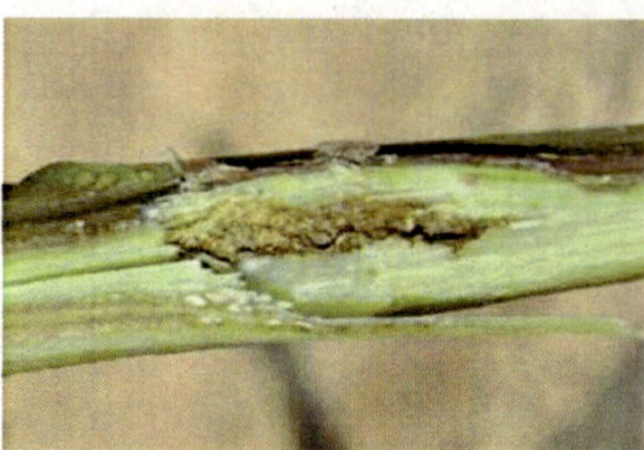

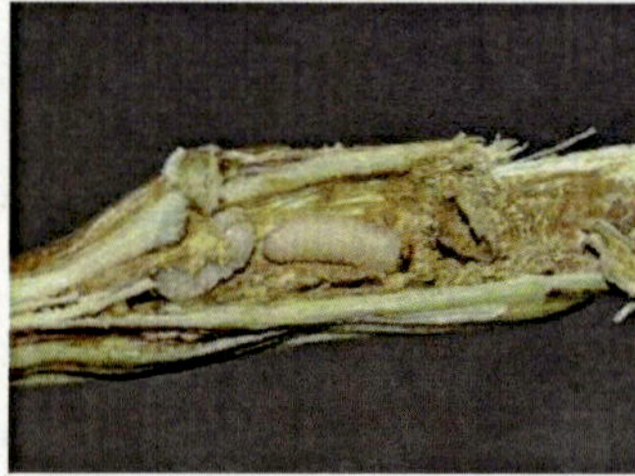

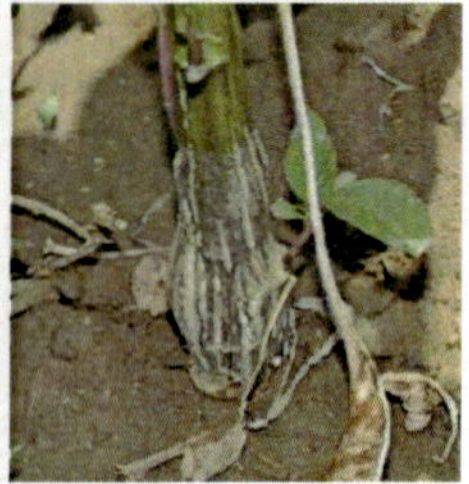

Symptoms of damage by *Hypolixus truncatulus*

Management

- Destroy the wild amaranthus seen near the field as these act as alternate hosts to the weevil.

- Destroy the affected plants along with the grubs and pupae to reduce the intensity of the pest attack.
- If the infestation is severe apply malathion 50EC @ 2 ml/l

Semilooper : *Plusia / Argyrogramma signata* F.

Family : Noctuidae

Order : Lepidoptera

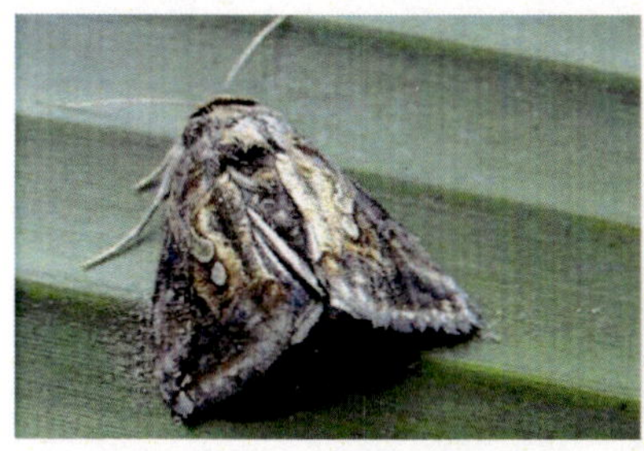
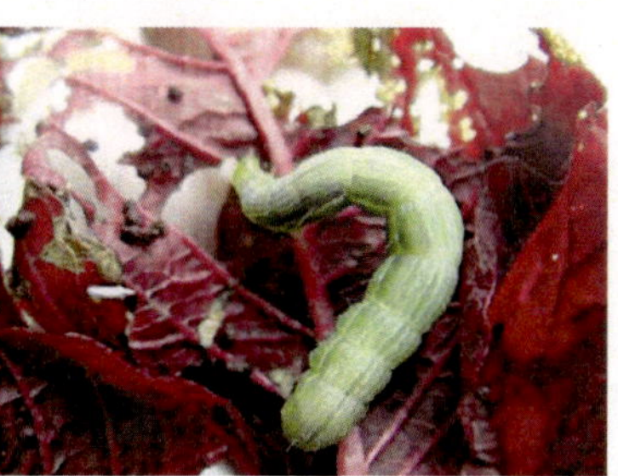

Adult and larva of *Plusia signata*

Hairy caterpillar : *Spilosoma /Diacrisia obliqua* Walker

Family : Erebidae

Order : Lepidoptera

Biology: Polyphagous pest. The moth is yellowish in colour. The head thorax and under side of the body are dull yellow. The antennae and eyes are black. The female lays 400 to 1000 eggs. Eggs are spherical and are laid in clusters. Egg period is 8 to 12 days.

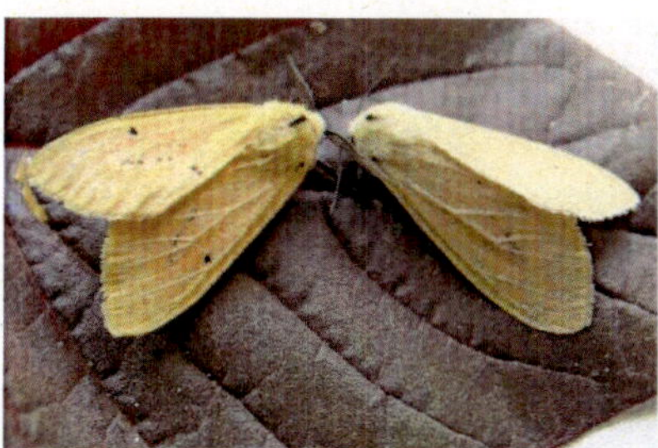
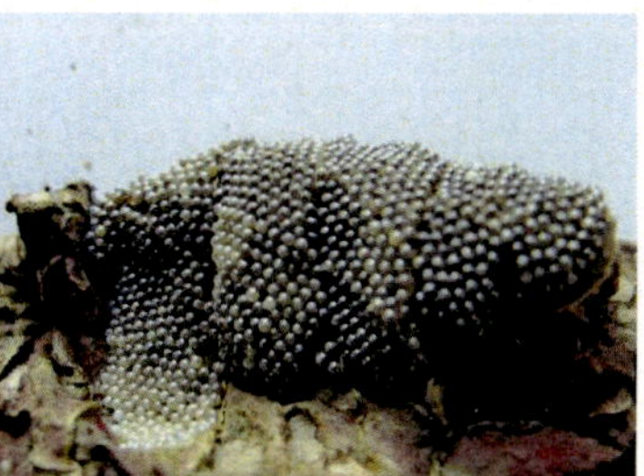

Adults and eggs of *Spilosoma obliqua*

Emerging caterpillars feed gregariously. When grown they disperse widely in search of food. They undergo 7 instars within a period of 4 to 8 weeks. The caterpillar is profusely covered with long grayish hair. When full grown, caterpillar spin loose silken cocoon for pupation. Pupal period is 1 to 2 weeks. Moth lives for about a week. The life cycle is completed in 6 to 12 weeks and the pest passes through 3 to 4 broods in a year.

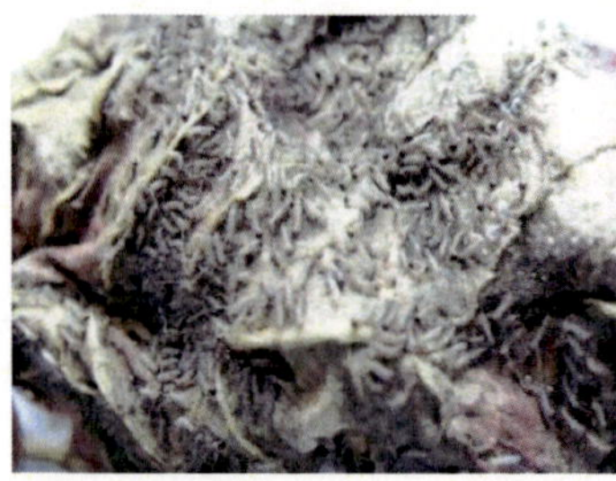
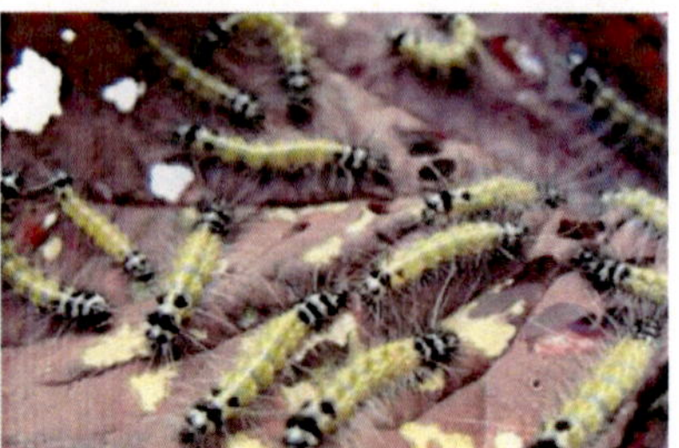

Larvae of *Spilosoma obliqua*

Nature of damage

The caterpillar eats leaves and soft portions of stem and branches. In severe infestation complete defoliation may occur.

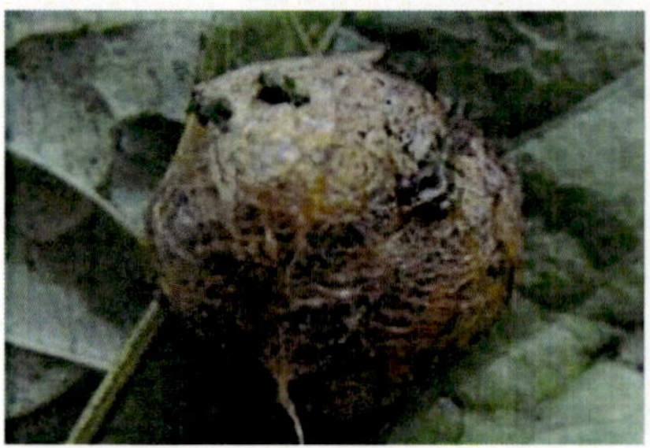

Pupation in silken cocoon

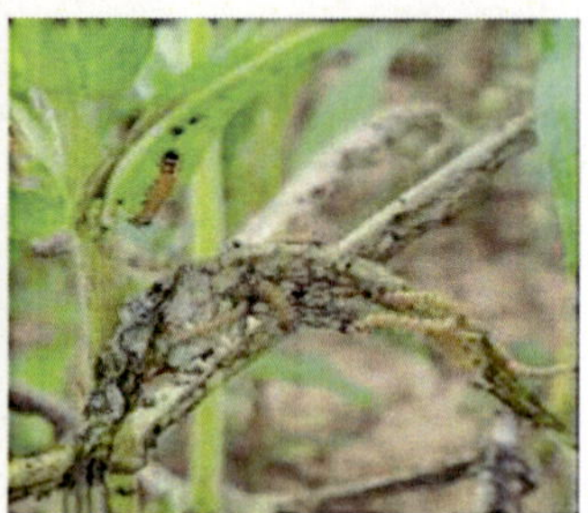

Damage symptoms of Spilosoma obliqua

Symptoms

- Neonates (young larvae) feed gregariously especially from the inner surface of leaves
- Larvae feed on leaves and during severe infestation, it causes complete defoliation

Tobacco caterpillar	:	*Spodoptera litura* F.
Family	:	Noctuidae
Order	:	Lepidoptera

Biology: Polyphagous pest. The fore wings of the moth have beautiful golden and grayish brown patterns. The female lays about 300 eggs in clusters. The eggs are covered with brown hairs. Egg period is 3 to 5 days. The caterpillar feed gregariously for a few days and then disperse to feed individually. There are 6 instars with a larval period of 15 to 30 days. The caterpillar is velvety black with yellowish green dorsal stripes and lateral white bands. The fully grown larva enters the soil for pupation. Pupal period is 7 to 15 days. Moth lives for 7 to 10 days.

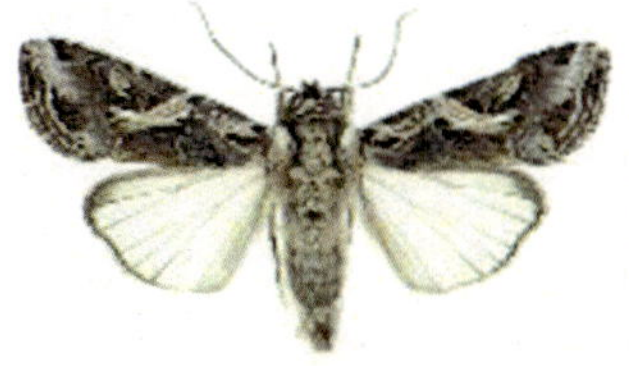 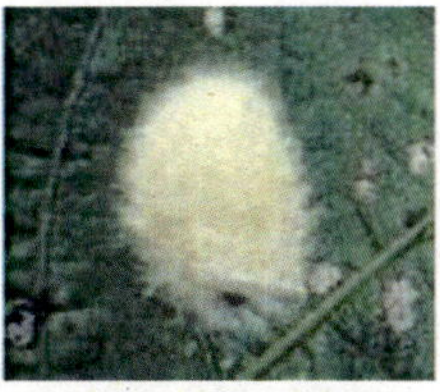 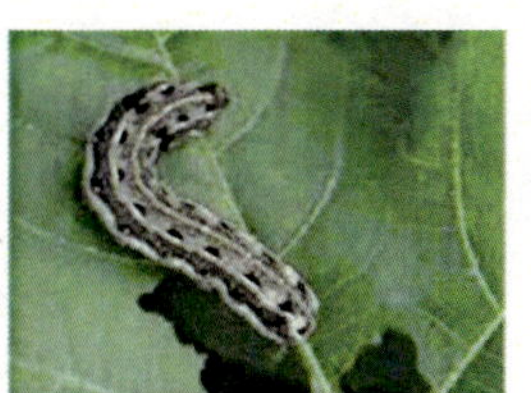 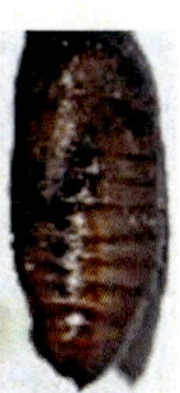

Adult egg mass, larva and pupa of *Spodoptera litura*

Nature of damage

The caterpillar feed on leaves, stem and flowers. They are active at night and cause extensive damage.

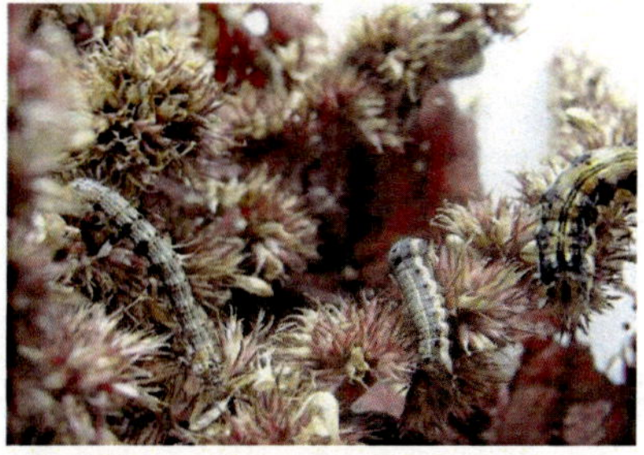

Damage of *Spodoptera litura*

Symptoms

Neonates feed on the foliage, and the matured larvae feed on the leaves, tender stems, flowers and grains, especially if the amaranth is grown for seed purposes.

Management of defoliators

- Collection and destruction of affected plant parts
- Summer ploughing to expose pupae to natural enemies and hot sun
- As far as possible avoid use of chemical insecticides
- If the infestation is severe cases apply malathion 50EC @ 2 ml/l

Amaranthus leaf miner : *Hypurus* sp.

Family : Curculionidae

Order : Coleoptera

Biology: Adult is brownish black with yellowish setae on elytra. Eggs are laid within the leaf tissues. Egg period - 3 days. Grubs mine the leaves and become full grown in 5 days. Pupation in soil for 9 to 10 days (Nair and Visalakshi, 1999).

Nature of damage

Adults damage leaves by eating them and creating holes. Grubs mine the leaves, causing blisters, and may also affect the tender stem and petiole.

Leaf-footed bug : *Cletus bipunctatus* Herrich-Schaffer

Nature of damage and symptoms

Bugs can cause severe damage to flowering head and seeds, and may be particularly damaging to grain amaranth when present in large numbers during the critical seed fill stage. They are usually of minor importance in vegetable amaranth.

References

Nair M. R.G.K. and Visalakshi, A. 1999. A Monograph on Crop pests of Kerala and their control KAU Publishers p. 227.

Rajeshkanna, S., Sivaraga, N. and Mikunthan, G. 2017. Biology and management Of Amaranthus stem borer (Hypolixus truncatulus) (Coleoptera: Curculionidae). Annals of Sri Lanka Department of Agriculture. 19: 258– 266.

Srivastava K. P. and Butani, D. K. 2009. Pest management in vegetables Vol I. Studium Press (India) Publishers p. 381.

Questions

1. What is a characteristic symptom of amaranthus weevil infestation?
   a) Webbing of leaves
   b) Skeletonized leaves
   c) Gall-like swellings on the stem with longitudinal white markings
   d) Leaf curling and distortion
2. Why is it important to destroy wild amaranthus near the field?
   a) It competes for nutrients with the main crop
   b) It serves as an alternate host for the amaranthus weevil
   c) It attracts beneficial insects that harm pests
   d) It promotes soil fertility
3. How does the larvae of leaf webber damage the leaves?
   a) By tunneling inside the stem
   b) By sucking sap from leaves
   c) By webbing and skeletonizing the leaves
   d) By boring into petioles and roots
4. What is a characteristic feature of the *Spodoptera litura* caterpillar?
   a) Yellowish caterpillar with red head
   b) Velvety black caterpillar with yellowish green dorsal stripes and white lateral bands
   c) Green caterpillar with faint black dots
   d) Hairy caterpillar with long white bristles
5. What is the egg-laying capacity of a *Spilosoma obliqua* female moth?
   a) 100 to 300 eggs
   b) 200 to 500 eggs
   c) 400 to 1000 eggs
   d) 1000 to 1500 eggs
6. Which of the following statements about Spilosoma obliqua is TRUE?
   a) The caterpillars feed individually throughout their life cycle.
   b) The adult moth has bright green forewings with black dots.
   c) The larvae feed gregariously when young and later disperse widely.
   d) The moth lays eggs singly on the underside of leaves.

7. Which control measure is common for both Hairy Caterpillar and Leaf Caterpillar infestations?
   a) Spray neem oil at 1% concentration
   b) Collection and destruction of affected plant parts
   c) Application of *Bacillus thuringiensis* (Bt) formulation
   d) Use of pheromone traps
8. Which of the following statements about *Cletus bipunctatus* is TRUE?
   a) It is a major pest in vegetable amaranth.
   b) It causes severe damage to amaranth stems and petioles.
   c) It is particularly harmful during the seed fill stage of grain amaranth.
   d) It primarily mines leaves and creates blisters.
9. Which of the following is a characteristic symptom of Amaranthus Leaf Miner infestation?
   a) Wilting and yellowing of leaves
   b) Blisters on leaves due to mining
   c) Webbing of leaves
   d) Gall formation on stems
10. Where does the maaranthus leaf miner lay its eggs?
   a) On the soil near the plant base b) Within the leaf tissues
   c) Under the bark of stems d) On flowers and seed heads

Assertion-Reasoning Questions

11. **Assertion (A):** The amaranthus weevil (*Hypolixus truncatulus*) causes damage by both adult and grub stages.

    Reason (R): The adult weevil feeds on leaves, whereas the grubs bore into stems, causing yellowing and wilting.
   a) Both A and R are true, and R is the correct explanation of A.
   b) Both A and R are true, but R is not the correct explanation of A.
   c) A is false, but R is true.
   d) A is true, but R is false.

12. **Assertion (A):** *Spodoptera litura* caterpillars pupate in loose silken cocoons.

    Reason (R): The larvae of *Spodoptera litura* burrow into the soil for pupation.

    a) Both A and R are true, and R is the correct explanation of A.

    b) Both A and R are true, but R is not the correct explanation of A.

    c) A is false, but R is true.

    d) A is true, but R is false.

13. **Assertion (A):** The larvae of leaf webber (*Psara / Herpetogramma basalis*) skeletonize the leaves completely.

    Reason (R): The larvae web the leaves and feed from within the webbings, leaving only the veins intact.

    a) Both A and R are true, and R is the correct explanation of A.

    b) Both A and R are true, but R is not the correct explanation of A.

    c) A is true, but R is false.

    d) A is false, but R is true.

14. **Assertion (A):** The Leaf Webber (*Hymenia/Spoladea recurvalis*) lays its eggs in the soil.

    Reason (R): The eggs of Leaf Webber are laid on leaves and hatch in 3 to 4 days.

    a) Both A and R are true, and R is the correct explanation of A.

    b) Both A and R are true, but R is not the correct explanation of A.

    c) A is false, but R is true.

    d) A is true, but R is false.

15. **Assertion (A):** The pupation of Hairy Caterpillar (*Spilosoma / Diacrisia obliqua*) occurs inside the soil.

    Reason (R): The full-grown caterpillar of Hairy Caterpillar spins a loose silken cocoon for pupation.

    a) Both A and R are true, and R is the correct explanation of A.

    b) Both A and R are true, but R is not the correct explanation of A.

    c) A is false, but R is true.

    d) A is true, but R is false.

Answer Key

1	c	2	b	3	c	4	b	5	c	6	c	7	b
8	c	9	b	10	b	11	a	12	c	13	a	14	c
15	c												

2

Pests of Cucurbits

Cucumbers, muskmelons, watermelons, squashes, gourds, and pumpkins are commonly grown cucurbits in most parts of the world. Cucurbitaceous crops are the most important summer vegetables grown all over the world and it includes 118 Genera and 825 Species. Production and productivity of cucurbits are affected by the incidence of pests and diseases. Important pests attacking cucurbits are fruit fly, snake gourd semilooper, red pumkin beetles, hadda beetles/ epilachna beetles, pumkin caterpillar, vine borer/ clear winged moths, gall fly, serpentine leaf miner, shield bug, snake gourd bug and plume moth.

Sl. No.	Common name	Scientific name	Family and Order	Site of oviposition	Site of pupation
1	Melon fly	*Bactrocera cucurbitae*	Tephritidae, Diptera	Fruits	Soil
2	Snake gourd caterpillar	*Anadevidia peponis*	Noctuidae, Lepidoptera	Tender leaves	Leaf folds
3	Epilachna beetle	*Henosepilachna septima, H. implicata, H. vigintioctopunctata*	Coccinellidae, Coleoptera	Lower side of leaves	Leaf surface
4	Pumpkin beetle	*Aulacophora spp.*	Chrysomelidae, Coleoptera	Moist soil	Earthern chambers in soil
5	Pumpkin caterpillar	*Diaphania indica*	Pyralidae, Lepidoptera	Under surface of leaves	On leaves
6	Vine borer	*Melittia sp.*	Sessidae, Lepidoptera	Tender stem	Soil
7	Gall fly	*Lasioptera falcata*	Cecidomyidae, Diptera	Tender shoots or buds	Galls
8	Serpentine leaf miner,	*Liriomyza trifolii*	Agromyzidae, Diptera	Plant tissue	Soil
9	Shield bug	*Aspongopus janus*	Pentatomidae, Hemiptera	Underside of leaf	-

10	Snake gourd bug,	*Leptoglossus australis*	Coreidae, Hemiptera	Stem, leaf, fruit	
11	Plume moth	*Sphenarches caffer*	Pterophoridae, Lepidoptera	Bud and leaves	Pod

Melon fly : *Bactrocera cucurbitae* Coquillett.

Family : Tephritidae

Order : Diptera

The melon fruit fly is distributed widely in temperate, tropical and subtropical regions of the world. It has been reported to damage 81 host plants and is a major pest of cucurbitaceous crops. The extent of loss varies between 30 –100 per cent depending on the cucurbit species and season. The adult is reddish brown with lemon yellow curved vertical markings on the thorax and fuscous shading on the outer margin of wings.

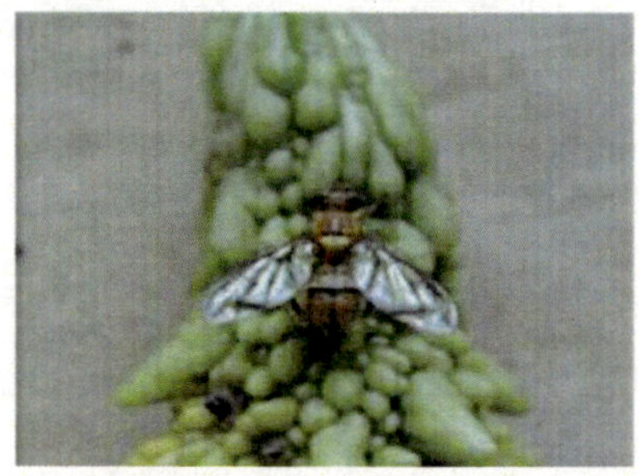

Oviposition by adult female

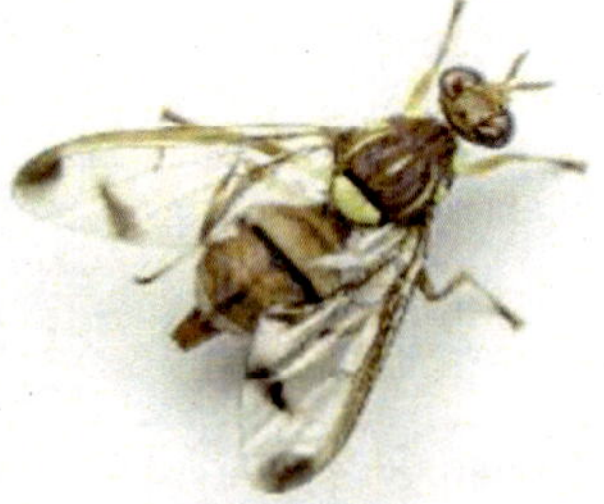

Bactocera cucurbitae adult

Biology: Eggs are white and cylindrical and laid singly or in clusters in cavities made with the ovipositor of the females on the fruits. The holes are sealed with gummy secretions, which solidify to form a shiny brown resinous material. Egg period is 1 to 2 days. The emerging maggots are apodous, dirty white, thicker at one end and tapering at the other and are seen within the fruits. Larval period is 7 days. The mature larvae emerge from the fruits and pupate in soil for a period of one week. Life cycle is completed in 15 to 20 days.

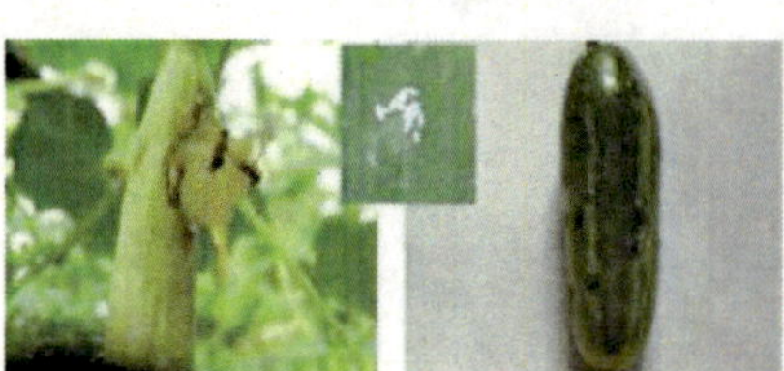

Gummy exudation followed by oviposition

Ovipositional scars on ivy gourd

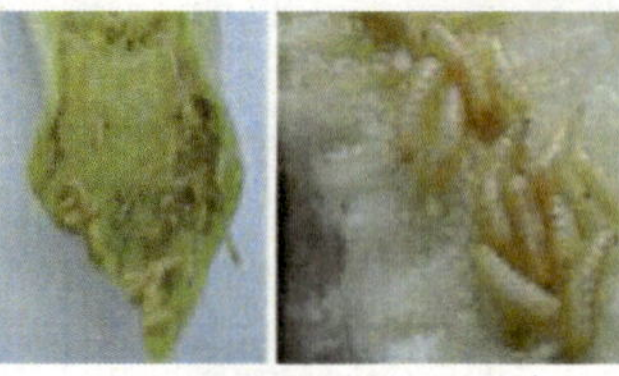

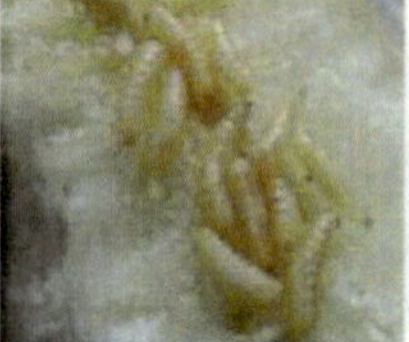

Maggots

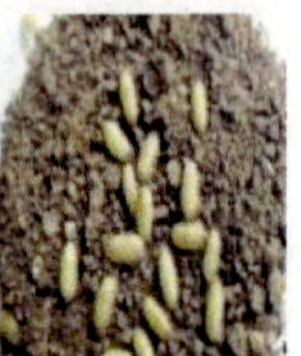

Pupae

Nature of damage and symptom

The maggots bore into the pulp of the fruit and feed within. The fruits become distorted and malformed initially. Later, the fruits rot and drop. A brown resinous fluid is seen oozing from the fruit.

Management

- Adjust the time of planting as the fly population is low in hot dry conditions and peak during rainy seasons
- Collect and destroy infested fruits
- Rake up the soil under the plants to destroy the puparia
- Dispose affected fruits promptly
- Protect fruits with paper, cloth or polythene bags in homestead gardens
- Spray 2% neem oil emulsion to suppress oviposition
- Spray 3000 ppm azadirachtin@ 5mL/L
- Spray 0.2 % malathion emulsion containing sugar or Jaggery
- Use bait traps and cue lure traps (Sruthi *et al*., 2023)
- Hang the cue lure traps @ 10-15 traps per hectare to attract male fruit flies

Snake gourd caterpillar	:	*Anadevidia peponis* F.
Family	:	Noctuidae
Order	:	Lepidoptera

Anadevidia peponis is a species of moth belonging to Noctuidae. It is primarily found in Southeast Asia, including countries such as Japan, India, Taiwan, and the state of New South Wales in Australia. Adult is a shiny stout dark brown moth with dark patches on the forewings. Eggs are laid singly on tender leaves. Caterpillars are green semiloopers with black warts on the body later they become white. Pupation is in leaf folds within a thin cocoon.

Nature of damage and symptom

Caterpillars defoliate the plants. Complete defoliation seen in young plants and this may even result in the death of the plant. The caterpillars may also feed on flowers and young fruits.

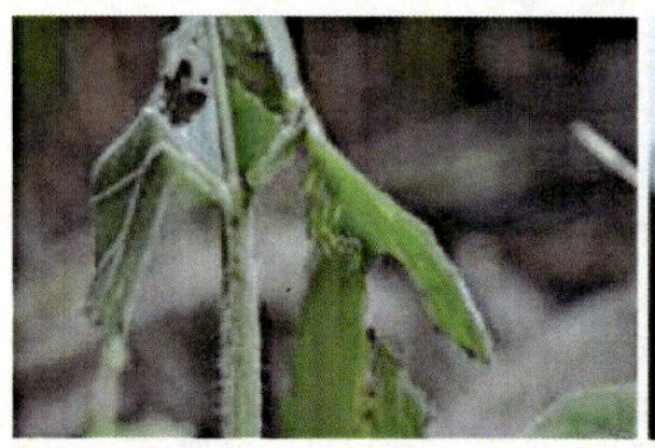

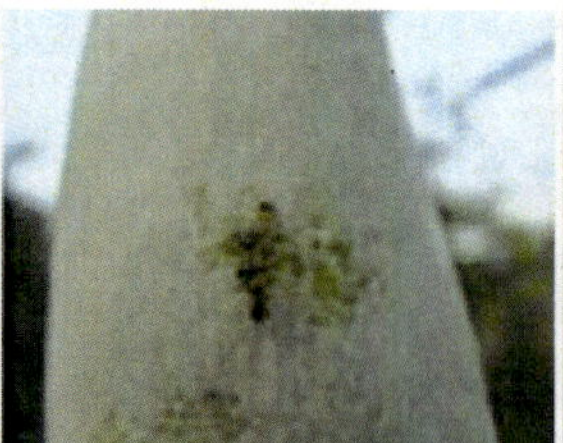

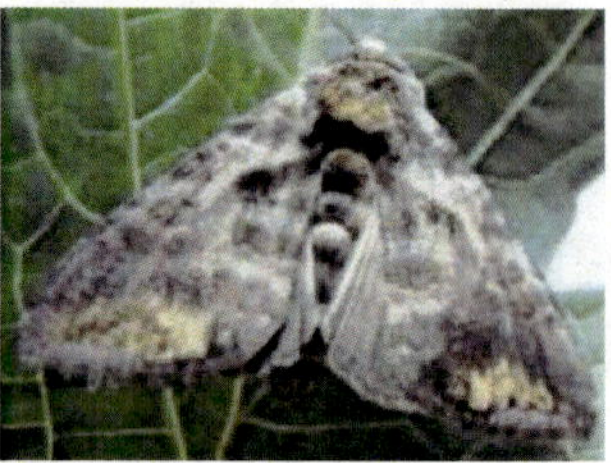

Caterpillar feeding on the leaf and fruit

Adult

Management

- Collect and destroy the caterpillars
- Crop rotation should be followed
- *Bacillus thuringiensis* (Bt) @ 1-2 g/L water – safe for pollinators and natural enemies.
- *Beauveria bassiana* or *Metarhizium anisopliae* @ 1×10^7 conidia/mL – effective under high humidity.
- The larvae is parasitised by *Apanteles taragamae*, *A. plusiae*, and pupae are parasitised by *Brachymeria marginata*, *Tetrastichus* sp. *Trichospilus pupivora*
- Pathogenic fungus *Pencillium purpurogenum* infects the caterpillar
- Foliar spray with spinosad 45 SC @ 3.3 ml/101 or emamectin benzoate @ 5 SG @ 4 g/10L or quinalphos 0.05% when infestation is severe.

Epilachna beetle : *Henospilachna septima* Dieke, *H. implicata* Mulsant, *H. vigintioctopunctata* F.

Family : Coccinellidae

Order : Coleoptera

The epilachna beetle, commonly known as the squash beetle, is a significant pest of cucurbitaceous plants. This species feeds on a variety of plants in the cucurbit family, such as cucumbers, pumpkins, melons, and squash. The adult beetles and their larvae damage the leaves, stems, and fruits, leading to stunted plant growth and reduced crop yields. Despite its destructive impact on crops, the epilachna beetle is often mistaken for a ladybug or a cucumber beetle due to its similar appearance (Uikey *et al.*, 2016).

Biology: Beetle is hemispherical and reddish brown with 12-28 black spots dorsally. Yellowish cigar shaped eggs are laid in erect clusters on the lower side of leaves. Grubs are yellow, fleshy and covered with hairs and spines. Pupation on the leaf surface.

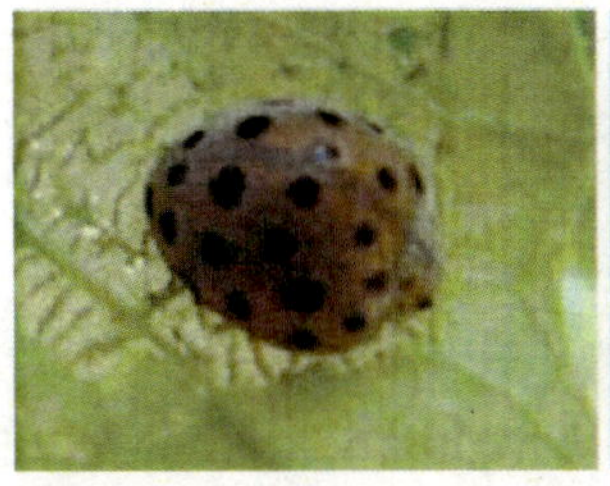
Adult

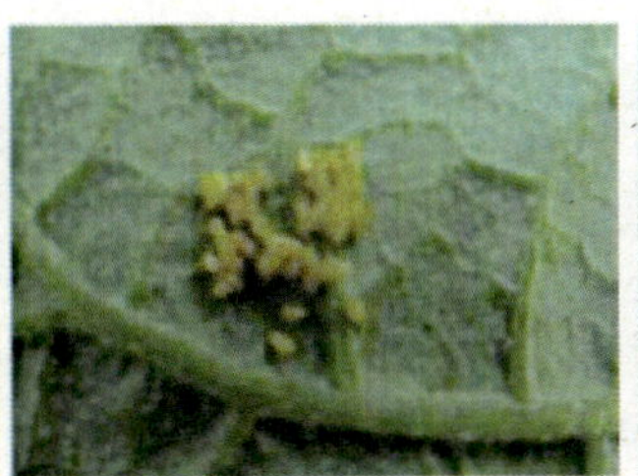
Egg mass

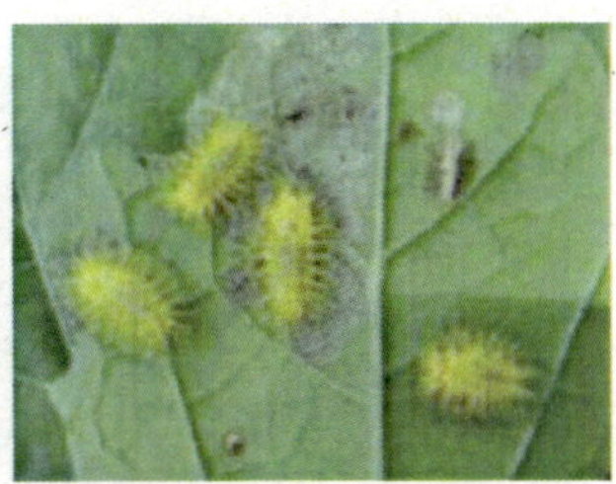
Grubs

Nature of damage and symptoms

Beetles and grubs scrape the green matter from leaves and feed on it. The leaves are skeletonised. Maximum damage is caused when young plants are attacked.

Management

- Collect and destroy adults and immature stages
- Spray persistent contact insecticide like quinalphos 0.05% @ 2mL/L when attack is severe

Pumpkin beetle : *Aulacophora* spp.

Family : Chrysomelidae

Order : Coleoptera

Aulacophora species, including *Aulacophora foveicollis*, commonly known as the red pumpkin beetle, are significant pests of cucurbitaceous plants.

A. foveicollis belongs to the family Chrysomelidae and is a foliage pest that primarily affects pumpkins but can also infest other cucurbit crops like cucumbers, melons, and squash. These beetles cause damage by feeding on the leaves, leading to defoliation, which can stunt plant growth and reduce yields. Beyond cucurbits, *A. foveicollis* is also known to be a pest of millets in India.

Biology: The beetles are red, blue or grey coloured. Eggs are orange brown laid singly or in groups in moist soil around the base of the plant. The eggs hatch in 6 to 15 days. The grubs creamy yellow with brownish prothorax. They remain below the soil, near the roots, underground stem and fruits lying in contact with soil. They full grown in 13 to 25 days and pupate in thick walled earthen chambers in the soil. Pupal period lasts for 7 to 17 days and the beetles on emergence, begin to fed and breed. Freshly hatched grubs are dirty white and fully grown creamy yellow.

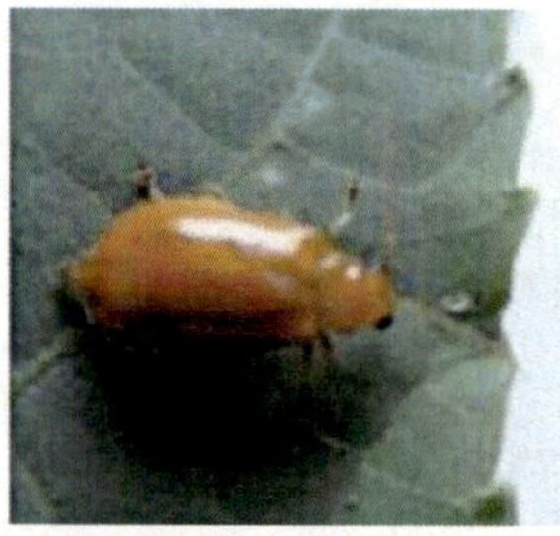
A. foevicollis

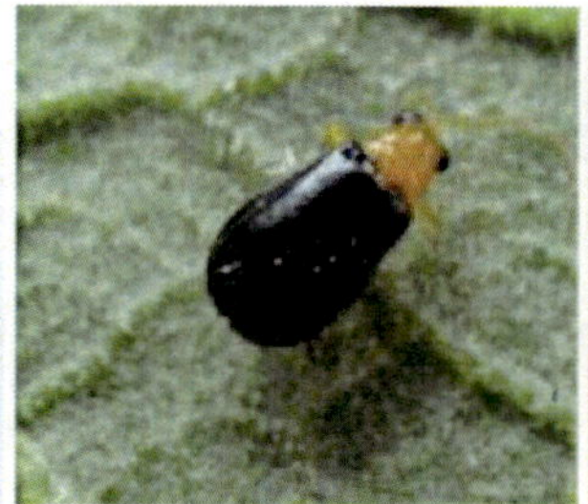
A. lewisii

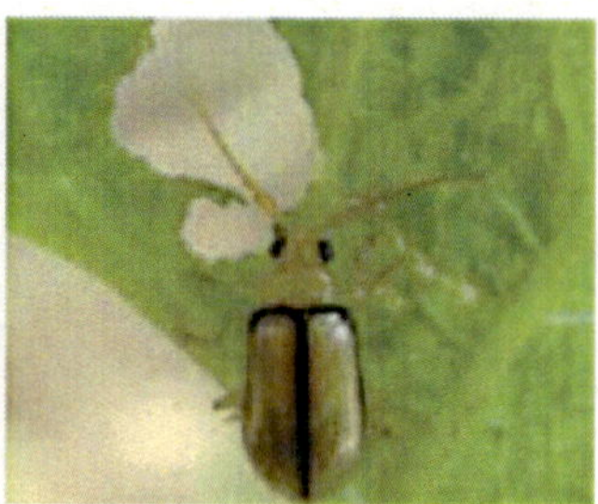
A. cincta

Nature of damage and symptoms

The beetles feed extensively on the leaves, flowers and fruits. The seedlings when attacked are completely destroyed. The grubs feed on the roots, stem and fruits touching the soil.

Management

- Collect and destroy adult beetles
- Crop rotation should be followed
- Keep the field clean - after harvesting, plough the field deep to expose grubs and pupae to predatory birds and other natural enemies
- Foliar spraying with neem seed kernel extract (NSKE) 5% to deter feeding by adults
- *Metarhizium anisopliae* or *Beauveria bassiana* @ 1×10^7 spores/mL as soil drench to target grubs and pupae
- Incorporate fipronil 0.5G granules in pits @3.5to5g/pitbefore sowing the seeds to destroy grubs and pupae
- Foliar spray with quinalphos 25 EC @ 2mL/L
- In case of severe infestation, foliar spray with spinosad 45SC @60gai/ha coupled with soil application with fipronil 0.5G@30gai/ha is effective in reducing the infestation (Singh *et al.*, 2023)

Pumpkin caterpillar : *Diaphania indica* Saunders

Family : Crambidae

Order : Lepidoptera

Diaphania indica, commonly known as the tropical pumpkin borer or the melon worm, is a significant pest of cucurbitaceous crops. It belongs to the grass moth family Crambidae, specifically the large subfamily Spilomelinae. Although native to southern Asia, *D. indica* has spread to many tropical and subtropical regions outside the Americas. This moth is occasionally a major pest of cucurbits, particularly affecting pumpkins, melons, cucumbers, and squash. The larvae of *D. indica* bore into the stems and fruits of these plants, causing wilting, reduced fruit quality, and potentially significant crop losses. Due to its widespread presence and the damage it can cause, effective pest management strategies are crucial for protecting cucurbit crops from this destructive pest.

Biology: Adult is a fragile moth. Forewings are hyaline with broad black marginal patches. Abdomen carries anal tuft of orange coloured hairs. Eggs are laid on the under surface of leaves. Egg period is 3 to 4 days. The caterpillar is bright green with a pair of thin white longitudinal lines mid dorsally. Larval period is 10 days. Pupation is on the leaves in a cocoon. Pupal period is one week (Hosseinzade *et al.*, 2014).

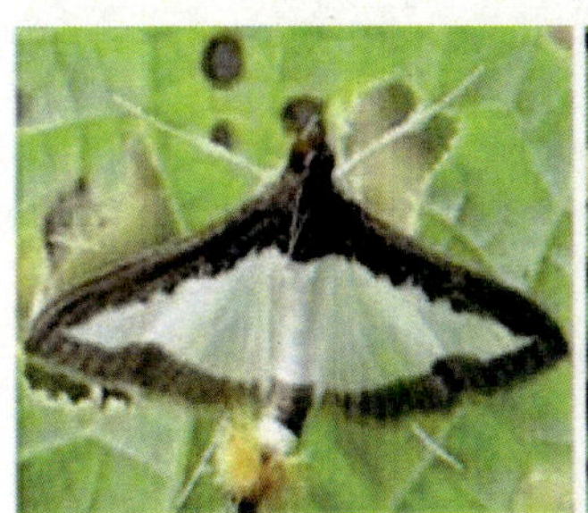
Adult moth

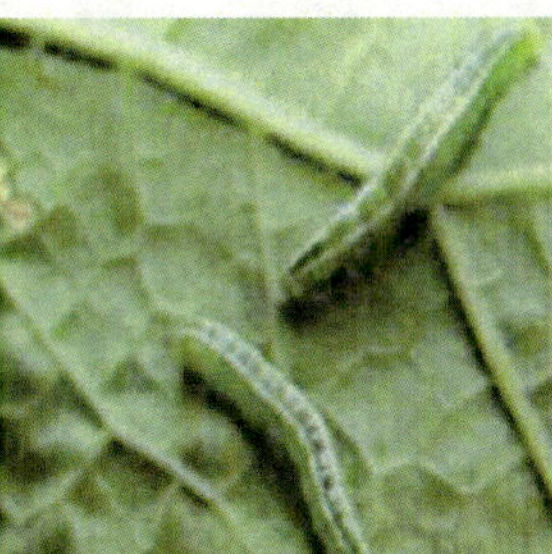
Larvae

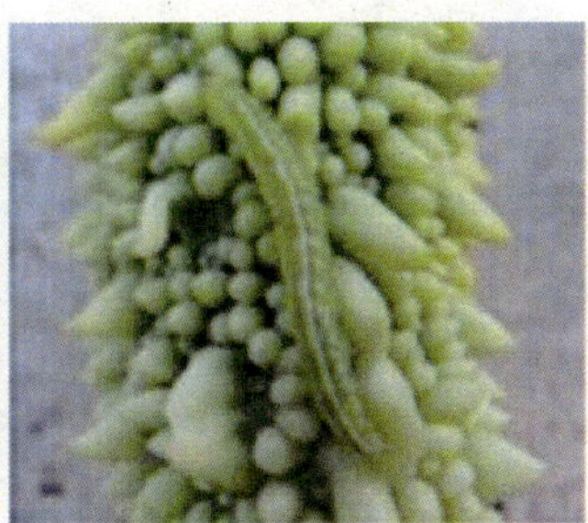
Larva feeding on the fruit

Nature of damage and symptoms

The caterpillar binds together the leaves and feed on them. Larvae scrape the chlorophyll and later webs leaves. Also feeds flowers and bores into developing fruits.

Management

- Collect and destroy early stage caterpillars
- Encourage activity of parasioid: *Apanteles* spp.
- *Bacillus thuringiensis* (Bt) @ 1–2 g/L – effective on young larvae.
- *Beauveria bassiana* or *Metarhizium anisopliae* @ 1×10^7 spores/mL – spray in the evening or under high humidity.
- Neem Seed Kernel Extract (NSKE) 5% spray or Azadirachtin 1% EC @ 2–3 mL/L
- Spray insecticides like quinalphos 25EC @ 2 mL/L of water or flubendiamide 480SC @ 2mL/10L is effective

Vine borer : *Melittia* sp.
Family : Sessidae
Order : Lepidoptera

Melittia spp. is a genus of moths that includes several species known as pests of cucurbitaceous crops. These moths are often referred to as "clear wing moths" due to the transparent wings of the adult insects, which distinguish them from other moth species. The larvae of *Melittia* spp. species are particularly harmful to cucurbits like pumpkins, cucumbers, and melons.

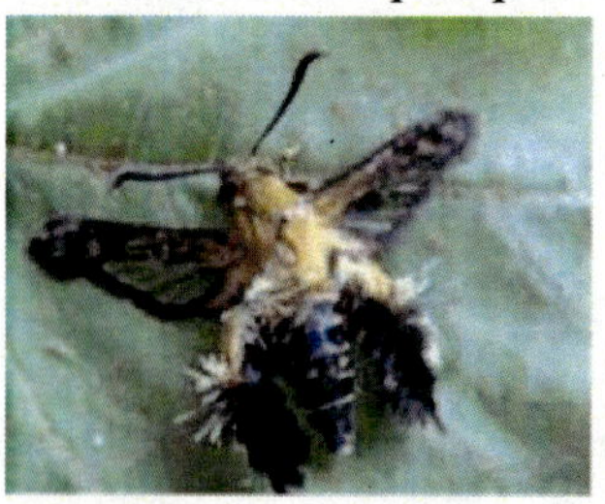
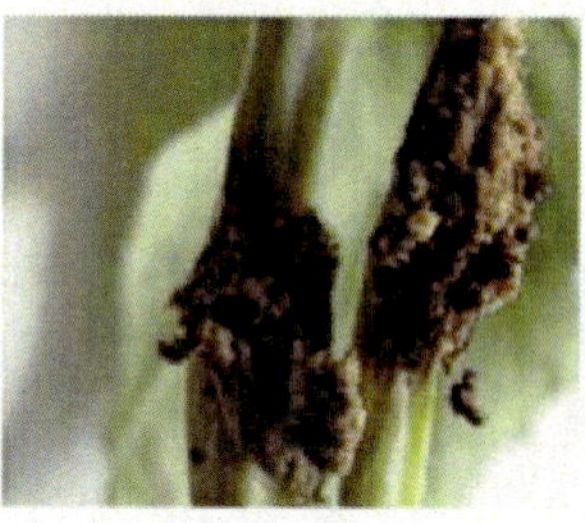
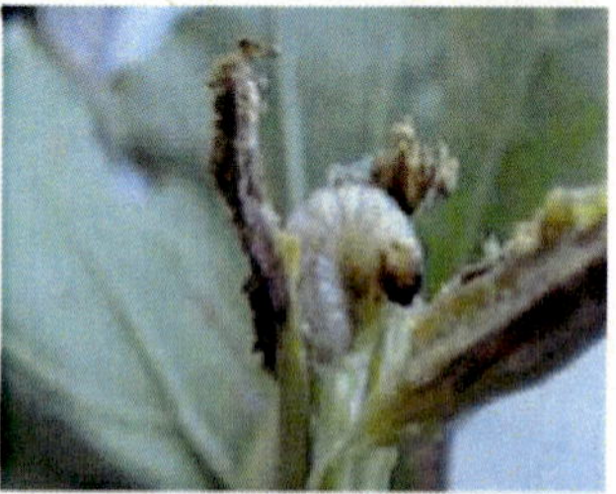

Nature of damage and symptoms

The adult moths lay their eggs on the plants, and the larvae, upon hatching, burrow into the plant tissues. Larvae tunnel through the vine, forming galls. Continuous feeding of stem tissues can lead to wilting and weakening of the plants, potentially resulting in significant crop losses. A single caterpillar can be seen in a gall. Pupation occurs inside a cocoon in soil.

Gall fly : *Lasioptera falcata* Felt
Family : Cecidomyidae
Order : Diptera

Gall fly, *L. falcata* is a notable pest of cucurbit crops, particularly affecting members of the Cucurbitaceae family, such as pumpkins, cucumbers, and melons. This pest is a type of gall midge, with its larvae causing damage by feeding on the plant tissues, often leading to the formation of galls or abnormal growths on the affected plants. The presence of *L. falcata* can severely impact plant health, causing stunted growth, deformed fruits, and reduced yields. Its small size and ability to cause damage within the plant tissues make it difficult to detect and control.

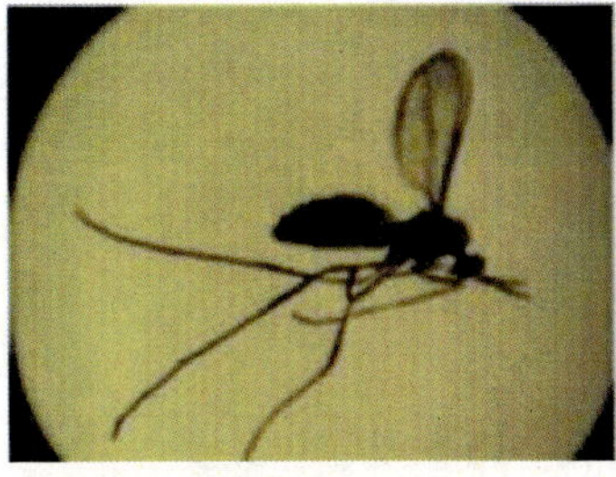
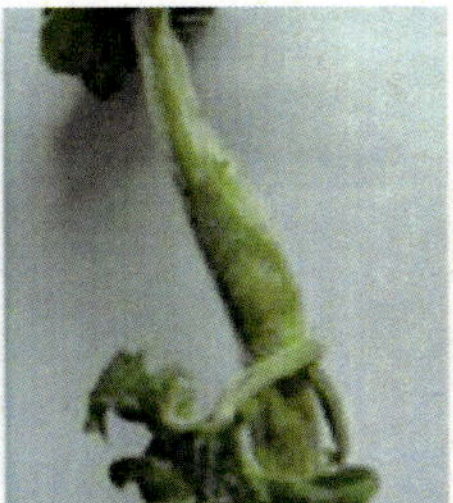
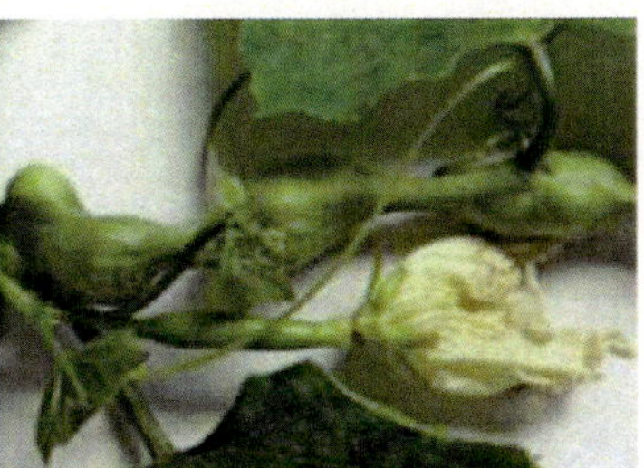

Adult Symptoms on the terminal shoot

Nature of damage and symptoms

- Maggot feeds within distal stems of bitter- gourd, ribbed and smooth gourds causing formation of elongated galls in between nodes.
- Gall formation causes stunting of plants.
- Maggots feed within the distal stem causing formation of elongated galls

Serpentine leaf miner : *Liriomyza trifolii* Burgess
Family : Agromyzidae
Order : Diptera

Liriomyza trifolii, commonly known as the vegetable leaf miner, is a significant pest of cucurbit crops, including cucumbers, melons, pumpkins, and squash. This small, leaf-mining fly belongs to the family Agromyzidae, and its maggots are responsible for the damage. The maggots burrow into the leaves of the plant, creating distinctive winding tunnels or mines, which can impair the plant's ability to photosynthesize, leading to weakened growth, reduced yields, and even plant death in severe cases. The adult flies lay their eggs on the undersides of the leaves, and upon hatching, the maggots feed on the internal tissues, causing characteristic damage. Due to its ability to rapidly reproduce and spread, *L. trifolii* can become a major problem for cucurbit growers.

Biology: Eggs are pale, white, oval thrust into the plant tissue. Yellow maggots with black mouthparts emerge and mine the leaves. Pupa is silky brown, pupation in soil. It causes liner to blotch leaf mines in the leaves or cotyledons (Akash *et al*., 2025).

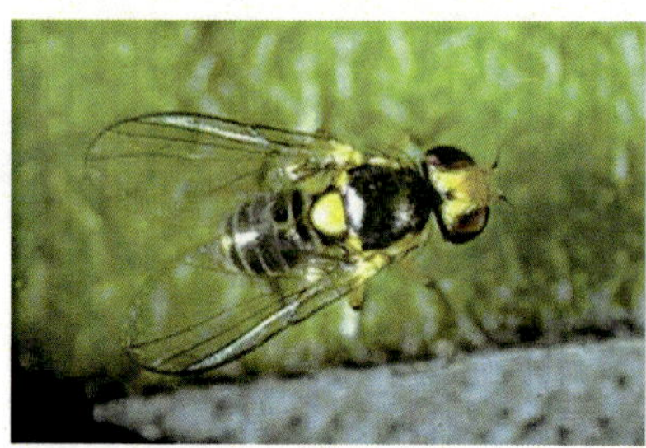

Adult fly

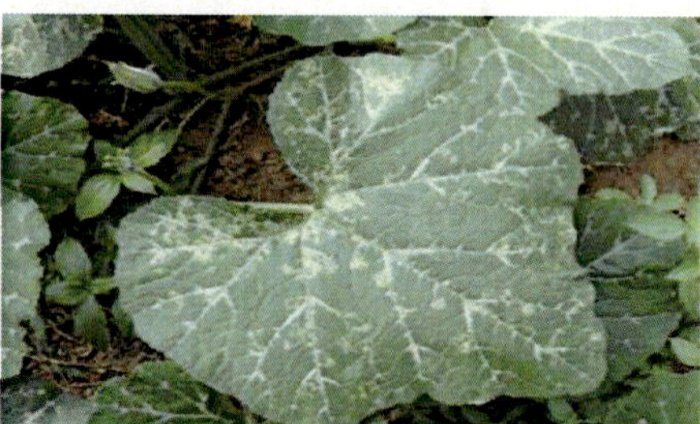

Mining symptoms on the leaf

Management

Since parasitoids can effectively control leaf miners in the field when disruptive insecticides are avoided, there has been interest in releasing these parasitoids into crops. This occurs principally in greenhouse-grown crops, but is also applicable to field conditions. Destruction of weed plants as well as infested senile plants will reduce the population and damage. Deep ploughing of crop residues is recommended. Adults experience difficulty in emerging if they are buried deeply in soil. In case of severe infestation, foliar spray with spinosad 45SC @ 3.3mL/10L or fipronil 5SC @2mL/L effectively reduce leaf miner damage.

Shield bug : *Aspongopus janus* F.

Family : Pentatomidae

Order : Hemiptera

Aspongopus janus is a destructive pest of cucurbit crops, including cucumbers, pumpkins, and melons. This species is easily identifiable by its striking appearance: the pronotum and base of the hemelytra are bright red, while the ventral side, legs, and head are black. *A. jamus* typically forms colonies on cucurbit plants, where it feeds by sucking sap, particularly from the veins of leaves. This feeding activity can weaken the plants, causing yellowing, stunted growth, and reduced yields. The damage from these sap-feeding insects can also make plants more susceptible to secondary infections and environmental stress.

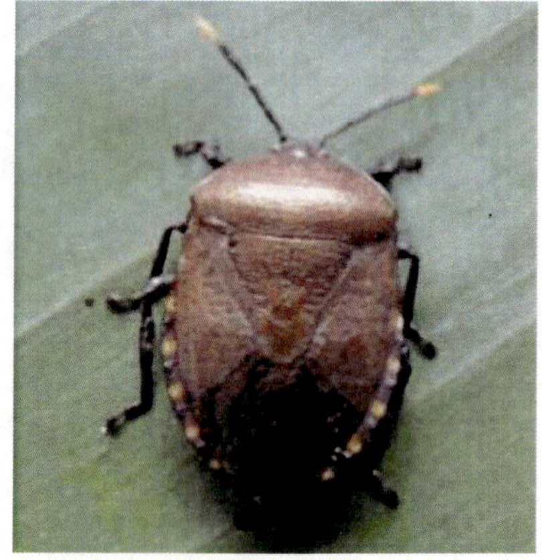

Aspongopus janus - adult

Nature of damage

- Nymph and adult suck sap from the leaf veins, retarding the plant growth

Snake gourd bug : *Leptoglossus australis* F.

Family : Coreidae

Order : Hemiptera

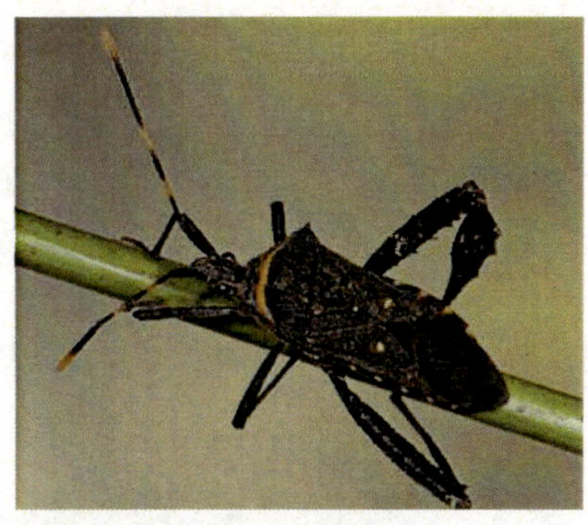

Leptoglossus australis-adult

Leptoglossus australis is a significant pest of cucurbit crops, such as pumpkins, melons, and cucumbers. This elongated bug is easily recognized by its dull black body, adorned with a distinctive transverse red band behind the head and several red spots on the underside. One of its most notable features is the swollen and flat tibia of its hind legs. Snake gourd bug sucks sap from the cucurbit plants, particularly targeting the fruit and stems. Its feeding causes damage to the plant tissue, leading to deformities, discoloration, and reduced fruit quality. This pest can also make the plant more vulnerable to secondary infections.

Biology: The eggs are laid in chains of 16-17. They are brownish in colour, cylindrical in shape. Nymphs are similar in shape to the adults but without wings. They are reddish in colour in the early stages. There are some black spines on the head and thorax. The eggs are laid on vines, frequently along the tendrils. They hatch in six to seven days. The nymphs cluster soon after emergence then move onto the tender parts of the plant to feed. The total nymphal period is around 50 days, but may vary with the host being fed on. Adults can live for several weeks.

Nature of damage and symptoms

The adults and nymphs suck sap from the fruits, producing sunken spots making it unmarketable. This insect usually feeds on flowers or green-mature fruit. The nymphs often cluster on fruit while feeding. Infested fruits develop dimple-like surface blemishes at the feeding sites.

Management

- Remove plant debris after harvest to eliminate overwintering sites
- Crop rotation should be practiced
- Handpick bugs and egg clusters in early morning when they're sluggish
- Application of insecticidal soap is effective against nymphs

- In case of severe infestation apply synthetic pyrethroids insecticides viz lamda cyhalothrin 2.5EC@ 5-6mL/10L or cyfluthrin 2.5EC @ 4ml/10l will reduce the pest population and damage
- Continuous application of synthetic pyrethroids should be avoided
- Application of spinosad 45SC @ 3.3mL/L as foliar spray reduce bug infestation

Plume moth : *Sphenarches caffer* Zeller

Family : Pterophoridae

Order : Lepidoptera

Sphenarches caffer, commonly known as the bottle gourd plume moth, is a significant pest of cucurbit crops, particularly bottle gourds, pumpkins, cucumbers, and melons. This moth belongs to the family Pterophoridae and is found in regions including India, Malaysia, Mauritius, the Seychelles, and South Africa.

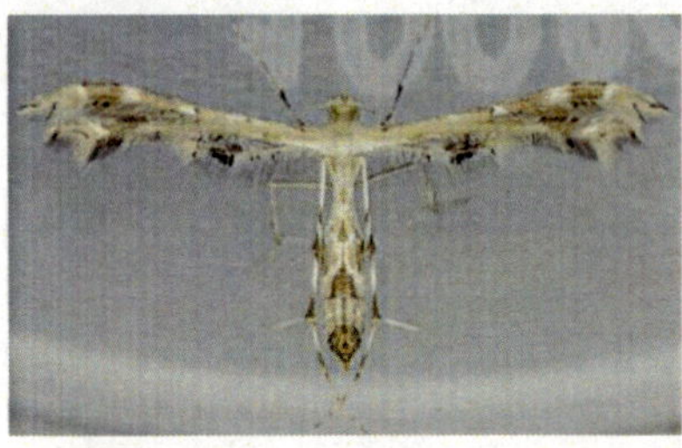

Adult moth

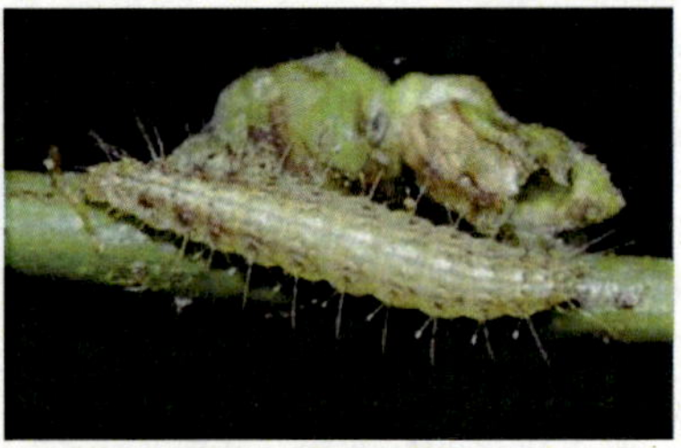

Larva feeding on pod

Biology: Eggs are laid singly on buds and leaves. Larva is small, cylindrical and yellowish green with short spines all over body. Pupa is greenish brown pupa. Adult are lender moth with lobed wings, fringed with scales (Sujithra *et al.*, 2010).

Symptoms of damage

Larva feeds on leaves making small holes

Management

- Collect and destroy larvae and pupae
- Crop rotation should be followed
- Spray Dimethoate 30 EC @1.5 ml/l

Helmet scale/coffee brown scale: *Saisettia hemispherica* (Targ.)

Family : Coccidae

Order : Hemiptera

Nature of damage and symptoms

The coffee brown scale is a major pest of coccinia. Both nymphs and adults suck sap from the mature vines initially and then spread to all parts of the plant resulting in loss of vigor, deformations of affected plant parts and finally leads to the death of the plant. During severe cases of infestations, an yield loss upto 100% was reported (Vijayasree, 2006).

Green citrus aphid : *Aphis spiraecola* (Patch)

Family : Aphididae

Order : Hemiptera

Nature of damage and symptoms

Highly polyphagous pest infesting more than 278 species/subspecies under 68 plant families. Green citrus aphid or apple aphid infests almost all cucurbitaceous crops including coccinia. Severe infestation and population build up occurs during summer period. Population of both nymphs and adults can be seen on almost all the tender plant parts including tender vines, flower buds, flowers, tender fruits and leaves. Both nymphs and adults suck plant sap and continuous desapping results in stunted growth, premature flower drop, crinkling, curling and malformations of infested plant parts, reduction in fruit set and there by yield loss.

Management

- Severely infested plant parts should be clipped off and destroyed
- Follow crop rotation with non-host crops
- In case of severe infestation, foliar application of imidacloprid 0.005% is very effective against both scales and aphids

References

Akash, M.S., Deepthy, K.B., Sruthi, A.B., Kannan, E.G. 2025. Invasive insect species: Challenges and management strategies. In B.C. Anu, F. Rasool, K.V. Chaudary, V.V. Birari (Eds.), Agricultural entomology: Advances in pest management and ecosystem balance (pp.126-163). Stella International Publications.

Hosseinzade, S., Izadi, H., Namvar, P., and Samih, M. A. (2014). Biology, temperature thresholds, and degree-day requirements for development of the cucumber moth, Diaphania indica, under laboratory conditions. Journal of Insect Science, 14, 61.

Singh, S., Rajak, R. K., Tiwari, S., Dwarka., Mansion, H., and Chandra, U. (2023). Management of red pumpkin beetle, Aulacophora foveicollis L. in Bottle gourd (Lagenaria siceraria M.) crop. The Pharma Innovation Journal, 12(9): 286-288.

Sruthi, A. B., Kavitha, Z., Shanthi, M., and Beaulah, A. 2023. Role of protein and food baits in attraction of melon fruit fly Zeugodacus cucurbitae in bitter gourd. Indian Journal of Entomology 85(2): 455-458.

Sujithra, M., Srinivasan, S., & Krishna, T. M. (2010). Bionomics and Seasonal occurrence of Plume moth, Sphenarches caffer on Field bean. Annals of Plant Protection Sciences, 18(1), 241-243.

Uikey, B. L., Bhupendrakumar, T. G., Jha, S., & Kekti, R. K. (2016). Incidence pattern and biology of epilachna beetle, Henosepilachna septima dieke on bottle gourd in Gangetic new alluvial zone of West Bengal. Indian society for the advancement of insect science, 29(1), 63-66.

Vijayasree, V. (2006). Pests of coccinia (cocinia grandis (L) voigt) and their management Ph.D thesis, Kerala Agricultural University p.146.

Questions

1. Which of the following is the primary pest of cucurbits?
   a) Fruit fly
   b) Shield bug
   c) Plume moth
2. What type of damage do melon fly larvae cause to the fruit?
   a) They cause the fruit to ripen prematurely.
   b) They cause the fruit to rot and drop.
   c) They cause wilting of plant.
3. Which pest is known as the 'red pumpkin beetle'?
   a) *Diaphania indica*
   b) *Epilachna septima*
   c) *Aulacophora foveicollis*
4. Where do *Aulacophora foveicollis* larvae pupate?
   a) In the fruit
   b) On the leaves
   c) In the soil
5. Which pest's larvae are green semiloopers with black warts on the body?
   a) Vine borer
   b) Pumpkin caterpillar
   c) Snake gourd caterpillar
6. Where do *Liriomyza trifolii* larvae create damage on cucurbits?
   a) Roots
   b) Leaves
   c) Flowers
7. **Assertion**: The *Epilachna* beetle is a significant pest of cucurbits.

   Reason: This beetle scrapes the green matter from leaves, causing them to skeletonize.

   a) Both assertion and reason are true, and the reason is the correct explanation for the assertion.
   b) Both assertion and reason are true, but the reason is not the correct explanation for the assertion.
   c) The assertion is true, but the reason is false.
   d) The assertion is false, but the reason is true.

8. **Assertion**: The *Diaphania indica* larvae bore into the stems and fruits of cucurbits.

   Reason: The larvae feed on leaves and create distinctive mines inside them.

   a) Both assertion and reason are true, and the reason is the correct explanation for the assertion.

   b) Both assertion and reason are true, but the reason is not the correct explanation for the assertion.

   c) The assertion is true, but the reason is false.

   d) The assertion is false, but the reason is true.

9. Which of the following is true about *Lasioptera falcata* (gall fly)?

   a) *Lasioptera falcata* larvae feed on the flowers of cucurbits.

   b) *Lasioptera falcata* larvae cause the formation of galls in the leaves and stems.

   c) *Lasioptera falcata* does not affect cucurbit crops.

   d) The gall fly feeds exclusively on cucumbers.

10. Which of the following statements about the *Sphenarches caffer* (plume moth) is correct?

    a) The larvae feed on the roots of cucurbits.

    b) *Sphenarches caffer* is only found in tropical regions of the Americas.

    c) The larvae of *Sphenarches caffer* feed on the leaves, making small holes.

    d) The adult moths of *Sphenarches caffer* do not harm cucurbits.

Answer Key

1	a	2	b	3	c	4	c	5	c	6	b	7	a
8	c	9	b	10	c								

3

Pests of Cowpea / Pulses

Cow pea is an important vegetable crop in Kerala. The crop was originated in Africa and is the major source of plant proteins in the diet of rural populations in Africa. The grains contain 25% protein and several vitamins and minerals. Insect pests pose the greatest threat to cowpea production. The crop is severely attacked at every stage of its growth by insects. High pest densities occur at many locations with complete loss of grain yield if no control measures are taken.

Sl no	Common name	Sc. name	Family and Order	Site of oviposition	Site of pupation
			Borers		
1	Spotted pod borer	*Maruca testulalis / Maruca vitrata*	Crambidae, Lepidoptera	Floral buds, flower, tender leaves, shoots and pods	Within or near surface of the ground
2	Gram pod borer	*Helicoverpa armigera*	Noctuidae, Lepidoptera	Near flower buds and pods	Soil, leaf, pod and crop debris.
3	Pod borer / Lima bean pod borer	*Etiella zinckenella*	Phycitidae, Lepidoptera	On pods	Soil
4	Field bean borer	*Adisura atkinsoni*	Noctuidae, Lepidoptera	On pods or flower buds	Soil
5	Pod caterpillar/ pea blue butterfly	*Lampides boeticus*	Lycaenidae, Lepidoptera	Single egg on flower buds and pods	Leaf, twig or pods
6	Grass blue butterfly	*Euchrysops cnejus*	Lycaenidae, Lepidoptera	Under the leaves	Soil or plant debris
7	Plume moth	*Exelastis atomosa*	Pterophoridae, lepidoptera	Singly on the tender parts of the plant	Soil of plant debris
8	Noctuid moth	*Eublemma dimidialis*	Noctuidae, Lepidoptera		At junction of leaf lamina and petiole

			Defoliators		
9	Dead hawk moth	*Acherontia styx, Agrius convulvuli*	Sphingidae, Lepidoptera	On leaves	In soil
10	Bihar hairy caterpillar	*Spilosoma obliqua*	Arctidae, Lepidoptera	Underside of leaves	In soil
11	Groundnut red hairy caterpillar	*Amsacta albistriga*	Arctidae, Lepidoptera	Underside of leaves	In soil
12	Stem fly / bean fly	*Ophiomyia phaseoli*	Agromyzidae, Diptera	on the upper leaf surfaces, often near the midrib close to the petiole	beneath the epidermis of the stem near the soil surface
13	Pod fly	*Melanagromy-za obtusa*	Agromyzidae, Diptera	Singly within the pods	Inside larval grooves
14	American serpentine leaf miner	*Liriomyza trifolii*	Agromyzidae, Diptera	Thrusted on the leaf surface	In soil
			Sucking pests		
15	Cowpea aphid	*Aphis craccivora*	Aphididae, Hemiptera	On leaves or parthenogenisis	-
16	Flower thrips	*Megaluro-thrips distalis, M. sjostedti*	Thripidae, Thysanoptera	In flower buds	In soil
17	Mites	*Tetranychus spp*	Tetranychidae, Acari	Underside of leaves	-
18	Leaf hopper	*Empoasca spp*	Cicadellidae, Hemiptera	On underside of leaves	-
			Pod bug complex		
19	Green bean bug	*Riptortus pedestris Clavigralla gibbose, C. horrens*	Coreidae, Hemiptera Coreidae, Hemiptera	Leaves and pods	-
20	Lablab bug / stink bug	*Coptosoma cribraria*	Coptosomati-dae, Hemiptera	Underside of leaves, stem or loose soil	-
21	Green shiled bug/ Southern green stink bug	*Nezara viridula*	Pentatomidae, Hemiptera	Underside of leaves	-
22	Bruchids	*Callobruchus chinensis, C. maculatus*	Bruchidae, Coleoptera	On the grain or pod	Soil

Pod borer complex in cowpea

Spotted pod borer : *Maruca testulalis / M. vitrata* F.

Family : Crambidae

Order : Lepidoptera

Spotted pod borer also known as legume pod borer/bean pod borer, is one of the most important pests of cowpea, field bean, groundnut and other pulse crops causing a yield loss of about 20-80 %. The larvae feed on the buds and flowers and bore into the pod to eat the developing seeds. Moths are active during night and shelter within the plant canopy during day time.

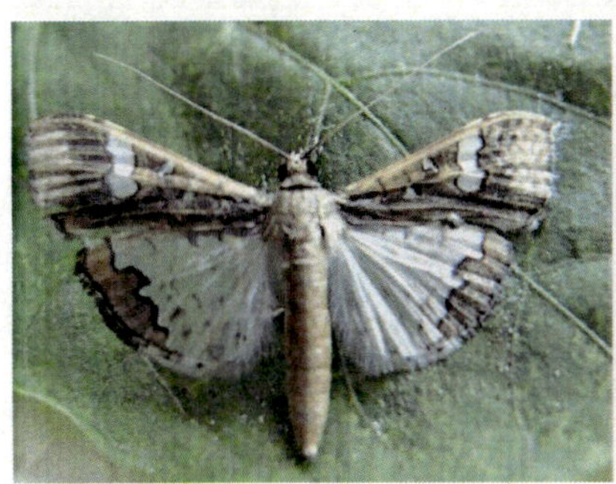

Adult moth

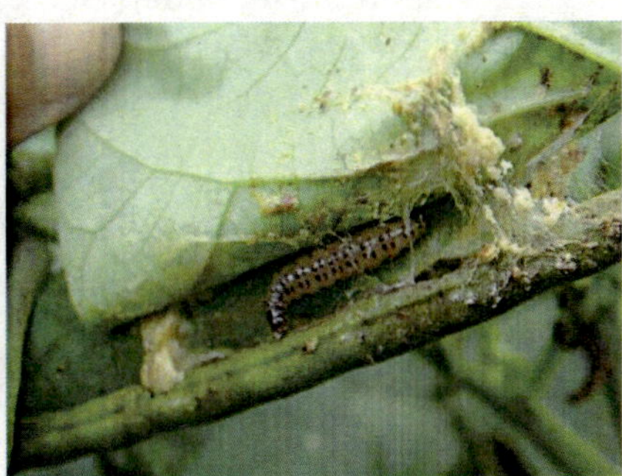

Larva within the silken webbings

Moth has greyish brown forewings with large transverse hyaline band and a few smaller spots. Hind wings are hyaline with brown outer margin. The female moth lays eggs on or near flower buds. Caterpillars are brownish green with black warts. The young caterpillars bore into the buds, flowers or pods. Pods with bore holes may be seen. The infested flowers and pods may be webbed together. Flower drop may occur in severe cases. Caterpillars may bore into the stem also (Mahalakshmi *et al.*, 2016).

Host range

Soybean, blackgram, greengram, Groundnut, common bean, lima bean, chickpea, mung bean, broad bean, pigeon pea.

Distribution

All over tropical and sub-tropical regions of the world.

Biology: The adults tend to lay their eggs on flowers, flower buds, young shoots, and tender pods. The total larval duration was 16-17 days. The duration of pupal period was 6-7 days and moths emerged generally during dusk or night hours between 6 pm to 11 pm. The average adult duration was about 7-8 days and the pest took 36 -37 days to complete the life cycle. Pupation within debris or near surface of ground.

Symptoms of damage

1. Bore holes on the buds, flower or pods.
2. Infested pods, leaves and flowers are webbed together and larvae feed from inside.
3. Damage occurs mainly during flowering and podding stages, since young larvae feed mainly on flowers, whereas mature larvae attack fruits and pods in beans (Rekha and Mallapur, 2007).

Natural enemies

Braconids: *Apanteles taragamae* Viereck, *Bassus asper* Chou & Sharkey and *Dolichogenidea* sp., ichneumonids: *Trichomma* sp., *Triclistus* sp., and *Plectochorus* sp. The egg parasitoid reported was *Trichogramma evanescens* Westwood (Sharma 1998)

Gram pod borer : *Helicoverpa armigera* Hubner.

Family : Noctuidae

Order : Lepidoptera

Helicoverpa armigera, commonly known as the cotton bollworm or the gram pod borer, is a highly destructive polyphagous pest that affects a wide range of crops, including cotton, pulses, tomatoes, and corn. The larvae of *H. armigera* are notable for their distinctive appearance. They are typically green with dark broken grey lines and dark and pale bands. The larvae show significant colour variation, ranging from greenish to brown, depending on their developmental stage and the environment.

The larvae exhibit polyphagous feeding habits, meaning they can feed on various plant species. In the early stages of development, they primarily consume the foliage of the host plant. However, in later stages, as they grow larger, the larvae shift to feeding on the seeds, particularly in crops like pulses and cotton. This feeding behaviour severely reduces crop yields, as it damages both the leaves and the reproductive parts of the plants.

One of the characteristic signs of *H. armigera* infestations is the presence of round holes in the pods of affected plants. The larvae can often be seen feeding with only their head inside the pod, while the rest of their body hangs outside. This feeding pattern is a typical behaviour of the larvae as they burrow into the pods to consume the seeds, making it an important indicator of the pest's presence.

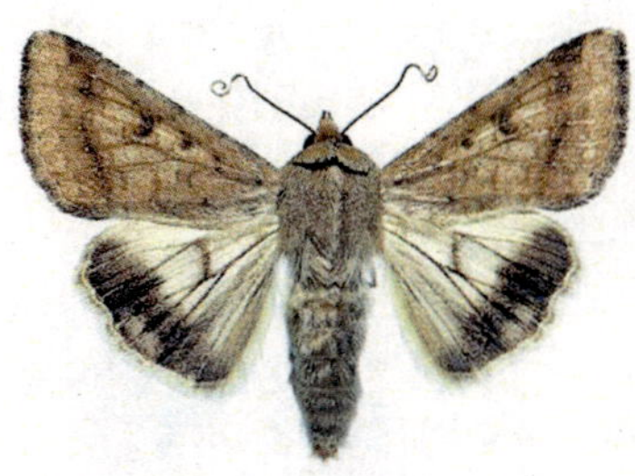
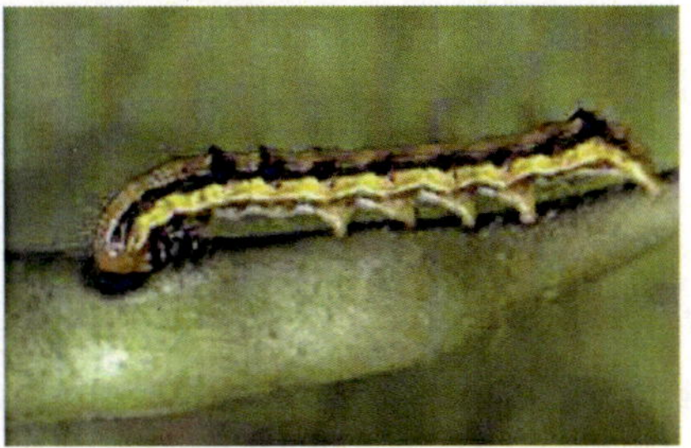

Host range

Gram pod borer is a polyphagous pest infesting a wide array of crops like cotton, tomato, chickpea, soybean, peas, maize, groundnut, sunflower, lentils, mung bean, crucifers, okra, popper, rice, apple, papaya, citrus.

Distribution

Wide distribution prevailing in majority of cropping systems in Asia, Africa, Europe, Australia, America etc.

Biology: Eggs are sculptured and creamy white in colour, laid singly, hatches in three – ten days. Larva has six growth stages and shows colour variation from greenish to brown. It has dark brown grey lines on the body with lateral white lines and also has dark band. Pupa is brown in colour, occurs in soil, leaf, pod and crop debris. Adult females are light pale brownish-yellow stout moths, and males are pale greenish moths with V-shaped specks. The forewings are olive green to pale brown with a dark brown circular spot in the centre, and the hindwing is pale smoky white with a broad blackish outer margin. The moths live for about 10 days. The entire lifecycle takes 4-5 weeks at an average temperature of 28°C.

Nature of damage and symptom

- Larvae cause damage by feeding on the pods
- Neonates cause defoliation
- Larvae thrust head alone inside the pods and rest of the body is outside.
- Pods with round holes

Spiny pod borer / Lima bean pod borer	:	*Etiella zinckenella* Treitschke
Family	:	Pyralidae
Order	:	Lepidoptera

Etiella zinckenella, commonly known as the pulse pod borer, is a significant pest of pulse crops, particularly affecting legumes like chickpeas, lentils, and beans. The larvae of *E. zinckenella* are initially greenish in colour and undergo a colour change as they approach pupation, turning pink. One distinguishing feature of the larva is the presence of five black spots on the prothorax.

The adult moth is a brownish-grey insect, with its forewings displaying dark marginal lines and a distinctive white stripe running along the anterior margin. These moths are typically nocturnal, and the females lay their eggs on the pods of pulse plants, where the larvae eventually hatch and begin feeding.

Host range

Chickpea, lentils, beans

Biology: Eggs are laid on the pods. Egg period is 5 days. Newly emerged larva enters the pods and feed on the internal parts. The full-grown larva is rosy with purplish tinge. Larval period is 10 to 27 days. Pupation takes place in soil and pupal period is 10 to 15 days.

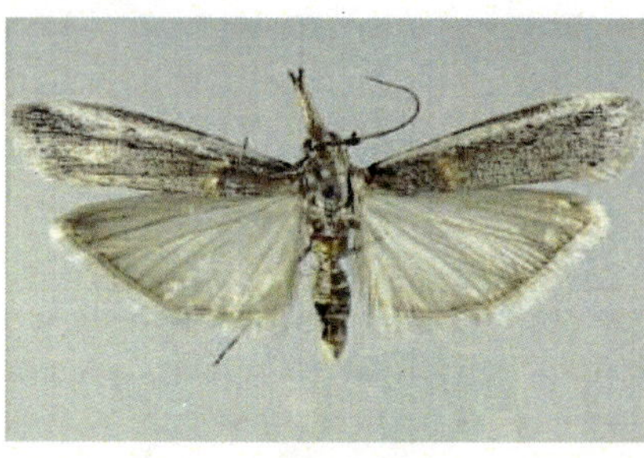

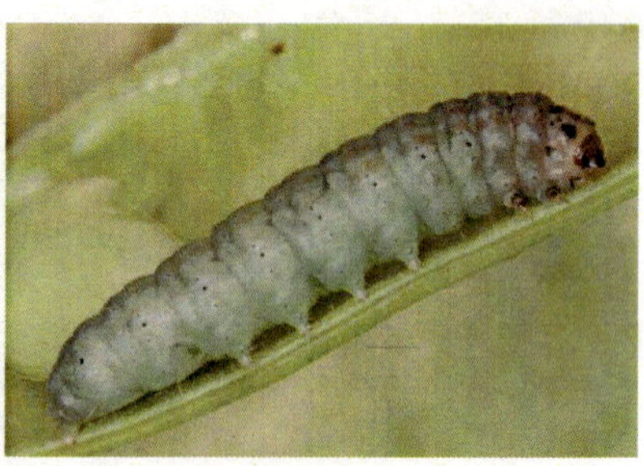

Symptoms of damage

- Dropping of flowers and young pods
- Older pods marked with a brown spot where a larvae has entered
- Larvae cause damage by feeding on the developing pods of pulse crops, leading to significant yield loss if infestations are left uncontrolled.

Field bean borer	:	*Adisura atkinsoni* Moore
Family	:	Noctuidae
Order	:	Lepidoptera

Adisura particularly *A. atkinsoni* is a specific, locally adapted, economically important pod borer on cowpea, lablab, beans and other pulse crops. The life cycle of the pod borer appears to have co-evolved with the life cycle of the plant. In Karnataka, South India, *A. atkinsoni* is attracted to the specific odour that emanates from the plant and its parts. Thus, 'local cultivar' is highly susceptible to this pod borer. In some Lablab varieties, which secrete the so-called fragrant oil on the surface of pods is preferred for consumption by humans and insects as well.

The moths start emerging by middle of October from the pupae of previous season, formed inside the soil. During the season, insect completes two generations and third generation caterpillars pupated in the soil and remains till the next season of the crop. The egg laying by *A. atkinsoni* started in the month of October and appeared to be three generations, the fourth generation larvae hibernate in the soil as pupae, till the next season. The second generation of the pest appeared to be most damaging

Host range

Field bean, soybean, chickpeas, lentils, peas etc.

Distribution

Wide distribution from tropical to subtropical regions of the world.

Biology: The entire life cycle is about 44 days. The fecundity vary from 150 to 180 eggs. Eggs are opalescent white spherical eggs are laid singly either on the pods or on the flower buds. The incubation period lasts for three to four days. Tender leaves were preferred only when flower buds and pods were absent.

A. atkinsoni have five larval instars with 3, 2, 2, 2 and 6 days, respectively. A fully grown 5th instar caterpillar measures 27-28 mm long. A great variation is seen in the colour of the later stages of the larva depending on the nature of food available. Especially in the third generation, brownish green-coloured larvae were seen than in the earlier generations. The caterpillar enters the soil, prepares an oval earthen chamber underground and pupates. However, even in the absence of soil the larvae pupate in individual receptacles. Pupae measures 18 mm long and appear thick and red brown. The pupal period varied from 15 to 18 days.

Nature of damage and symptoms

- Bore into the pods and eat the seeds.
- Pods have round holes and seeds inside may be partially or completely eaten.

Pea blue butterfly: *Lampides boeticus* L.,Lycaenidae , Lepidoptera

Pea blue butterfly also called peacock pansy is a pest of fabaceae Family. Adult is a fragile blue butterfly. Eggs are laid singly on flower buds and pods. Caterpillars are flat and pale green. Caterpillars burrow into the tender pods feeding on the seeds or into buds destroying them. The caterpillars are seen partly exposed at the entrance of the bore hole. Adult moth is greyish blue with prominent black spots in the hind wings and a long tail; Ventral side of wings with numerous stripes and brown spots.

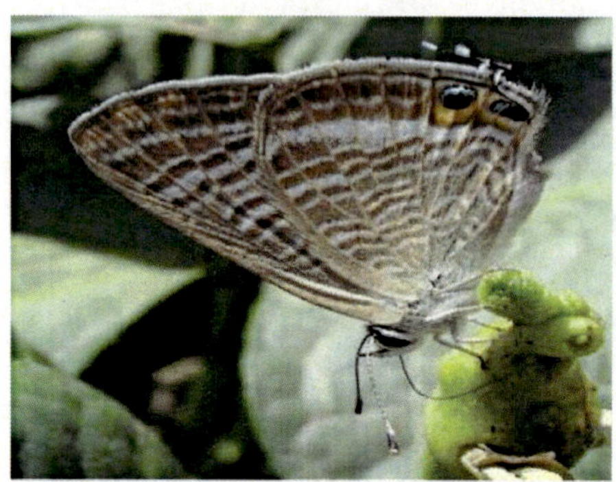
Adult

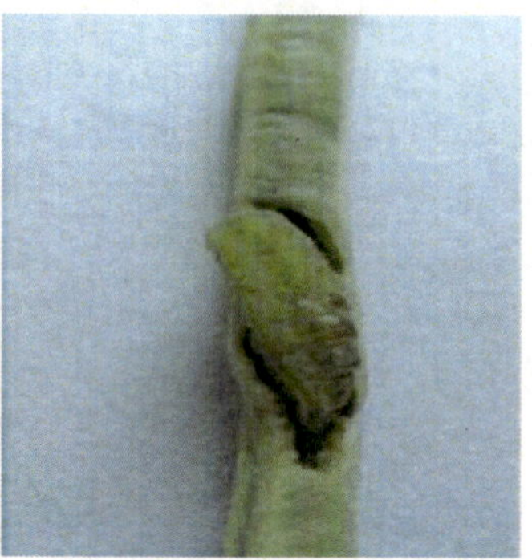
Larva feeding on the pod

Host range

Crotalaria sp., *Sesbania* sp., *Phaseolus* sp., *Vigna* sp.

Distribution

Tropical and sub-tropical region of Asia – India, Srilanka, Bangladesh, Thailand, Indonesia

Biology: *Lampides boeticus* completes its life cycle in 15-22 days. Eggs are laid on flower buds and pods, egg period is 2-3 days, larval period is 8-12 days, pre- pupa period is for 2-3 days and pupal period is 3-4 days.

Nature of damage and symptoms

- Defoliation
- Feeding results in irregular holes and tattered edges
- Buds, flowers and young pods with boreholes Presence of slug like caterpillar.
- Honey dew secretion with black ant movements

Grass blue butterfly: *Euchrysops cnejus* F., Lycaenidae, Lepidoptera

Euchrysops cnejus, commonly known as the common silver line. The larvae of *E. cnejus* are typically pale green or yellow in colour, with a characteristic red line running along the body. The body is covered with minute white tubercles, there are also a few scattered white hairs. Adult butterfly is medium sized and blue coloured with 5 black spots in hind wings.

Host range

Crotalaria sp., *Sesbania* sp., *Phaseolus* sp., *Vigna* sp.

Distribution

Tropical and sub-tropical regions of Asia including India, Sri Lanka, Thailand, Indonesia

Biology: The eggs are laid singly under the leaves. There are 4 larval instars, prepupa and pupal stage. Total larval duration is 15-16 days, prepupa lasts for about 3 days and pupation for 7 days. Total life cycle will be completed within 23-30 days.

Nature of damage and symptoms

- Buds, flowers and young pods with boreholes and presence of slug like caterpillar.
- Larval entry hole on the pod is plugged with excreta.

Plume moth, *Exelastis atomosa* Wals., Pterophoridae, Lepidoptera

Plume moths, belonging to the Pterophoridae Family, can pose a significant threat as pests to pulse crops. These moths are characterized by their unique wing structure, where the wings are divided into narrow, feathery plumes, giving them an elegant but deceptive appearance. While they may seem delicate, the larvae of plume moths are known to cause considerable damage to pulses, such as lentils, chickpeas, and beans. The larvae feed on the leaves, flowers, and seeds of the plants, often causing stunted growth, reduced yield, and even plant death in severe infestations.

Host range

Chickpea, lentil, pigeon pea, green gram, black gram, pea, soybean, horse gram, lablab

Biology: Female moth lays egg singly on the tender parts of the plants. Egg period is 2 to 5 days. Larvae feed on the pods and become full grown within a period of 10 to 25 days. Pupal period is 3 to 12 days.

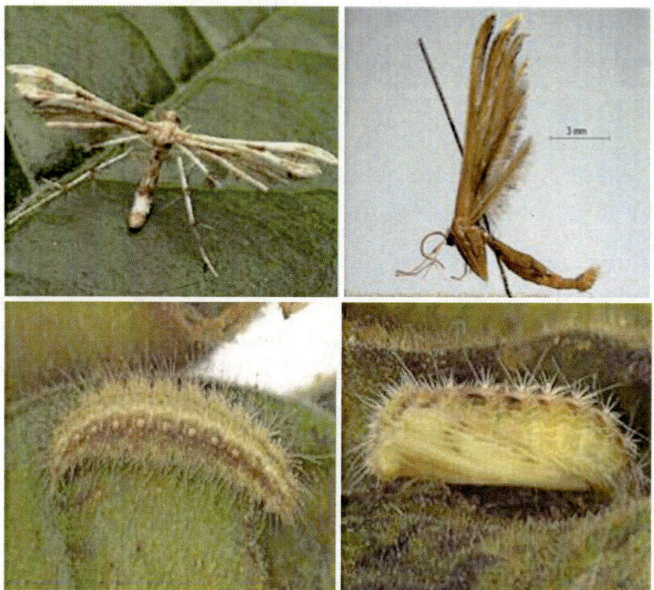

Nature of damage and symptoms

- The larvae first scrape the surface of the pods
- Mature larva make holes into them and feed on the seeds.

Eublemma (Polyorycta) dimidialis F., Noctuidae, Lepidoptera

The adult moth has forewings that have a pink marginal half containing a diffuse yellow band, and a basal pale brown half fading to pale yellow at the base. The hind wings are pale brown darkening toward the margins. Larva feed on flower as well as pods.

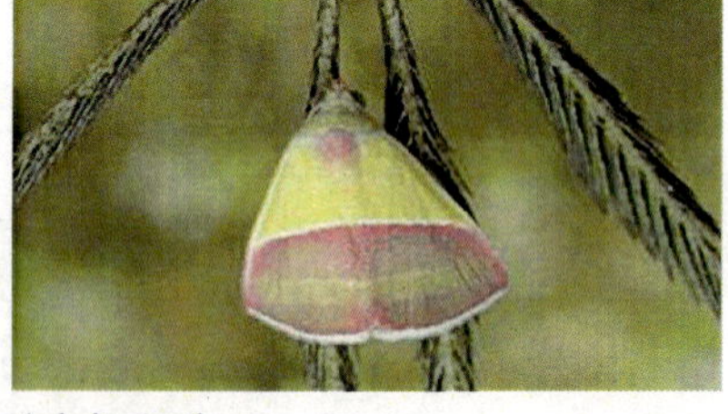

Adult moth

Management of pod borer complex in pulses

- Destruction of debris, crop residues, weeds & other alternate hosts
- Enhance the population of predatory birds by installing bird perches @ 50 / ha
- Set up light trap and collection and destruction of adult moths
- Frequent raking of soil beneath the crop to expose and kill the eggs, grubs & pupae
- Hand collection and destruction of infested leaves and fruits

- Adoption of proper crop rotation and avoid growing of same crops in sequence
- Use of resistant and tolerant varieties recommended by the State Agricultural Universities of the region
- ETL: 5-6 eggs or 2-3 small larvae / plant
- Spray *Bacillus thuringiensis* 2g/lit
- Release of egg parasitoids of *Trichogramma* species - *Trichogramma pretiosum* @ 1 lakh/ha/release at an interval of 7 days starting from flower initiation against *H. armigera* and 4-5 releases are needed
- Use pheromone traps Helilure @ 12 / ha for *Helicoverpa armigera*
- Intercropping with maize or sorghum reduce incidence of spotted pod borer
- Apply NPV @ 250 LE / ha + 0.1 % teepol for *H. armigera.*
- Spray NSKE 5%+ 1% soap solution for borers at flower initiation and then at 15 days interval
- Use of entomopathogenic fungi (EPF) like *Beauveria bassiana* or *Metarhizium anisopliae* talc formulation @20g/l
- In case of severe infestation, spinosad 45%SC / cypermethrin 10%EC / novaluron 10%EC/ fenvalerate 20 EC/ cypermethrin 10%EC / deltamethrin 28% EC/ cartap hydrochloride 50 SP
- Apply insecticides after harvesting the mature pods and pick pods only 5-7 days after application

Defoliators

Omiodes diemenalis (Nacoleia vulgaris) Guenee, Crambidae, Lepidoptera

Small day-active moth, yellow with dark brown wings; wings crossed with wavy lines. fore wings have 2 spots and 3 wavy lines. Hind wings have 1 thicker line crossing wings through the middle. Caterpillar lives in a shelter made of a rolled leaf and cause defoliation.

Dead hawk moth – *Acherontia styx* Medusa Moore, Sphingidae, Lepidoptera

Giant hawk moth, brownish with a characteristic skull marking on the thorax and violet and yellow bands on the abdomen. Hind wing yellow with black marking. Caterpillar stout green with yellowish oblique stripes and curved anal horn. Defoliator. Pupation in soil.

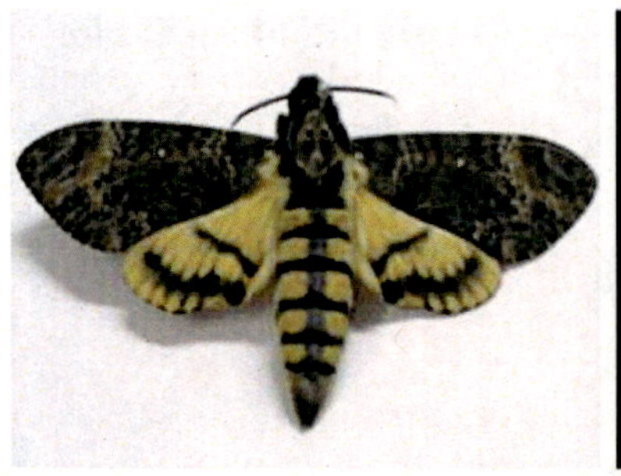
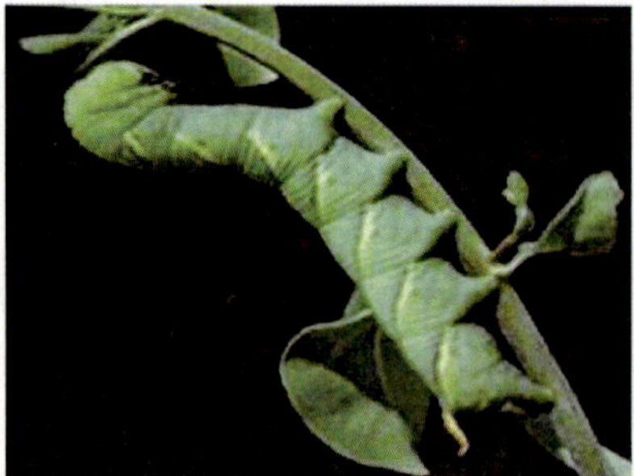
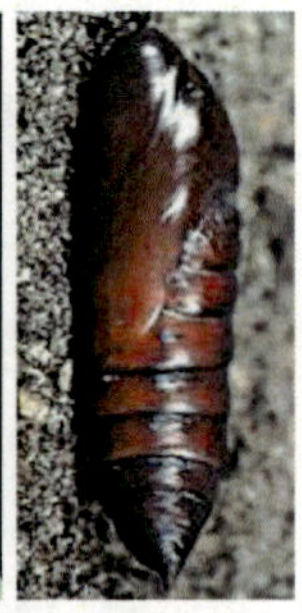

Adult Caterpillar Pupa

Agrius convolvuli L., Sphingidae, Lepidoptera

Eggs bright, glossy blue-green when laid, changing to yellowish green. Almost spherical, deposited singly on the leaves of the host plant. Larvae green with a prominent anal horn. The larval stages last from three to four weeks with 5 larval instars. All are extremely sluggish. Pupation in soil. Pupa very sensitive and mobile, twitching violently if disturbed. Formed in a smooth-sided, hollow, oval pupal chamber.

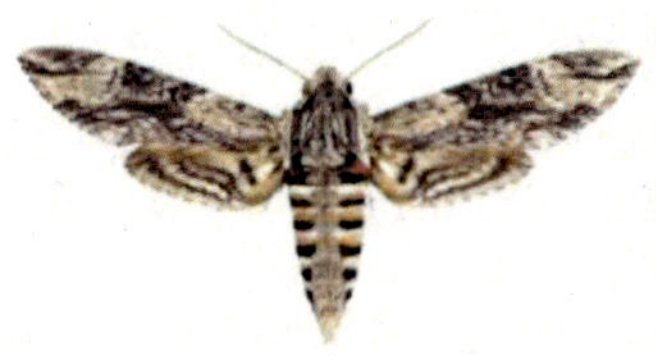
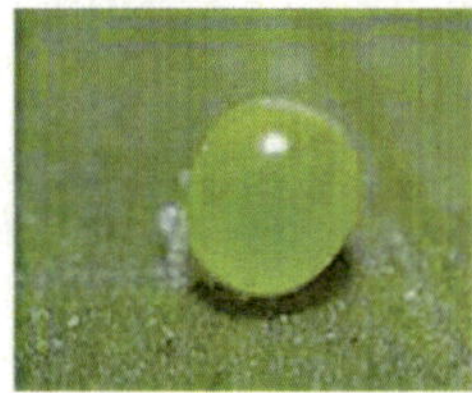
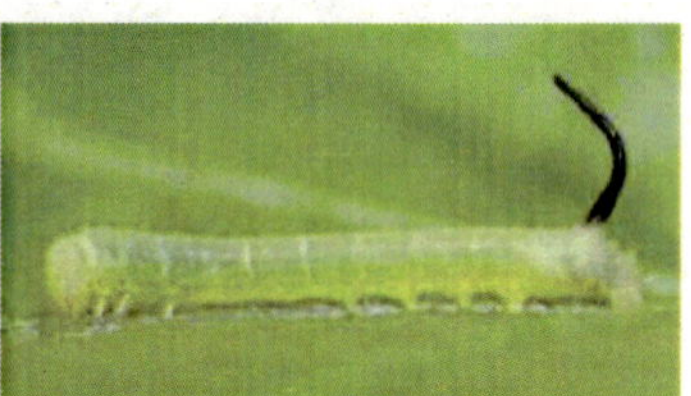

Adult moth Egg Larva

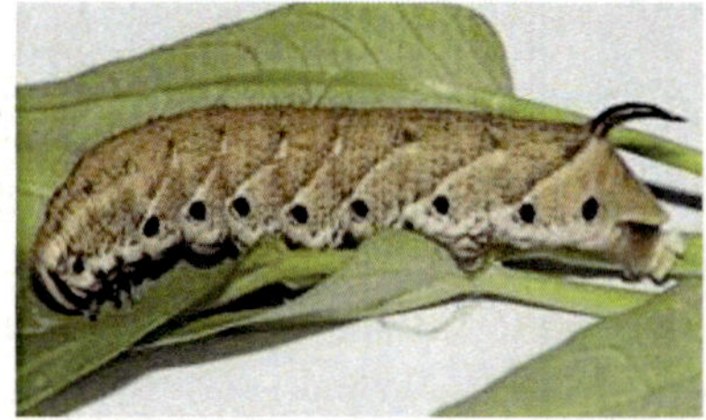
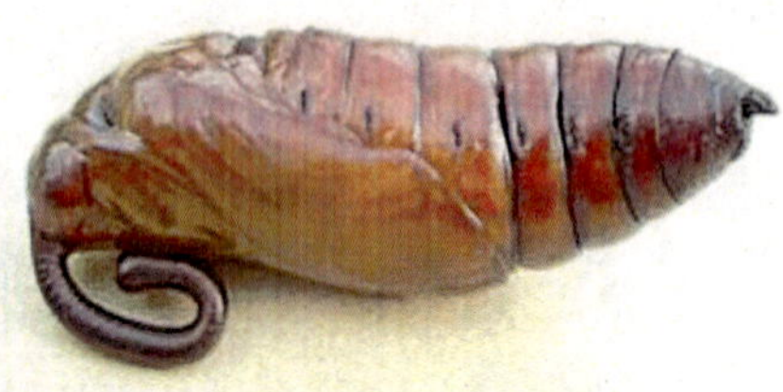

Matured larva Pupa

Bihar hairy caterpillar, *Spilosoma obliqua* Walker, Erebidae, Lepidoptera

Spilosoma obliqua, commonly known as the tussock moth or orange- tipped tussock moth. It is widely distributed across parts of Asia and the Indian subcontinent, where it is a pest of various crops. The eggs of *Spilosoma obliqua* are laid in clusters on the underside of leaves. The larval stage is distinctive, with caterpillars covered in long yellowish to black hairs. These larvae can cause considerable damage to crops as they feed on the leaves of plants. The adult moth is medium-sized with a brownish coloration and is characterized by its red abdomen. The moth's wings are typically pale with darker markings, and its presence is often noticed when it flies around vegetation at dusk or during the night.

Biology: Egg incubation period ranged from 5-6 days with an average of 5.75 days. Six larval instars with a mean duration of 20 days. Pupation occured in the soil, inside the hairy cocoon. Pupal duration is 8-9 days under optimal conditions.

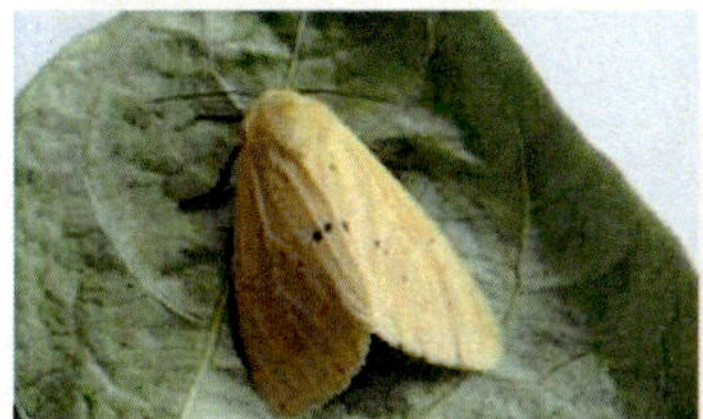
Adult moth

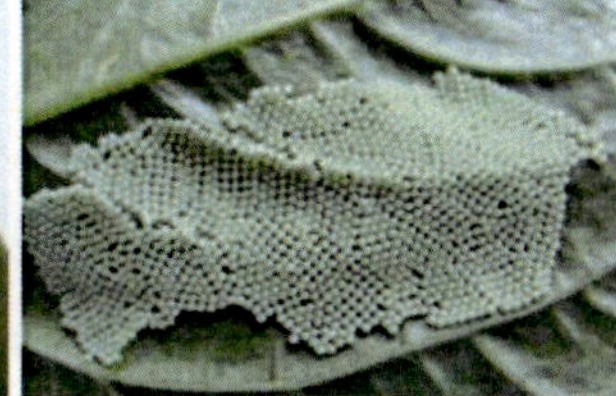
Egg mass

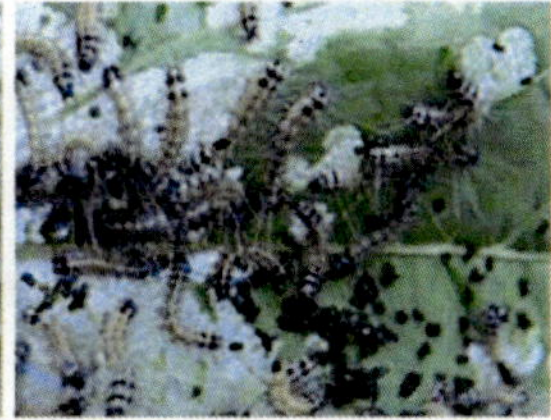
Larvae feeding on the leaves

Groundnut hairy caterpillar-*Amsacta albistriga* Walker, Erebidae, Lepidoptera

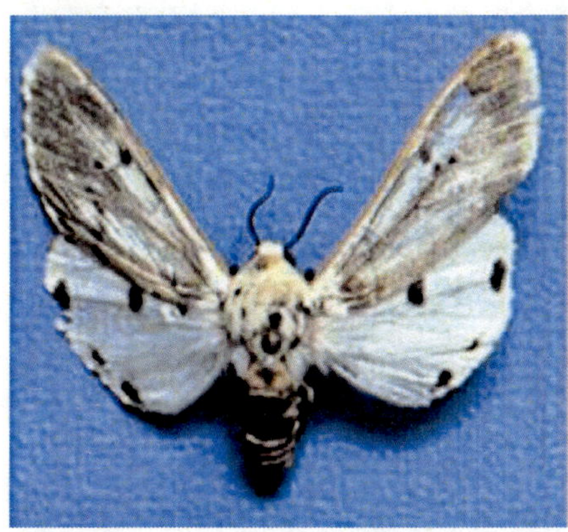
Moth

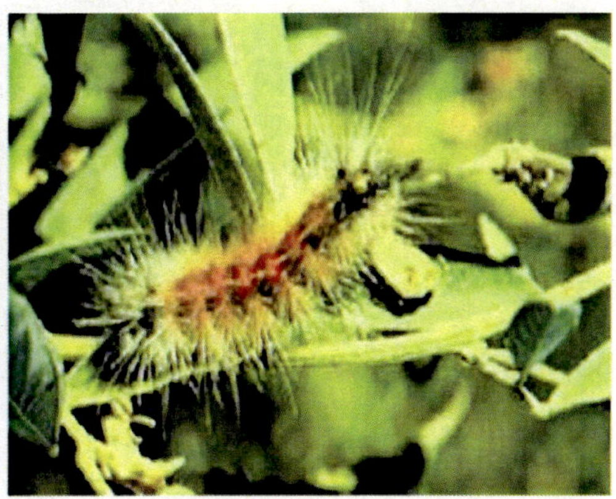
Larva

The adults emerge from the soil at the onset of the southwest monsoon (usually in June). Females lay 800-1000 eggs in clusters of 50-100 on groundnut and other host plants. The larvae are initially light brown, but turn reddish as they grow. Their 'hairiness' makes them conspicuous, especially the larger ones. They devastate groundnut foliage or other pulse crops and then migrate to the next groundnut field/ pulse field.

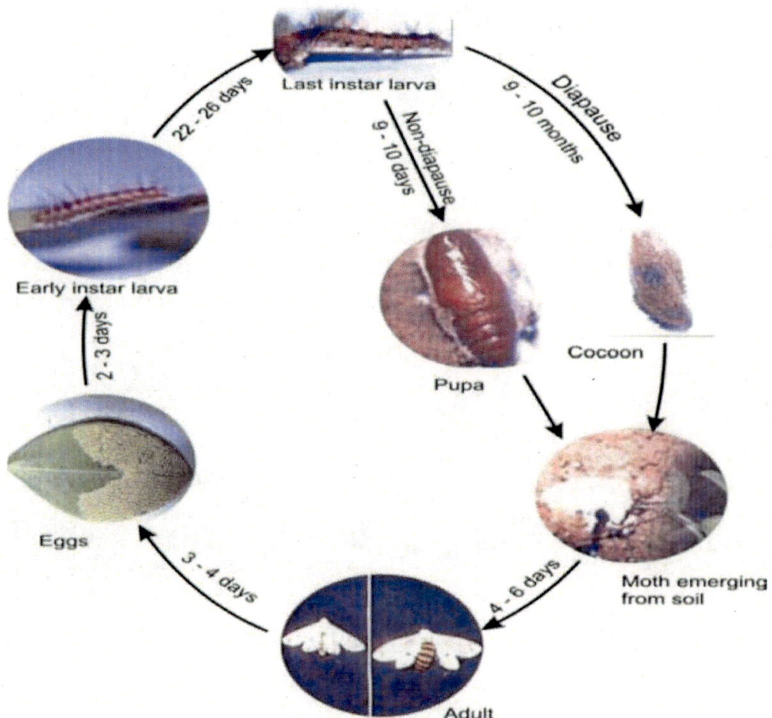

Symptoms of damage

- Young larvae feed gregariously on chlorophyll mostly on the under surface of the leaves, due to which the leaves look like brownish-yellow in colour.
- In later stages the larvae eat the leaves from the margin.
- The leaves of the plant give an appearance of net or web

Management

- Deep summer ploughing.
- Avoid pre monsoon sowing.
- Use optimum seed rate.
- Adequate plant spacing should be provided
- Intercrop soybean either with (early maturing) pigeon pea variety or maize or sorghum in the sequence of 4:2 should be practiced.
- Collect & destroy infested plant parts, egg masses and young larvae.
- Field Sanitation: Remove the infested plant parts at least once in 10 days and bury them in compost pit to monitor and reduce the population.

- Light Trap: Install one light trap (200W mercury vapour lamp) per hectare to catch the adults of some nocturnal pests such as hairy caterpillar (positively phototropic).

Stem fly/ Bean fly, *Ophiomyia phaseoli* Tryon, Agromyzidae, Diptera

Bean flies are one of the most destructive pests of food legumes, especially during the crops' seedling stage. They occur in Asia, Africa, Australia and Oceania. Larvae of these insects feed on legumes as internal feeders. *O. phaseoli* has the widest distribution and host range, and causes the maximum damage.

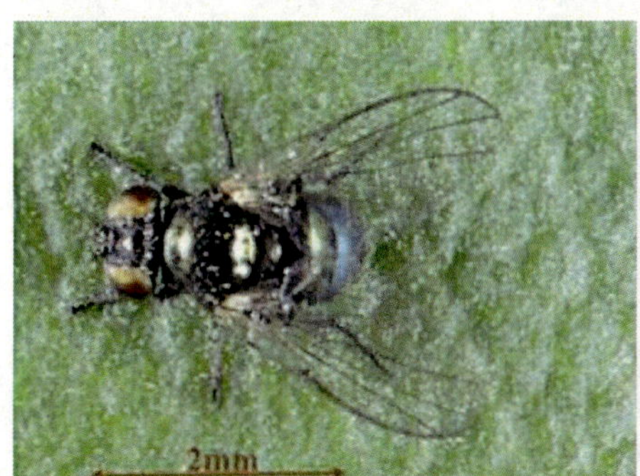

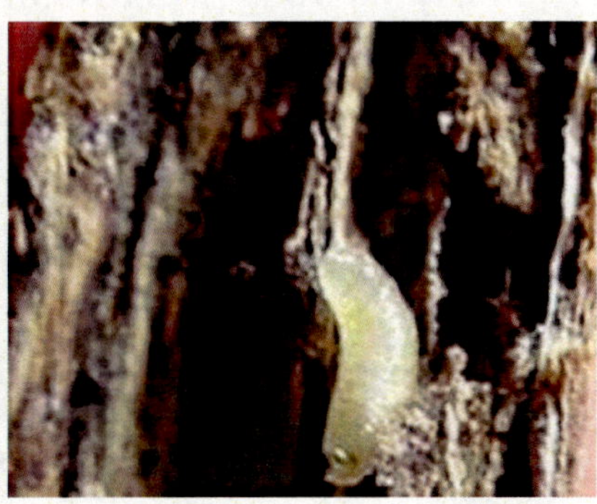

Biology: They usually lay the eggs on the upper leaf surfaces, often near the midrib close to the petiole. The eggs are inserted between the epidermis and spongy parenchyma. Each female lays about 300 eggs throughout its life. The egg period is 2 to 4 days depending on the temperature. Maggots are yellow in colour. The maggot of *O. phaseoli* has three instars. The newly hatched pale maggot remains motionless beneath the leaf epidermis in a cavity made by its mother during egg laying. One to two hours after emergence, it starts feeding inside a mine directed toward the vein of the leaf. On reaching the midrib, the larva constructs a tunnel in it and molts into the second instar. The yellowish white second instar larva moves its head constantly from side to side within the relatively straight mine built in the leaf vein. The light yellow-colored third instar larva actively feeds in the petiole or stem. In younger plants, the larva continues feeding inside the stem until or slightly below the soil level. However, it feeds only in the junction of petiole and stem until its pupation in older plants. The larval period is about 8 to 9 days. The maggot of *O. phaseoli* pupates on young plants beneath the epidermis of the stem near the soil surface. Under high larval density, pupation may also take place inside the stem pith. In mature plants, pupation takes place at the junction of the leaf lamina and petiole. The pupal period varies from 1 to 3 weeks depending on the temperature and altitude

Nature of damage and symptom

- The fly punctures the leaves with the ovipositor and the injured parts turn yellow
- The maggots bore into the stem as a result of which the plant withers, droops and dies
- The damage is more on seedlings than in grown up plants
- Attack on seedlings results in reduced stand of the crop

Pod fly – *Melanagromyza obtusa* Malloch, Agromyzidae, Diptera

Melanagromyza obtusa is a species of fly in the Family Agromyzidae and is recognized as a significant pest of cowpea (*Vigna unguiculata*), red gram and other pulse crops widely cultivated for its edible seeds and pods, especially in tropical and subtropical regions. This pest is known for its destructive impact on cowpea plants, leading to reduced yields and quality.

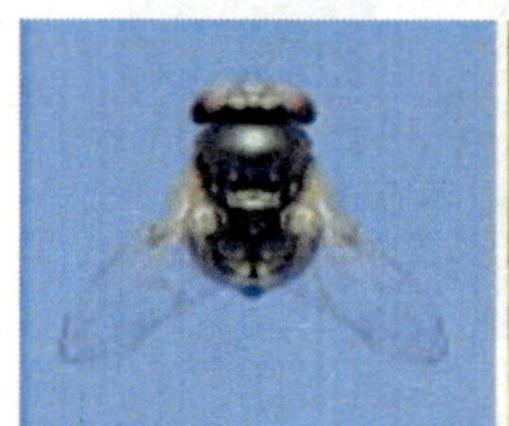
Adult fly

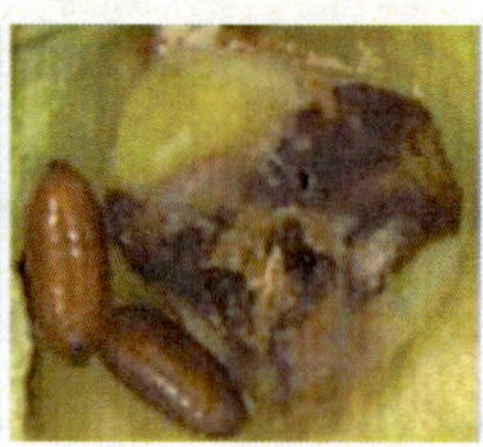
Pupae

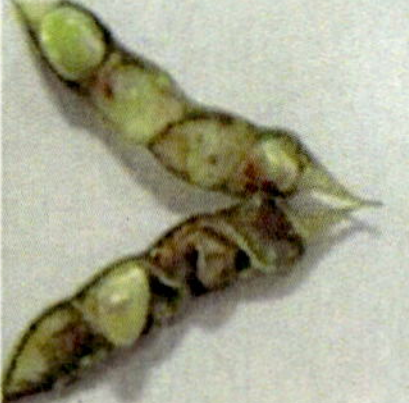
Infested pod

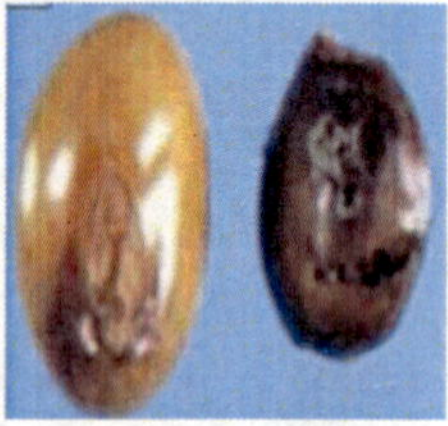
Damaged seeds

Biology: Adult is a small black fly. Needle shaped eggs are laid singly within the pods, can be seen projecting inwards from the walls of the pods. *M. obtusa* female lays eggs singly on the green pods. The freshly laid eggs are white and broad. The egg period is 3 to 10 days depending on the temperature. Maggots are small and white coloured and make galleries just below the epidermis of the seeds. The pupa is enclosed in a hard chitinous puparium that is attached to the inner side of the pod wall. The newly formed pupa is yellowish white and gradually turns to creamy yellow, reddish brown and darker. The pupal period varies from 1 to 3 weeks. Pupation is inside the larval groove.

Nature of damage and symptoms

- Maggots are causing damage.
- Initially, the maggots make galleries just below the epidermis of seeds.
- Later they feed deeper into the seeds.
- Seeds are partially eaten and become shriveled.
- Pods are undersized, become dry and show pin-head sized holes.

Management of both bean fly/ stem fly and pod fly

- Choose resistant or moderately resistant cultivars available in the region. For instance, accessions or varieties having purple stems, thinner stems and smaller pith diameter are resistant to bean flies
- Increase the seed rate by 25-30% - compensate for the loss of seedlings.
- Correct use of green manures and fertilizers. Improved fertility leads to vigorously growing plants which are able to tolerate infestation.
- Earth up the plants three days after the appearance of the cotyledons above ground, so that most of the plants can overcome bean fly infestation. Production of adventitious roots in the affected basal portion of the stem helps considerably in the resistance of the plant to bean fly / stem fly.
- Early sowing will reduce the infestation of bean fly.
- Mulching and earthing up promotes adventitious root establishment, providing recovery tolerance to stem.
- Foliar application of neem garlic emulsion 2%.
- Spraying dimethoate 2 ml/l.

American serpentine leaf miner, *Liriomyza trifolii* Burgess, Agromyzidae, Diptera

Liriomyza trifolii is a species of leaf miner fly in the Family Agromyzidae, recognized as a significant pest of cowpea (*Vigna unguiculata*), among many other crops. This pest is particularly problematic in warm, tropical, and subtropical climates, where it causes damage to various leguminous plants, including cowpea, through its larval feeding behavior.

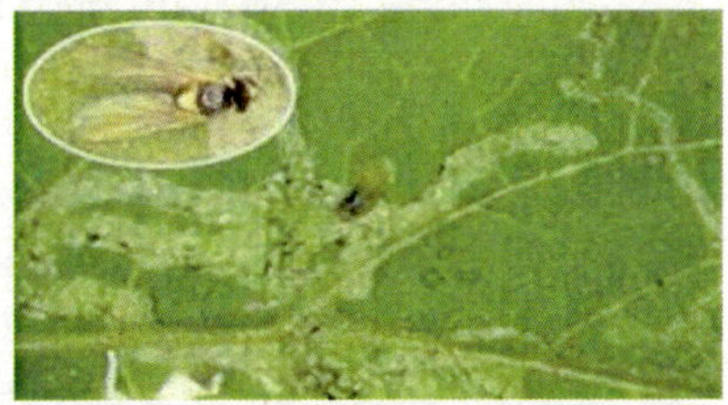

Serpentine mines on leaf caused by maggot

Biology: Eggs are thrust on the leaf surface. The emerging maggots are orange yellow and are seen in the mines on the leaves. The fully grown maggot comes out of the mine and pupates in the soil. Life cycle is completed in 20 to 30 days

Nature of damage and symptoms

- Maggots mine the leaves and feed on the mesophyll making serpentine mines on the leaves
- As the size of the maggot increases the breadth of the mine also increases and finally ends in a hood like blotch

- Several mines are seen on a leaf
- Severe infestation results in drying of the leaves

Management

- Neem cake application @ 200 kg/acre at the time of land preparation
- Spraying neem formulation @ 4 mL/L (azadirachtin 3000ppm)
- In severe conditions, spray spinosad @ 3.3 mL/10L or fipronil @ 2 mL/L

Sucking pest

Cowpea aphid, *Aphis craccivora* Koch, Aphididae, Hemiptera

Aphis craccivora is an important legume pest of Asia and recent observations suggest that aphids may also be seasonally important in parts of Africa. This species of aphid not only causes direct damage to its hosts (including groundnut as well as cowpea) but also transmits cowpea aphid-borne mosaic virus.

Biology: *Aphis craccivora* is a medium sized, shiny black aphid medium sized, shiny black aphid whose biology varies depending on climate and soil. Under favorable conditions a generation may take only 8-13 days. Adults live for 6 to 15 days and may produce over 100 progeny.

Nature of damage and symptoms

Colonisation by dark-coloured nymphs and adults can be observed on leaves, inflorescence stalks, and young pods. Due to honeydew excretion by the aphids, ants are commonly associated with them. On cowpea, aphids normally suck sap from young leaves, young stem tissue and young pods of mature plants. When present in large numbers, they cause direct feeding damage. The plants become stunted, leading to leaf distortion, premature defoliation, flower drop and malformation of pods. If seeedlings are infested, severe infestation can lead to their death. An indirect and generally more harmful effect, even of small populations, is the transmission of cowpea aphid-borne mosaic virus. The adults and nymphs suck sap from the underside of leaves, terminal shoots of stem and branches, flower stalks and pods. The plants are stunted with crinkled leaves. Pods are malformed.

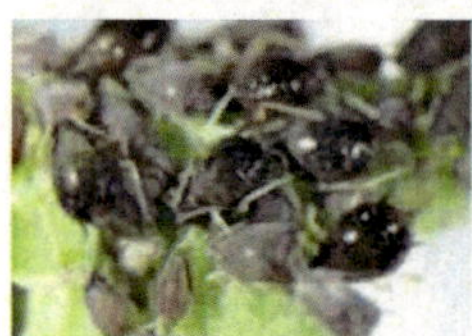
Aphis craccivora-adults

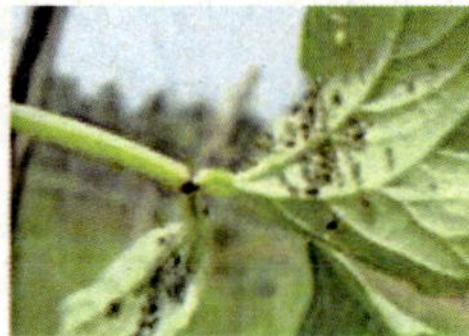
Population on leaves

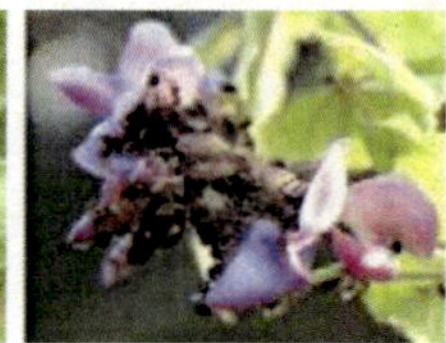
Flowers

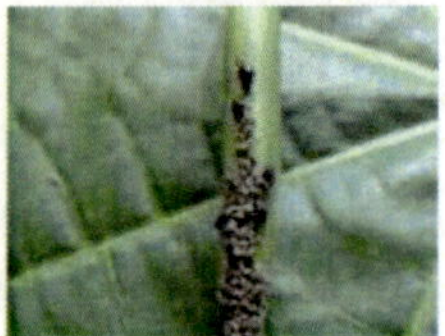
Stem

Management

- Hand collection and destruction of infested leaves and fruits.
- Avoid monoculture and follow crop rotation. The selected field should be located away from other legume crops and avoid growing of cucurbit crops in sequence
- Release green lace wings @ 2 grubs/plant against aphids.
- The ladybird beetles (*Menochilus sexmaculatus*, *Brumus suturalis*, *Harmonia dimidiate*, *Brumus suturalis* and *Coccinella septempunctata*) and green lacewings (*Chrysoperla zastrowii*) are efficient predators of aphids
- Application of neem seed kernel extract 5%
- Use entomopathogenic fungi (EPF) such as *Beauveria bassiana*, *Metarhizium anisopliae*, *Lecanicillium lecanii* and *Hirsutella thompsonii* at a concentration of 1×10^8 conidia mL/L and spraying should be repeated at 15 days intervals
- In case of severe infestation spraying of chemicals like imidacloprid @ 3 mL/10L or thiamethoxam @ 2g/10L or acetamiprid @ 2g/10L is recommended

Natural enemies

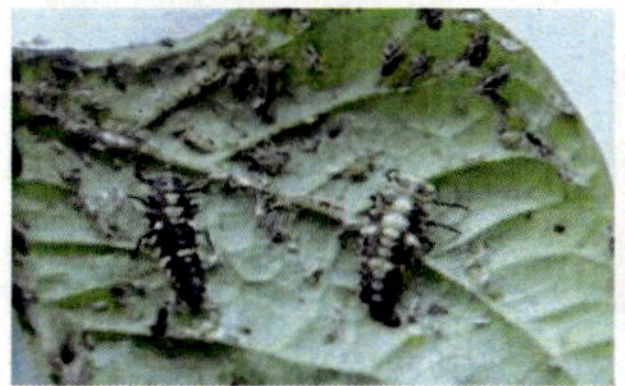

Coccinellid grubs

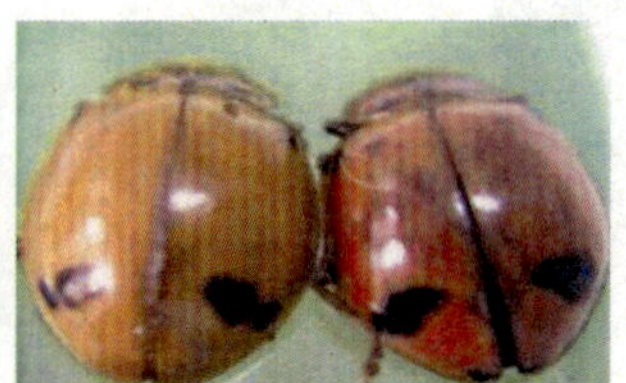

Harmonia octomaculata

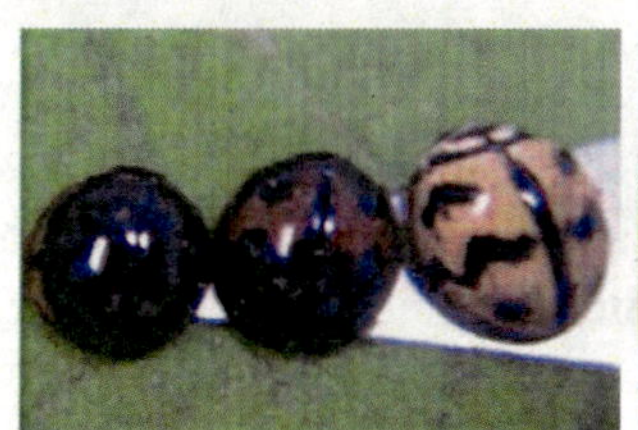

Menchilus sexmaculatus

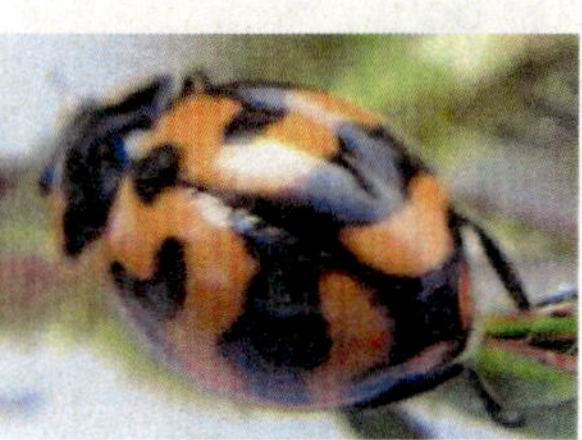

Coccinella transversalis

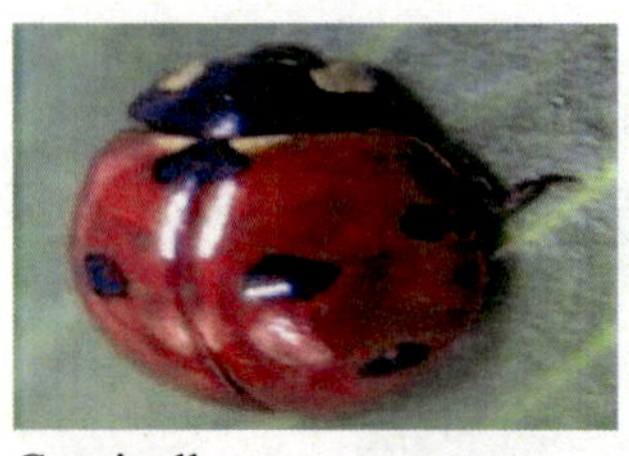

Coccinella septempunctata

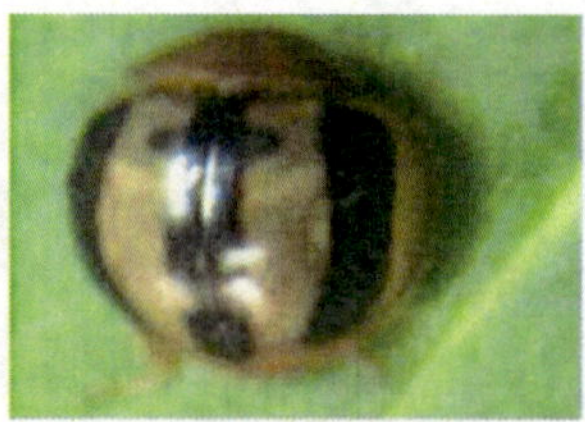

Brumoides suturalis

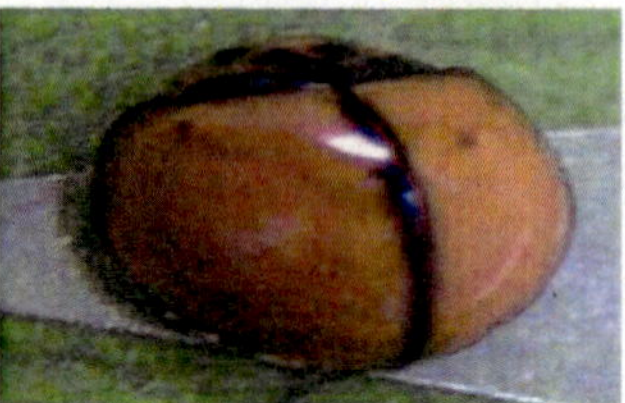

Micrapis discolor

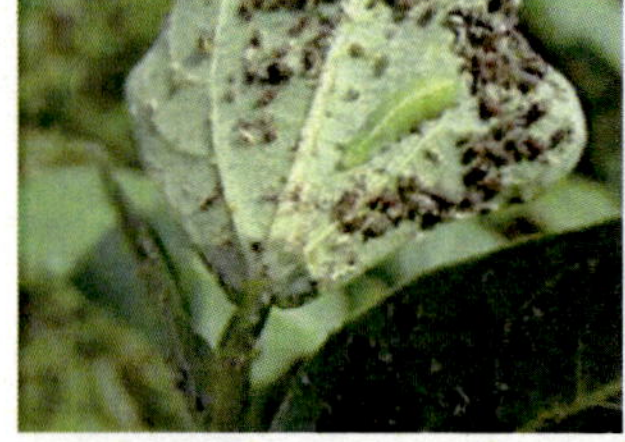

Syrphid maggot feeding on aphids

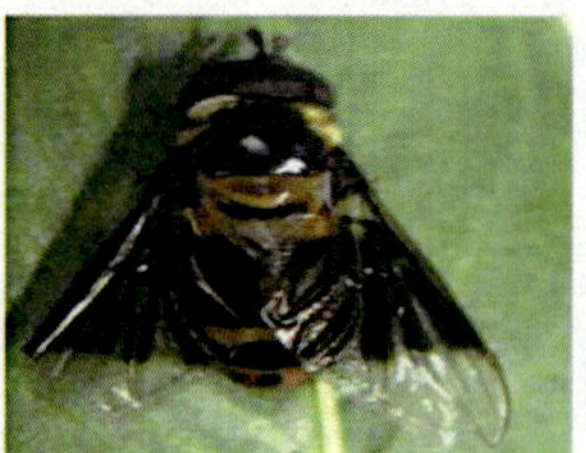

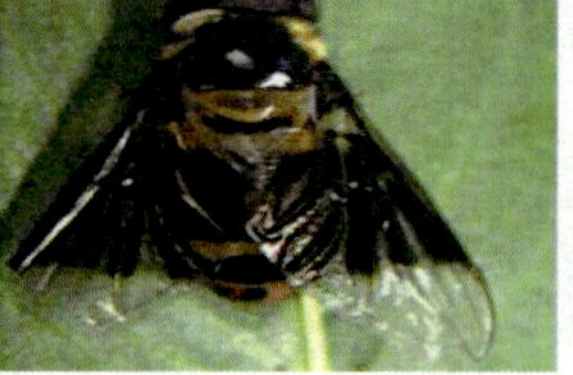

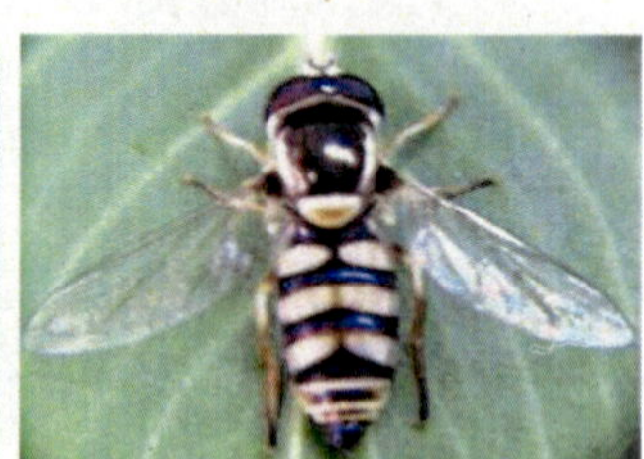

Syrphid adults

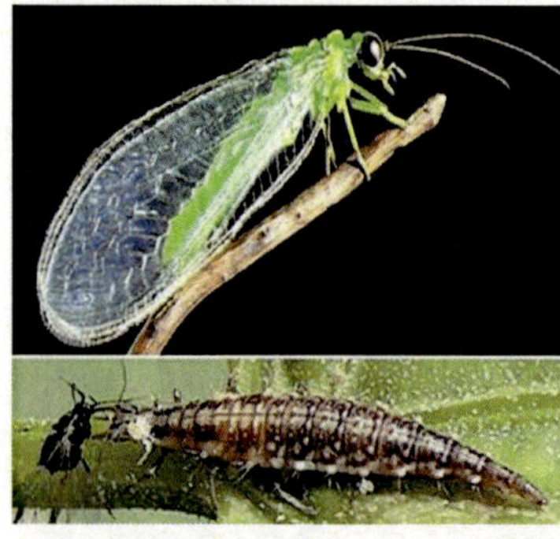

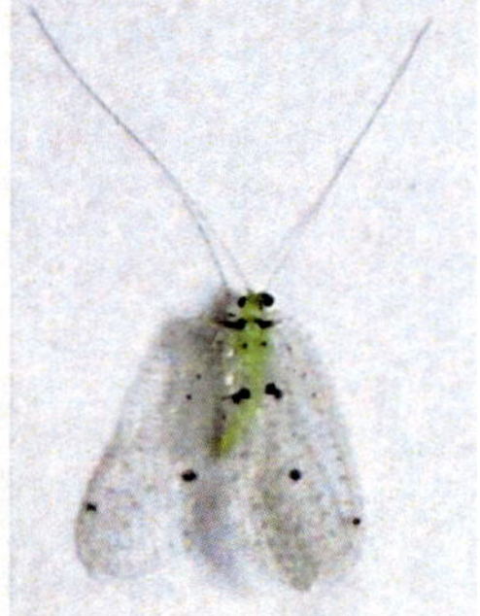

Chrysoperla zastrowii Zillemi

Flower thrips, *Megalurothrips distalis* Karny, *M. sjostedti (= Taeniothrips sjostedti*) Trybom

Flower thrips are one of the most important pests of cowpea. *M. distalis* and *M. usitatus* are widely distributed in South and Southeast Asia and Oceania; *M. sjostedti* predominantly occurs in Africa. They mainly feed on the flowers of legumes, and can cause 100% yield losses if left uncontrolled. In West Africa, they are frequently responsible for total crop loss.

Biology: The entire life cycle takes 14-18 days. Eggs are laid in the flower buds and nymphs lacerate the flower tissues and suck the exuding sap and cause extensive damage. Pupation in soil.

Nature of damage and symptoms

Adult thrips, which are shiny black, minute insects, and nymphs are found sucking sap from flower buds and flowers. Severely infested plants do not produce any flowers. Thrips remain hidden inside the flower buds and flowers. Slightly infested leaves exhibit silvery feeding scars. In severe infestations on the flowers, the open flowers are discolored and distorted showing elongated brownish streaks; they dry out, and fall prematurely without forming pods. Infested pods are scarred and deformed.

Management

- Application of *Metarhizium anisopliae* @ 10^8 spores / mL reduce the infestation of thrips
- Use mulch and reflective materials in vegetable legume fields to reduce the incidence of thrips
- In case of severe infestation chemicals like imidacloprid @ 3mL/10L or spinosad 3.3 mL/10L is recommended

Mites – *Tetranychus* spp.

Spider mites emerged as a serious pest of vegetable crops including vegetable legumes, eggplant, tomato, cucumber, and other field crops in South and Southeast Asia, Africa, Europe and Mediterranean countries. Low relative humidity favors the multiplication of mites and precipitation is the only important abiotic factor that restricts spider mite populations.

Biology: Eggs are round, white, or cream colored; egg period is 2 to 4 days. Upon hatching, spider mites will pass through a larval stage and two nymphal stages (protonymph and deutonymph) before becoming adults. The lifecycle is completed in 1 to 2 weeks. There are several overlapping generations in a year. The adult lives up to 3 to 4 weeks.

Nature of damage and symptoms

Both nymphs and adults are causing damage by sucking sap from the undersurface of leaves. Spider mites usually extract the cell contents from the leaves using their long, needle-like mouthparts. This results in reduced chlorophyll content in the leaves, leading to the formation of white or yellow speckles on the leaves. In severe infestations, leaves will completely desiccate and drop off. The mites also produce webbing on the leaf

Management

- Predatory mites such as *Phytoseiulus persimilis* and several species of *Amblyseius*, especially *A. womersleyi* and *A. fallacies* can be used to control spider mites

- Green lacewings (*Chrysoperla zastrowii*) also are effective generalist predators of spider mites
- Spraying Spiromesifen @ 8mL/10L or sulfex @ 3g/L is effective.

Leaf hoppers - *Empoasca* spp., Cicadellidae, Hemiptera

Empoasca species, commonly known as leafhoppers, are a group of sap-feeding insects that are significant pests of cowpea (*Vigna unguiculata*), particularly in tropical and subtropical regions. These insects are part of the Family Cicadellidae and can cause considerable damage to cowpea crops through their feeding behavior, which results in stunted plant growth and reduced yields.

Biology: Eggs, which are laid on the underside of leaves, hatch into nymphs within7-10 days. There are five stages (instars) in nymphal development which last about 10 days before the adult appears. The adults' life expectancy varies from 30 -60 days.

Nature of damage and symptoms

- Leafhoppers infest cowpeas at the seedling stage.
- The symptoms of damage are yellow discoloration of the leaf veins and margins, followed by cupping of the leaves
- Leave mottled and yellowish in colour
- Green colour insects found under surface of leaves
- Severely infested plants become stunted, and the symptoms developed will be similar to that of virus symptoms and may dry premature

Management

- In case of severe infestation, spraying dimethoate @ 1.5 mL/L

Pod bug complex in pulses

Green bean bug	:	*Riptortus pedestris* F.
Family	:	Alydidae
Order	:	Hemiptera

Biology: Egg period is 4 days. Nymphs resemble ants and are dark brown in colour. They undergo 5 instars during a nymphal period of 16 days

Nature of damage and symptoms

- Both nymphs and adults suck sap from the pods as well as seeds
- Pods with black spots initially and later malformation and drying of pods occur

- Shedding of green pods
- Poorly filled pods with shriveled grains inside

Tur pod bug : *Clavigralla gibbosa* S.
C. horrens S.

Family : Coreidae

Order : Hemiptera

C. gibbosa

The adult bugs are greenish brown in colour, having spines on pronotum and abdominal segments. The femur swollen at the apical end. The young nymphs are reddish and show prominent lateral spines on the prothoracic and abdominal segments.

Clavigralla horrens

Adult is brown and flat, bug with conspicuous lateral spines on the prothorax. Hind femur is enlarged. Eggs laid on pods and less frequently on leaves, or floral buds in cluster. Ep - 8 days. Nymphs gather together at a suitable feeding spot. Np - 17 days - five nymphal stages.

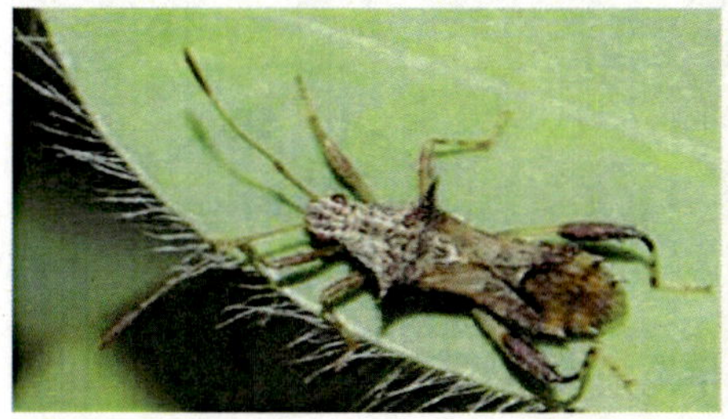

C. gibbosa

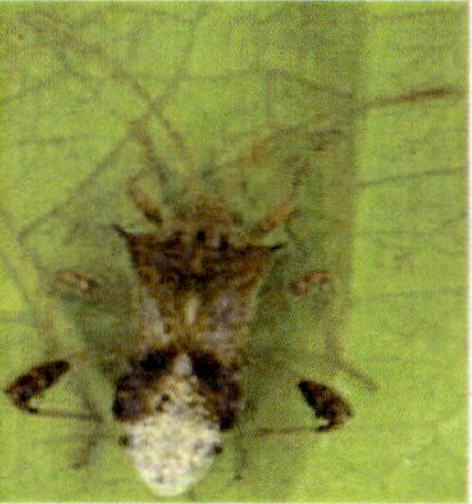

C. horrens

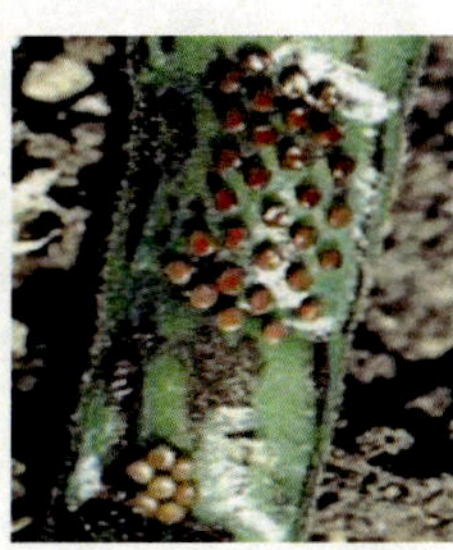

C. horrens egg mass

Lablab bug : *Coptosoma cribraria* F.

Family : Coptosomatidae

Order : Hemiptera

Adult bug is sub-globular oval and greenish with characteristic buggy smell. It lay creamy white sculptured egg in double rowed batches of 35 to 50 on the tender plant parts. The egg hatch in about 6 days. The life cycle is completed in about 7 weeks.

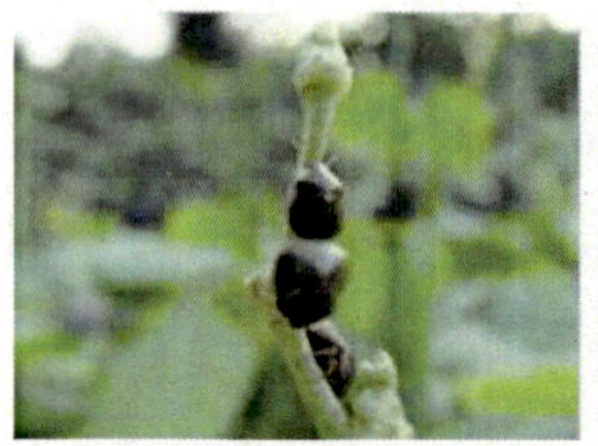
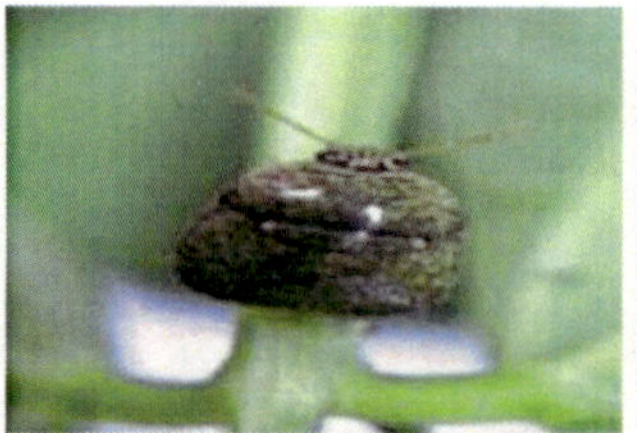
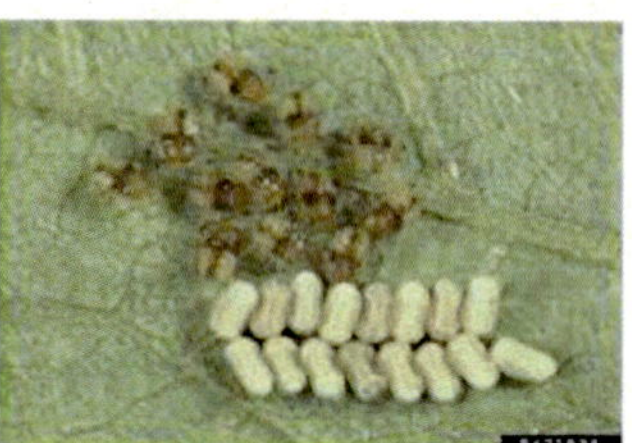

Green shield bug/ Southern green stink bug	:	*Nezara viridula* L.
Family	:	Pentatomidae
Order	:	Hemiptera

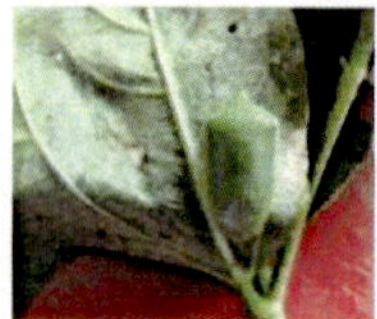
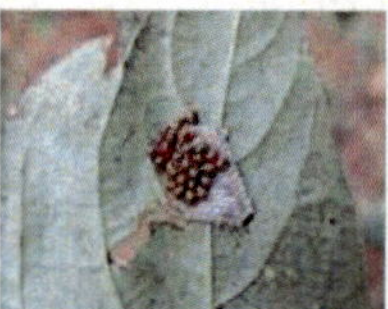
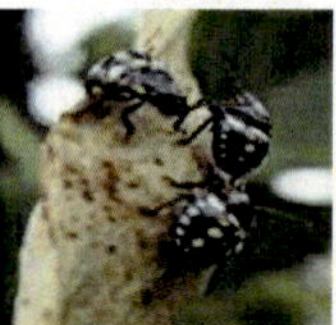
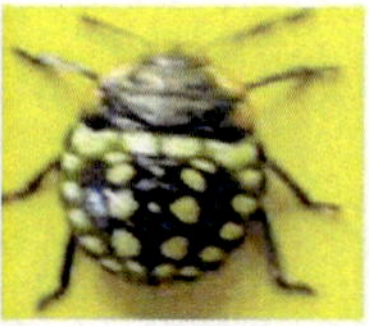
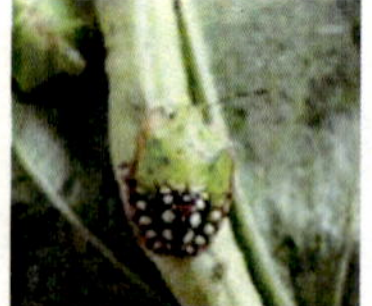

Large shield bug with green colour. All nymphs are about as broad as long, dark in color, with red, white or yellow markings on their body. The fourth and 5th nymphal stages with two colour phases - light to dark green or black - with characteristic yellow, red and green markings.

Nature of damage and symptoms

Adults and nymphs of pod bugs suck juice from the seeds as well as pods. The attacked seeds shrink and shrivel within the pods. Black spots are seen on infested pods. Severe infestation results in shedding of green pods.

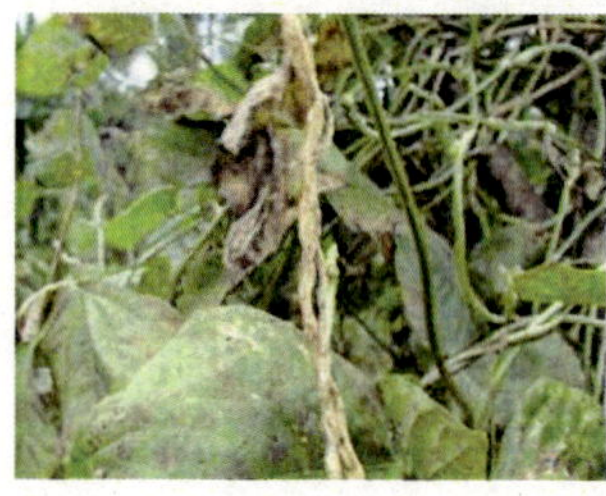
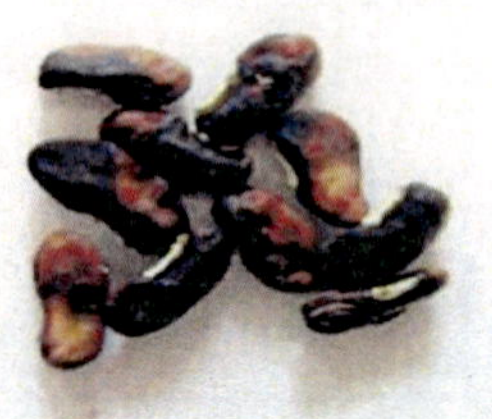

Damage symptoms on pods and seeds

Management

- Collect bugs with sweep nets and destroy
- Destroy alternate hosts
- Spray water, when the bugs are in the nymphal stage
- *Beauveria bassiana* 20g/L or *Verticillium / Lecanicillium lecanii* 20g/L

- Bird pepper extract (bird pepper 20g+cows urine 100mL in 1litre water) spray will help to ward off the pest
- Imidacloprid 0.003% @ 3 mL/10L / spinosad 45SC @3.3mL/10L effectively reduce pod bug infestation

Bruchids : *Callosobruchus chinensis* L.
C. maculatus L.

Family : Bruchidae

Order : Coleoptera

Bruchids have been reported from South and Southeast Asia, Africa, China, Taiwan and North America. They mainly attack grain legumes in storage, but also have been reported to attack corn, sorghum and cotton seeds.

Biology: The eggs are glued on to the surface of the grain in storage, or on green pods if the infestation starts in the field. Although the eggs are laid singly, several eggs may be seen on a grain or pod. The eggs are elongate, oval and scale-like. When freshly laid, the eggs are translucent. However, they turn to pale yellow before hatching. The egg period is about one week, but may take more than two weeks at low temperature. The grub period is 2 to 5 weeks depending on the temperature. The pupa is oval in shape and white in color. Pupal stage lasts for 1 to 4 weeks depending on the temperature.

Nature of damage and symptoms

- Both grubs and adults are causing damage
- The grub remains curved inside the grains and feeds, emptying out the seeds
- When multiple generations occur repeatedly in the same seed lot, almost the entire grain is damaged, leaving a foul-flavored flour
- The young grub feeds inside the grains, and completes its development
- Adults emerging from the initial infestation led to a secondary infestation in storage, which is much more damaging

Management

- Storage of legume grains or seeds in air-tight containers is an effective way to eliminate bruchids, as they are unable to survive without air. Triple bagging legume grains for storage can substantially reduce bruchid infestation
- Treating the legume grains with clays, sand, kaolin, and ash has been proven effective in controlling bruchid infestation in storage

- Vegetable oils (eg. olive oil or mustard oil at the rate of 15 ml/kg of seed) can also be used to treat legume grains and seeds to protect from bruchid infestation

References

Chethan, B. R., Rajappa, V., Hanchinal, S. G., Harischandra, N. R., Rao, Doddagouder S.R.,E. (2016). Incidence, bionomics and management of spotted pod borer [Maruca vitrata (Geyer)] in major pulse crops in India-), J. Exp. Zool. India Vol. 22, No. 1, pp. 233-237, 19-26.

Kunte, K. (2000). "Butterflies of Peninsular India." Oxford University Press

Madhusudan, M. D., & Suresh, R. (2007). "Peacock Pansy (Lampides boeticus) and its host plants in tropical ecosystems." Journal of Butterfly Research.

Mahalakshmi, M. S., Sreekanth, M., Adinarayana, M., Reni, Y. P., Rao, Y. K., & Narayana, E. (2016). Incidence, bionomics and management of spotted pod borer [Maruca vitrata (Geyer)] in major pulse crops in India-A review. Agricultural Reviews, 37(1), 19-26.

Nath, S., & Yadav, S. (2016). "Ecology and behavior of Euchrysops cnejus (Fabricius)." Indian Journal of Entomology.

Rekha, S., & Mallapur, C. P. (2007). Studies on insect pests of dolichos bean in northern Karnataka. Karnataka Journal of Agricultural Sciences, 2007, Vol. 20, No. 2, 407-409

Savde, V. G., Kadam, D. R., Ambad, R. B., & Patil, S. K. (2019). Management of Exelastis atomosa (Walsingham) based on spray schedule at different growth stages of pigeon pea.

Srinivasan, R., Tamò, M., and Malini, P. (2021). Emergence of Maruca vitrata as a major pest of food legumes and evolution of management practices in Asia and Africa. Annu. Rev. Entomol. 66, 141–161.

Questions

1. What is the primary damage caused by the spotted pod borer

   a) Feeding on leaves
   b) Boring into pods and flowers
   c) Defoliation
   d) Feeding on the roots

2. Which of the following pest has a highly polyphagous feeding habit?

   a) *Lampides boeticus*
   b) *Helicoverpa armigera*
   c) *Etiella zinckenella*
   d) *Exelastis atomosa*

3. **Assertion:** Pheromone traps can be used effectively for controlling *Helicoverpa armigera* in pulses.

   Reason: Pheromone traps attract the adult moths, reducing the number of eggs laid on crops.

   a) Both assertion and reason are true, and the reason is the correct explanation for the assertion.
   b) Both assertion and reason are true, but the reason is not the correct explanation for the assertion.
   c) The assertion is true, but the reason is false.
   d) The assertion is false, but the reason is true.

4. **Assertion:** *Maruca testulalis* larvae cause significant yield loss in pulse crops.

   Reason: *Maruca testulalis* larvae only attack the flowers and do not affect pods.

   a) Both assertion and reason are true, and the reason is the correct explanation for the assertion.
   b) Both assertion and reason are true, but the reason is not the correct explanation for the assertion.
   c) The assertion is true, but the reason is false.
   d) The assertion is false, but the reason is true.

5. Which of the following pests has a characteristic skull marking on the thorax?

   a) *Spilosoma obliqua*
   b) *Acherontia styx*
   c) *Omiodes diemenalis*
   d) *Maruca testulalis*

6. What is the preferred pupation site for *Agrius convolvuli*?

   a) Inside the soil b) Inside the host plant stem

   c) Inside a hollow stem chamber d) In a leaf roll

7. Which pest is responsible for the creation of serpentine mines on leaves?

   a) *Melanagromyza obtusa* b) *Liriomyza trifolii*

   c) *Ophiomyia phaseoli* d) *Spilosoma obliqua*

8. **Assertion:** Ophiomyia phaseoli maggots cause severe damage to seedlings.

   Reason: The maggots feed on the stem and petiole, leading to wilting of the seedlings.

   a) Both assertion and reason are true, and the reason is the correct explanation of the assertion.

   b) Both assertion and reason are true, but the reason is not the correct explanation of the assertion.

   c) The assertion is true, but the reason is false.

   d) The assertion is false, but the reason is true.

9. Which of the following is an effective biological control agent for Cowpea aphid (*Aphis craccivora*)?

   a) Green lacewings b) Nematodes

   c) Spinosad d) Dimethoate

10. Which of the following is true about the biology of bruchids (*Callosobruchus chinensis*)?

    a) Bruchids infest only fresh legumes in the field.

    b) Bruchids lay eggs on stored grains or pods.

    c) The grubs feed on the leaves of legumes.

    d) The pupal stage of bruchids lasts for 2 days.

Answer Key

1	b	2	b	3	a	4	c	5	b	6	a	7	b
8	a	9	a	10	b								

4

Pests of Crucifers

Crucifers, also known as Brassicas or cole crops, are a group of vegetables belonging to the family *Brassicaceae* (formerly *Cruciferae*). Common cruciferous vegetables include cabbage, cauliflower, broccoli, kale, mustard, turnip, and radish. These crops are widely grown around the world due to their nutritional value, economic importance, and adaptability to diverse climates.

However, crucifers are highly susceptible to a wide range of insect pests that can cause significant yield losses if not managed properly. These pests attack various parts of the plant, including leaves, stems, roots, and heads, leading to both quantitative and qualitative damage.

Cabbage leaf webber : *Crocidolomia binotalis*

Family : Crambidae

Order : Lepidoptera

Distribution

Crocidolomia binotalis is widely distributed in India and is particularly prevalent in regions where cruciferous vegetables are cultivated. The pest is active from the third week of November to the fourth week of December, with varying population densities depending on environmental conditions (Pawar *et al.,* 2010)

Biology and lifecycle

The moth has light brown forewings with distinct wavy lines and spots, and its hindwings are semi-hyaline. The larva is green with a red head and features longitudinal red stripes along its body, reaching a length of about 2 cm. Eggs are laid in clusters of 45-100 on the underside of leaves, and they hatch within 5-15 days. In the early stages, the larvae feed together on the leaf parenchyma, but as they mature, they disperse, web the leaves, and continue feeding. The larval stage lasts 25-30 days in summer and around 50 days in winter. Once fully grown, the larva descends to the ground and pupates in the soil, creating an earthen cocoon. The adult emerges after 14-40 days, with the full lifecycle taking 43-80 days. Multiple generations are completed during the season (Kumaranag *et al.,* 2014).

Nature of damage and symptoms

The larvae skeletonize the leaves by feeding on the undersides within webs. They also target flower buds and pods, often causing serious damage. This pest affects a range of cruciferous crops, including cabbage, cauliflower, radish, mustard, and others (Kumaranag *et al.,* 2014).

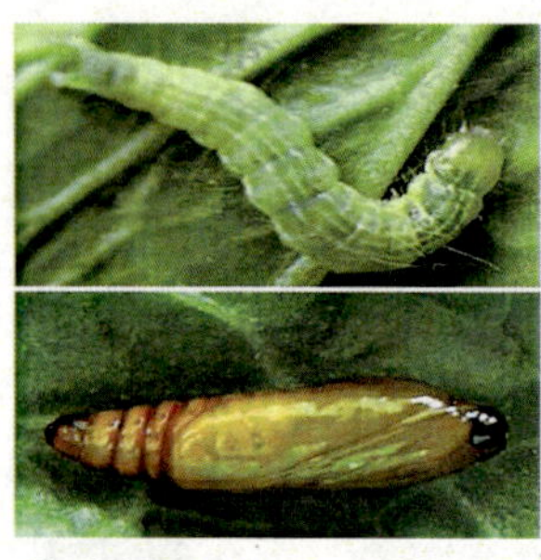
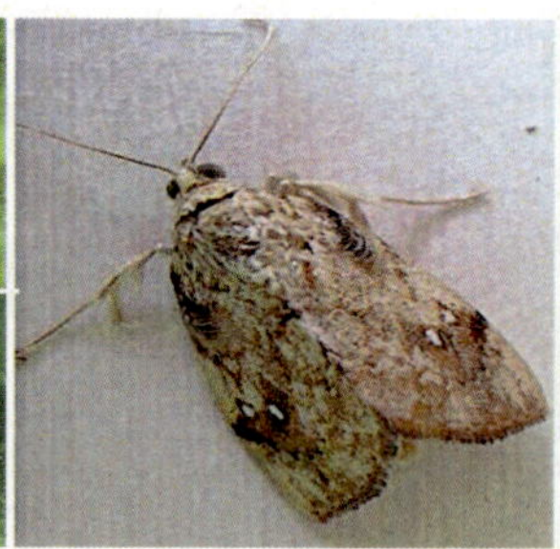
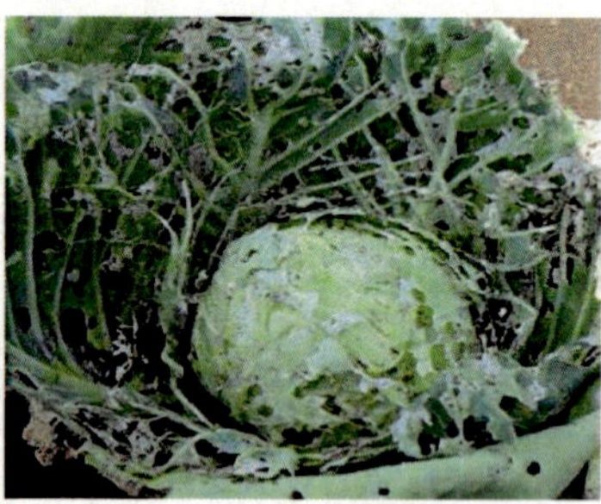

Cabbage caterpillar : ***Pieris brassicae***

Family : **Pieridae**

Order : **Lepidoptera Distribution**

Pieris brassicae, is a widespread pest of cruciferous crops across India. It has been reported in various regions, including northern states like Jammu and Kashmir, Himachal Pradesh, Punjab, Haryana, Uttar Pradesh, Uttarakhand, Delhi, and Rajasthan; eastern states like West Bengal, Bihar, and Odisha; northeastern states like Assam, Meghalaya, Manipur, and Sikkim; and southern states like Tamil Nadu.

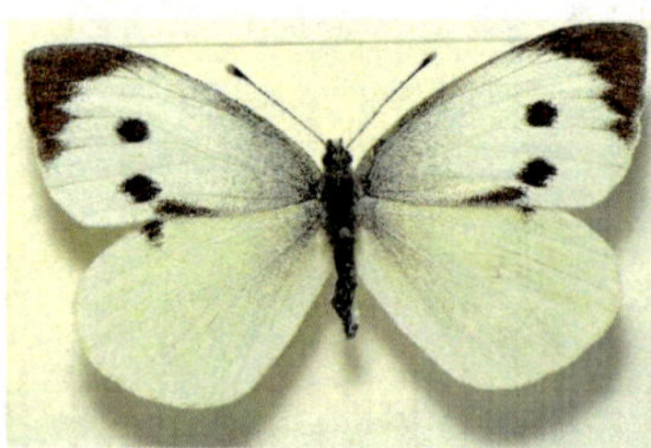

Adult – P. brassicae

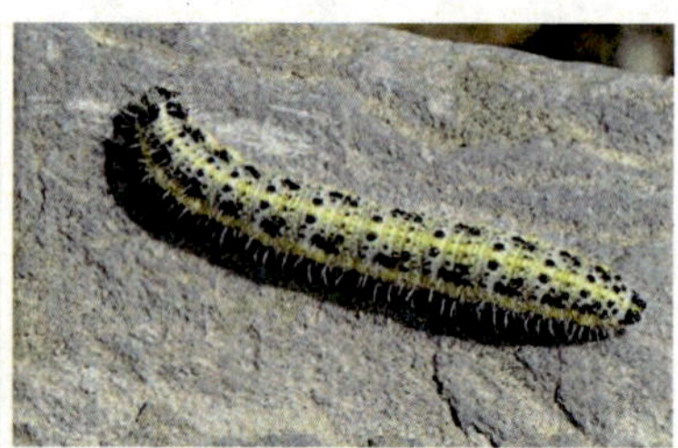

Larva

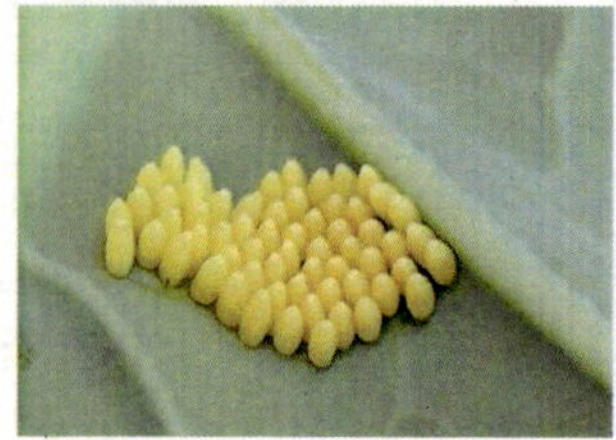

Egg mass

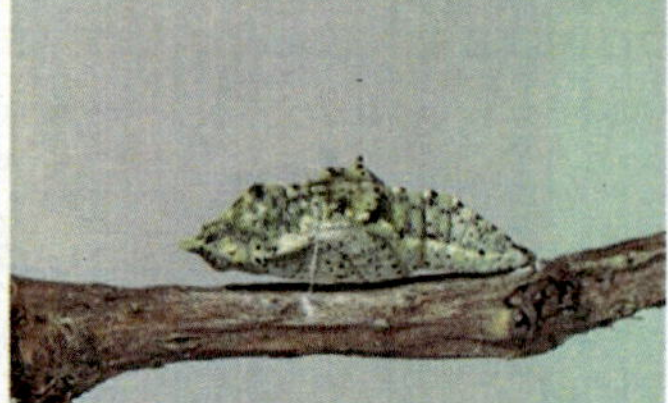

Pupa

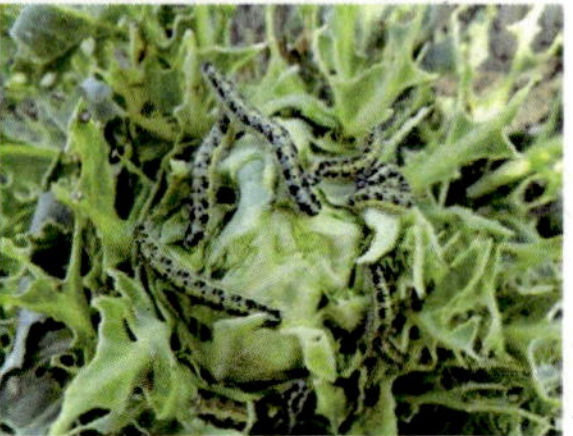

Larvae feeding on cabbage

Biology Egg stage: The female butterfly lays eggs in clusters, with the largest cluster having up to 116 eggs, while some clusters may have only 2-3 eggs. Initially yellow, the eggs turn greyish before hatching. They are attached to the leaves by a brownish secretion. The eggs typically hatch in 4-5 days, with an average hatching time of 4.60 days. The eggs measure about 1.28 mm in length and 0.49 mm in width (Bhowmik & Gupta, 2017).

Larval stage

The larvae of *P. brassicae* undergo four moults and pass through five instars. The first instar larvae are light yellow with shiny black heads, measuring 6.0-6.5 mm in length, and last about 4-6 days. The second instar larvae are greenish-yellow with black heads and short hairs, measuring 12.0-12.2 mm in length, and last about 4-5 days. The third instar larvae are green with black heads and black hairs on raised tubercles, measuring 23.6-23.7 mm in length, and last about 4-5 days. The fourth instar larvae are similar to the third instar but larger, measuring 32.0-32.2 mm in length, and last about 4-5 days. The fifth instar larvae are cylindrical and yellow with black heads and bright coloration, measuring 40.0-40.2 mm in length, and last about 6-7 days. The total larval duration ranges from 22 to 28 days, averaging 25.6 days (Bhowmik & Gupta, 2017).

Pupal stage

The pupa is pale green or greyish-white with black and yellow markings. It has a flattened ventral surface, lateral ridges along the sides, and several blunt spikes on the abdomen. The pupae vary in size, typically measuring 20.0 to 25.0 mm in length, with an average of 22.5 mm, and 3.0 to 3.2 mm in width, averaging 3.1 mm. The pupal stage lasts around 7.0 to 9.0 days, with an average duration of 7.9 days (Bhowmik & Gupta, 2017).

Adult stage

The butterflies are pale white with a smoky shade on their dorsal side. They have white wings with black tips on the forewings, larger in females with additional black spots. The undersides of the wings are pale yellow with grey dusting, except for the white center and base of the forewings. Females also have black dots on the undersides. The head, thorax, and abdomen are black with grey scales. Males live for about 6.8 days, and females for about 6.5 days. Males have a wingspan averaging 5.1 cm, while females average 5.5 cm (Bhowmik & Gupta, 2017).

Nature of damage and symptoms

The damage is caused exclusively by the caterpillars. Initially, the first instar caterpillars merely scrape the surface of the leaves. However, as they mature, they consume the leaves from the margins inward, leaving only the major veins intact (Kumaranag *et al.,* 2014).

Cabbage borer	:	*Hellula undalis*
Family	:	Crambidae
Order	:	Lepidoptera

Biology: The adult moth is slender, pale yellowish-brown, and has grey wavy lines on its forewings. The caterpillar is yellow with a pinkish tint, featuring seven purplish-brown longitudinal stripes. The female moth deposits its eggs on the growing point or older leaves, which hatch in 2-3 days. The caterpillars feed on the cabbage heart and grow to full size within 7-14 days, undergoing four moults. The fully developed caterpillar spins a cocoon among the leaves near the ground or inside the larval burrows. The pupal stage lasts about 7 days, and the entire life cycle takes 15-25 days to complete (Kumaranag *et al.,* 2014).

Nature of damage and symptoms

Initially, the caterpillars mine into the leaves. As they develop, they feed on the leaf surface while being protected within silken tunnels. When larger, they bore into the heads of cauliflower and cabbage. In severe infestations, the plants become infested with caterpillars, causing the heads to appear deformed (Kumaranag *et al.,* 2014).

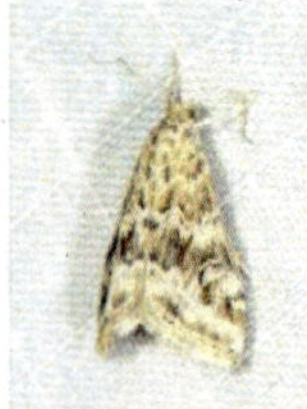
Adult

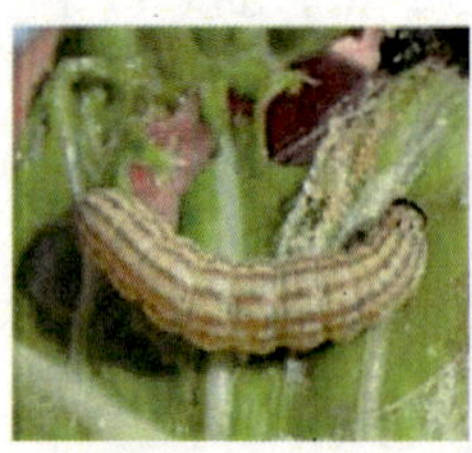
Larva

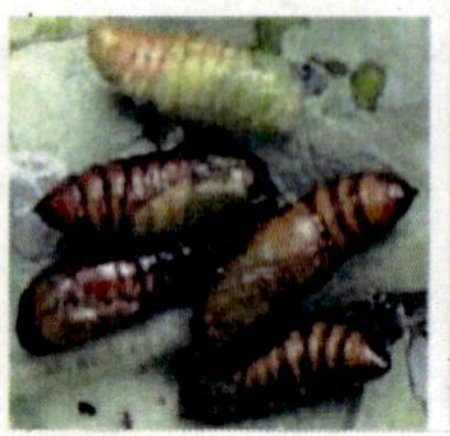
Pupae

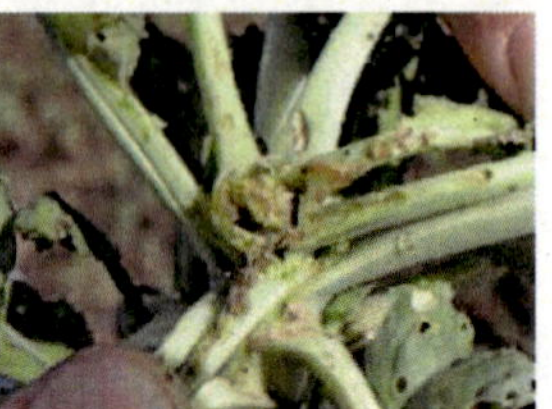

Diamond-back moth (DBM)	:	*Plutella xylostella*
Family	:	Plutellidae
Order	:	Lepidoptera

Biology: The moths are approximately 22 mm in length with a wingspan of about 40 mm. Their bodies are light down in color, with greyish-brown forewings that have white markings and white hindwings that feature a brown border. The adult female moth lays yellowish eggs either singly or in clusters of 5-57 on the undersides of leaves. Each female can lay between 20-358 eggs throughout her lifetime. The eggs hatch within 2-7 days, and the newly emerged caterpillars bore into the leaf tissue from below and feed within these tunnels. The third and fourth instar larvae feed on the undersides of leaves, leaving a transparent, parchment-like layer on the top surface. They reach full maturity in 14-21 days. Before pupation, the larvae construct barrel-shaped silken cocoons that are open at both ends and attached to the leaf surfaces. The pupal stage lasts 4-5 days, and the adult moths can live for up to 17 days. The entire lifecycle is completed in 15-18 days during September-October, and multiple generations occur within a year (Kumaranag *et al.,* 2014).

Nature of damage and symptoms

The larvae initially cause damage by tunneling through the leaves during the first and early second instars. As they progress to the second, third, and fourth instars, they create numerous small biting holes, leading to the complete destruction of the crop. This damage affects the foliage from the seedling stage to harvest, and their population can rapidly increase under favorable conditions such as hot and dry weather. The infestation significantly reduces yield and quality by contaminating the edible parts with their faecal matter (Kaur *et al.,* 2021).

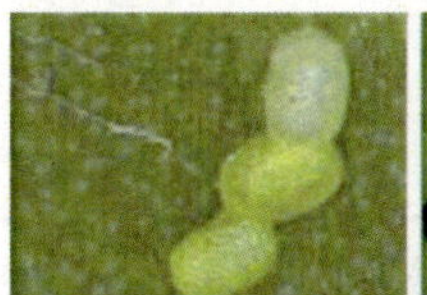 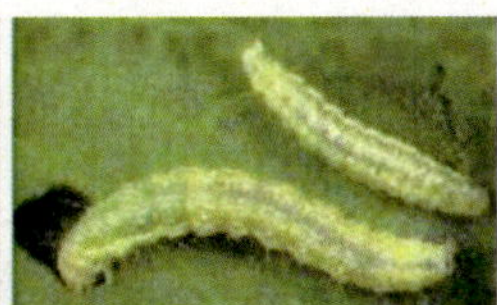 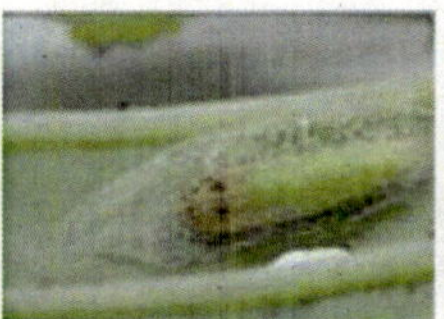 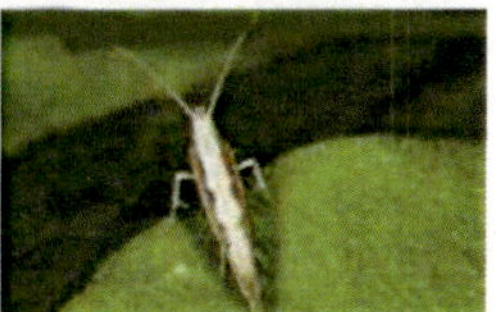

Cabbage semilooper : *Trichoplusia ni*

Family : Noctuidae

Order : Lepidoptera

Biology: The cabbage semilooper is a pale green caterpillar with white stripes along each side of its body. Adult moths are about 1 inch long, with wings folded over their backs when at rest. They are dark brown and gray, with a distinctive white "8" pattern in the middle of their wings. The female lays whitish, round eggs singly on the leaf surface. These eggs hatch in 3-7 days, and the larvae develop over 16 to 19 days before pupating. The pupa changes from green to dark brown, and the adult emerges 9 to 10 days later. The entire lifecycle lasts 32 to 37 days, allowing for one to two generations per season (Kumaranag *et al.,* 2014).

Nature of damage and symptoms

The larvae damage the leaves severely by biting holes and skeletonizing them (Kumaranag *et al.,* 2014).

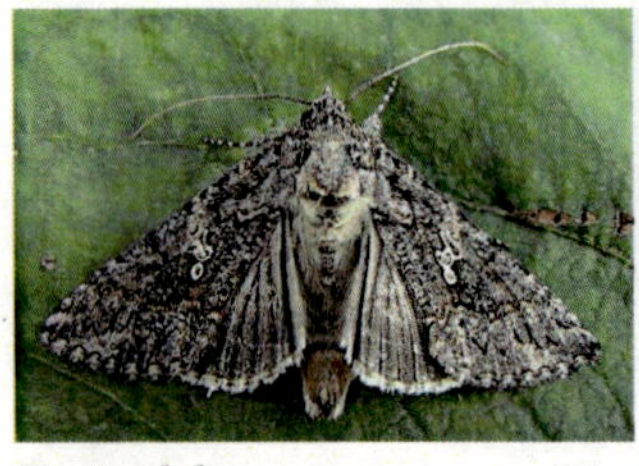
T. ni adult

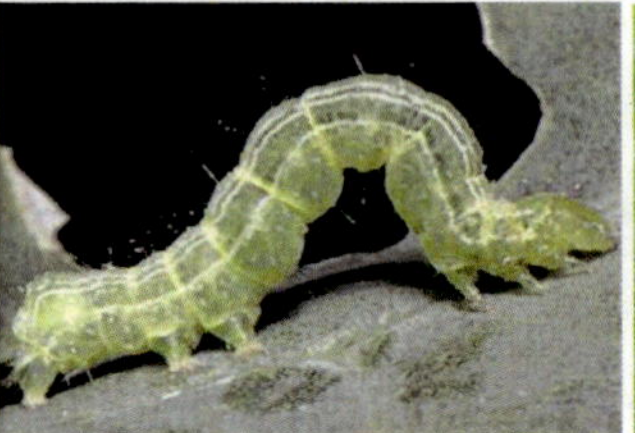
larva

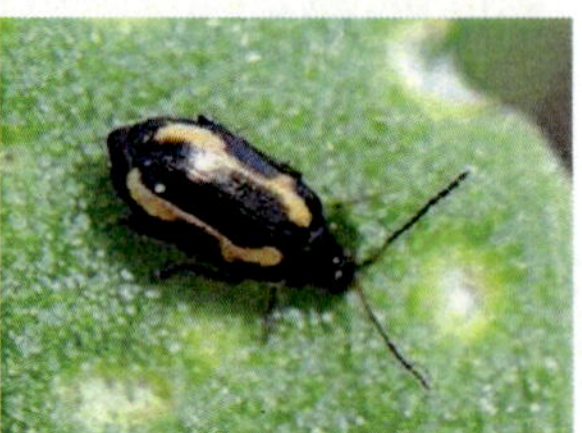
Flea beetle-adult

Flea beetles	:	*Phyllotreta cruciferae*
Order	:	Coleoptera
Family	:	Chrysomelidae

Biology: The small bluish-black beetles, measuring 2-3 mm (about 1/10 inch) in length and having enlarged hind femora, lay eggs in the soil. The eggs hatch in 12-5 days, depending on the temperature. The whitish larvae feed on the plant roots without causing significant damage. They complete their life cycle in 3-4 weeks, and the beetle produces one generation per year (Kumaranag *et al.,* 2014).

Nature of damage and symptoms

Adults consume the cotyledons and first true leaves of seedlings, resulting in bite holes and considerable damage. They also target the weed *Gynandropsis pentophylla.* Affected plants release a decaying odour (Kumaranag *et al.,* 2014).

Mustard sawfly	:	*Athalia lugens proxima*
Order	:	Hymenoptera
Family	:	Tenthredinidae

Biology and lifecycle: The larval stage is characterized by a dark green coloration and the presence of eight pairs of abdominal prolegs. Upon reaching full maturity, the larvae measure between 16 and 18 mm in length. The adult insects are small, with an orange-yellow body marked with black patterns, and feature smoky wings with distinct black veins. The female lays 30-35 eggs individually in slits along the underside of the leaf margin, which are created using a saw-like ovipositor. Egg hatching occurs within 4-8 days, with larvae reaching full growth in 16- 35 days before pupating in the soil. The complete life cycle spans 30-35 days, and the species typically completes 2-3 generations (Kumaranag *et al.,* 2014).

Damage symptoms

The larvae feed on the leaves by creating bite holes, primarily targeting the young growth, and ultimately cause the leaves to become completely skeletonized (Kumaranag *et al.,* 2014).

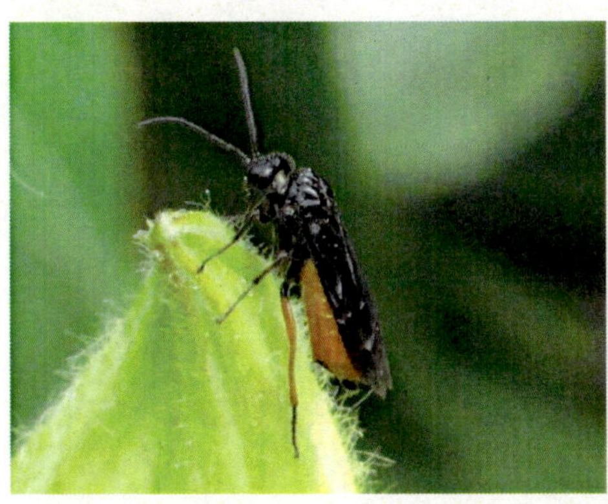

Adult

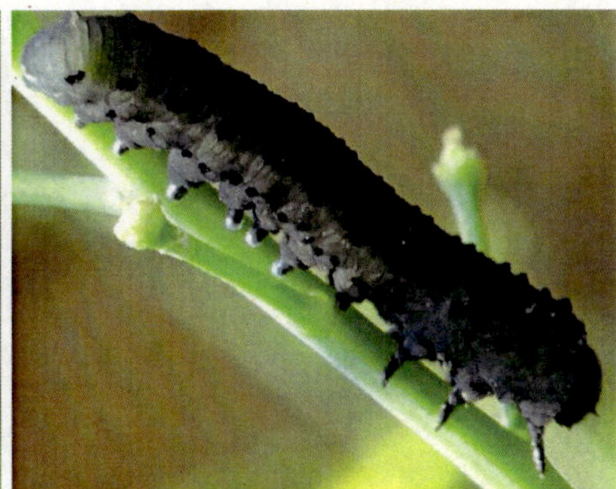

Larva

References

Bhowmik, M. and Gupta, M., 2017. Biology of Cabbage Butterfly Pieris brassicae Linn. (Lepidoptera: Pieridae). International Journal of Current Microbiology and Applied Sciences, 6(12), pp.3639-3644.

Kaur, M., Thakur, M. and Sharma, K.C., 2021. Biological and life table parameters of diamondback moth, Plutella xylostella (L.) (Lepidoptera: Yponomeutidae) from five different geographical regions of India. Phytoparasitica, 49, pp.819-827

Kumaranag, K.M., Kedar, S.C., Thodsare, N.H. and Bawaskar, D.M., 2014. Insect pests of cruciferous vegetables and their management. Popular Kheti, 2(1), pp.80-86

Pawar, V.R., Bapodra, J.G., Joshi, M.D., Ghadge, S.M. and Dalve, S.K., 2010. Incidence of leaf webber, Crocidolomia binotalis (Zeller) on mustard.

5

Pests of Okra

Okra, commonly known as lady's finger is a significant vegetable crops primarily grown in tropics and subtropics. Production and productivity of okra is affected by the incidence of pests and diseases. More than 70 insect pests have been recorded in okra (Ewete, 1978).

Sl. No.	Common name	Scientific name	Family and Order	Site of oviposition	Site of pupation
			Borers		
1	Shoot and fruit borer	*Earias vitella*	Nolidae, Lepidoptera	tender parts of the plant, leaf axils, bracts, leaf veins, buds, flowers & fruits	Plant parts
2	Fruit Borer	*Helicoverpa armigera*	Noctuidae, Lepidoptera		
			Defoliators		
3	Leaf roller	*Sylepta derogata*	Crambidae, Lepidoptera	On underside of leaves	Within leaf rolls
4	Green semilooper	*Anomis flava*	Erebidae, Lepidoptera	On leaves	Within the leaf folds
5	Semilooper Caterpillar	*Xanthodes graellsi*	Nolidae, Lepidoptera		In soil
6	Leaf caterpillar	*Spodoptera litura*	Noctuidae, Lepidoptera		In soil
7	Green semilooper	*Plusia/ Argyrogramma signata*	Noctuidae, Lepidoptera		
			Sucking pests		
8	Red Bug	*Dysdercus cingulatus*	Pyrrhocoridae, Hemiptera	In moist soil or plant debris	
9	Leaf Hopper	*Amrasca biguttula biguttula*	Cicadellidae, Hemiptera	within the leaf veins	
10	White fly	*Bemisia tabaci*	Aleyrodidae, Hemiptera	On leaf surface	

11	Aphids	*Aphis malvae, Aphis gossypii*	Aphididae, Hemiptera		
12	Dusky cotton bug	*Oxycarenus hyalinipennis*	Lygaeidae, Hemiptera		
13	Pink hibiscus mealybug	*Maconellicoccus hirsutus*	Pseudococcidae, Hemiptera		
			Other pests		
14	Petiole maggot	*Melanagromyza hibisci*	Agromyzidae, Diptera		
15	Flower beetles	*Oxycetonia* spp., *Popillio* spp.	Scarabaeidae, Coleoptera	In soil	In soil
16	Root knot nematode	*Meloidogyne incognita*	Heteroderidae, Tylenchida		
17	Red spider mite	*Tetranychus urticae*	Tetranychidae, Trombidiformes		

Shoot and fruit borer : *Earias vitella*

Family : Nolidae

Order : Lepidoptera

Biology: Forewings of the moth white with a pea- green wedge-shaped band running medially from base to outer margin of each wing. Eggs are laid on tender parts of the plant, leaf axils, bracts, leaf veins, buds, flowers and fruits singly or in two's or threes. Egg period - 3-4 days. Caterpillars are brownish with median longitudinal streak dorsally and pale yellow or green ventrally. Larval period is 2 weeks. Pupae are seen on the plant in dirty white boat shaped cocoons made of silk. Pupal period is one week. The life cycle is completed in about a month.

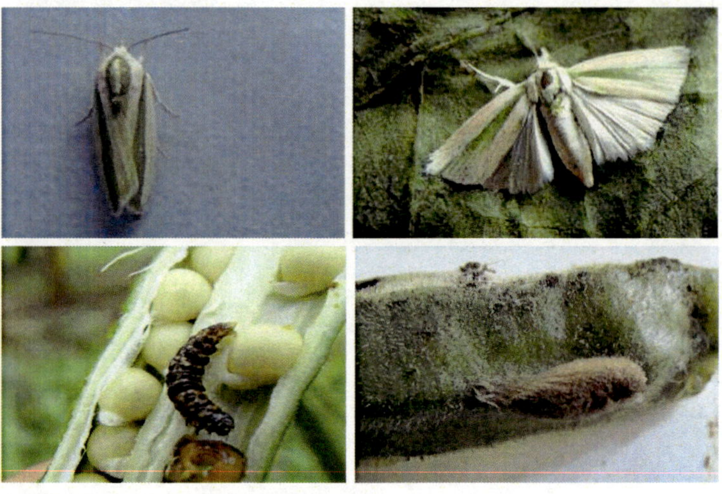

Adult, larva and pupa of *Earias vitella*

Nature of damage and Symptoms

The newly hatched larvae bore into the terminal shoots or fruits. The damaged shoots droop, wither and dry up. The infested fruits are deformed with holes on them plugged with excreta.

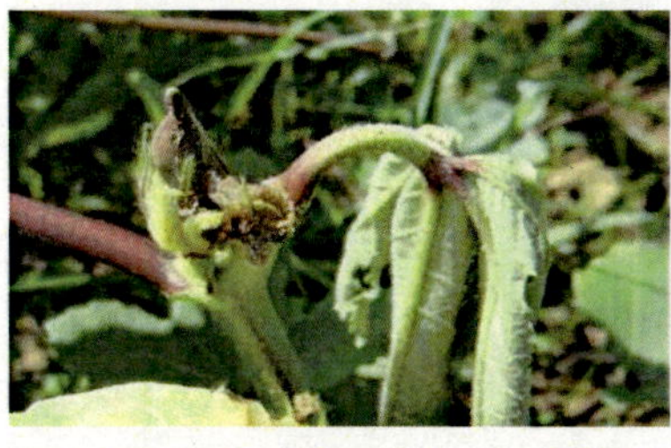
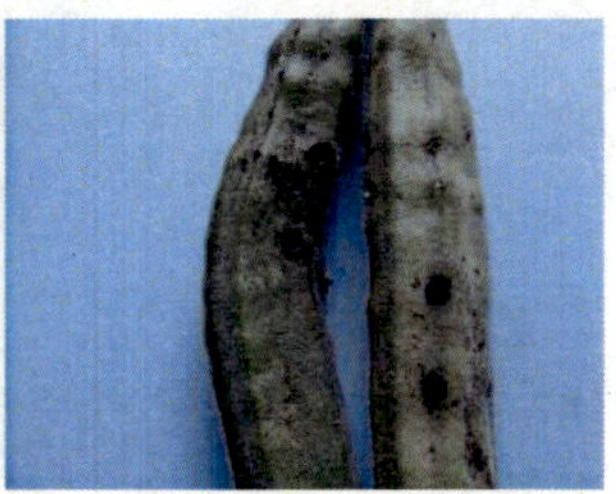

Damage symptoms of *Earias vitella*

Management

- Select less hairy or glabrous varieties
- Collect and destroy affected shoots and fruits
- Conserve egg parasitoids, *Trichogramma chilonis,* Egg-larval parasitoid *Chelonus blackburni.*
- Spray *Bacillus thuringiensis* (*B.t*) @ 2g/litre.
- In case severe infestation. Apply chlorantraniliprole 3 mL/10L
- Foliar spray of emamectin benzoate 4 g/10L or spinosad 3.3mL/L is effective

Fruit borer : *Helicoverpa armigera*

Family : Noctuidae

Order : Lepidoptera

Biology: The forewings are yellowish to orange in females and greenish-gray in males, with a slightly darker transversal band in the distal third. The external transversal and submarginal lines and the reniform spot are diffused. The hind wings are a pale yellow with a narrow brown band at the external edge and a dark round spot in the middle.

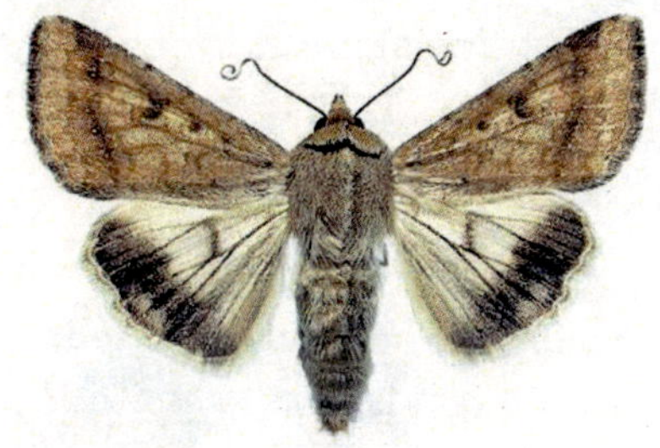

Adult of *Helicoverpa armigera*

Nature of damage and symptoms

They bore into the fruits making circular holes and eat the inner contents. Young larvae feed on tender leaves. Later instars attack the fruits. Larvae thrust only part of their body inside the fruit.

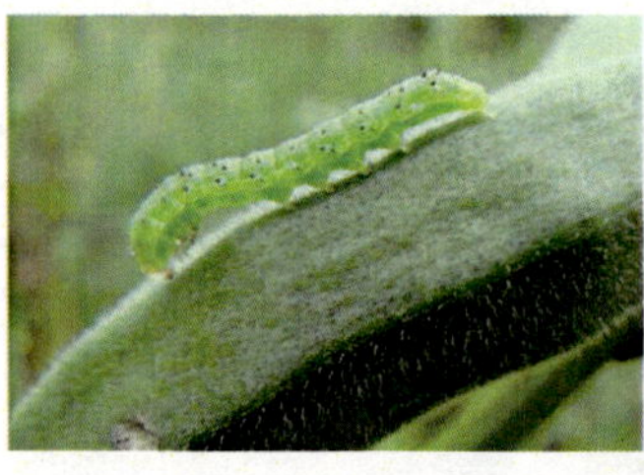

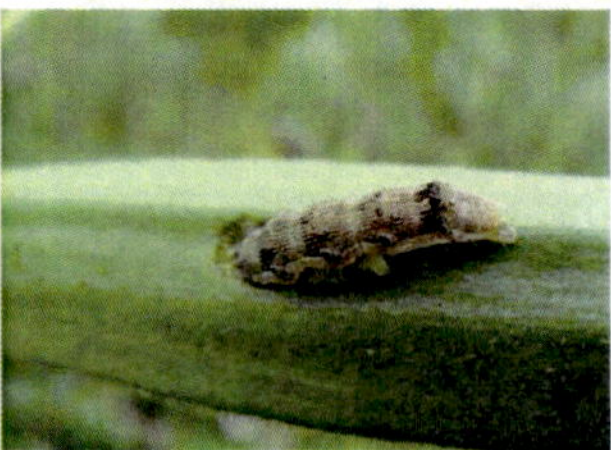

Larva and feeding symptoms of *Helicoverpa armigera*

Leaf roller : *Sylepta derogata*

Family : Pyralidae

Order : Lepidoptera

Biology: Moth is medium sized with yellowish wings having wavy brown markings. Eggs are laid singly on the underside of leaves. Egg period is 4 days. Caterpillars are bright green with dark head and prothoracic shield. Larval period is 2 to 3 weeks. Pupae are seen within leaf rolls. Pupal period is one week. The pest completes its life cycle in one to one and a half month

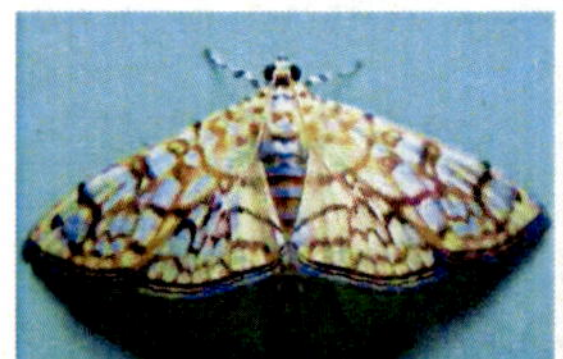

Adult of *S. derogata*

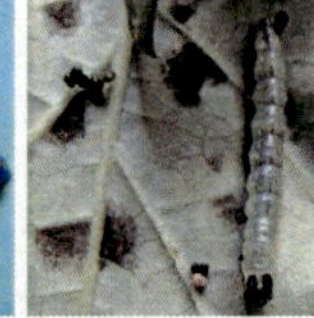

Larva

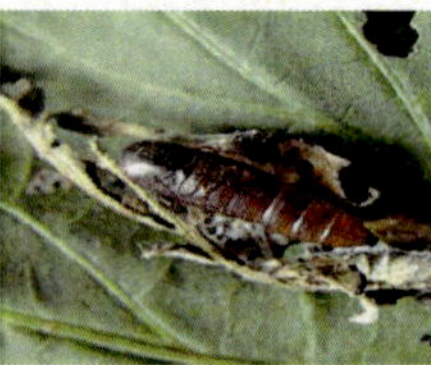

Pupa

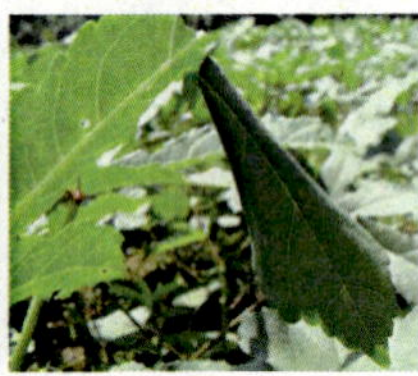

Leaf rolling by *S. derogata*

Nature of damage and symptoms

The caterpillar rolls the leaf and feeds on it from within. In severe cases of infestation almost the entire leaf lamina is cut and made into rolls

Green semilooper : *Anomis flava*

Family : Erebidae

Order : Lepidoptera

Biology: The moth with reddish brown fore wings tranversed by two darker zig zag bands. Hind wings are pale brown. Eggs are laid singly on leaves. Egg period - 5 days. Larva pale yellowish green with five white lines longitudinally on the dorsal surface. Larval period - 3 weeks. Pupation within the leaf folds. Pupal period - 8-9 days.

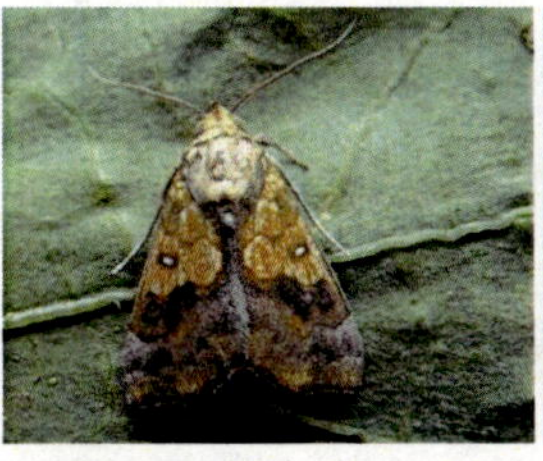
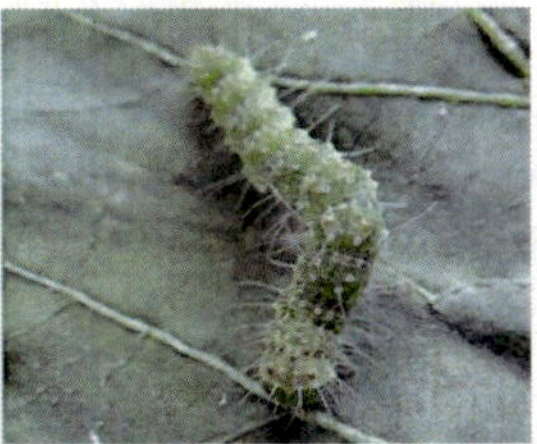

Adult and larva of *Anomis flava*

Nature of damage

The young larvae congregate in small groups and feed on leaf lamina making small punctures. The grown up larvae feed voraciously on the entire leaf, leaving only the main veins. The caterpillar also eat the tender shoots and fruit.

Yellow crab : *Pardoxia graellsii* Feisthamel.

Transverse moth : *Xanthodes transversa* Guene.

Family : Nolidae

Order : Lepidoptera

Biology: Moth has yellowish forewings with brown patches along the outer margins and curved lines. Caterpillar is green with a pair of horse-shoe shaped black mark on each segment. Pupate in the soil in a cocoon among dry leaves.

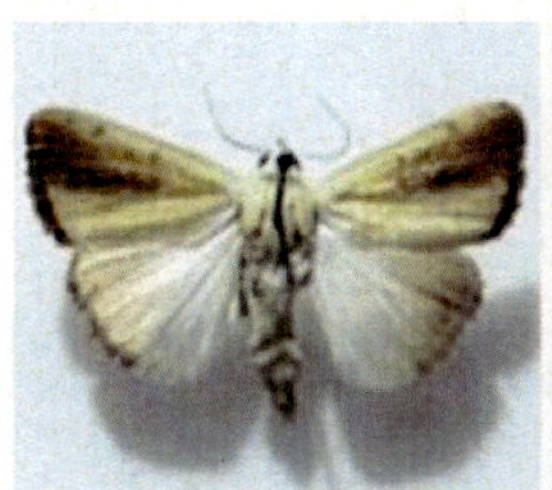
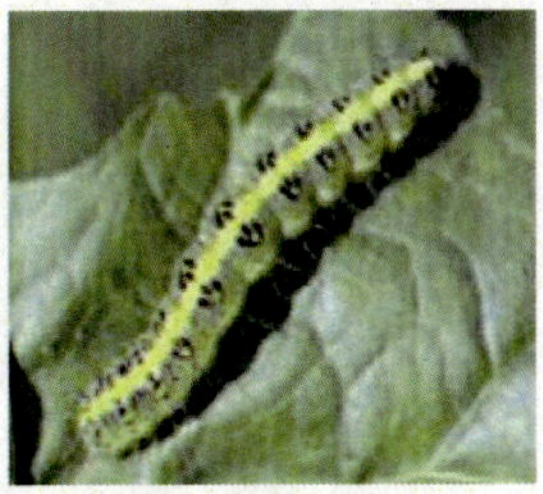

Adult and larva of *Pardoxia graellsii*

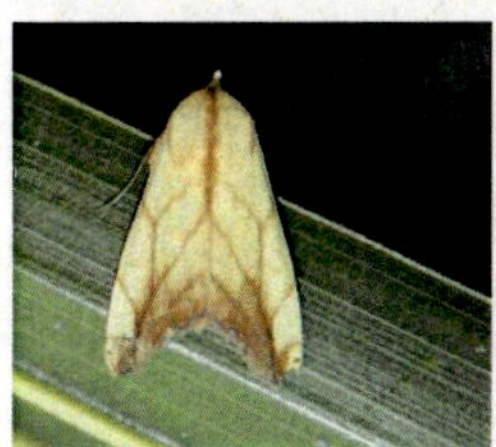
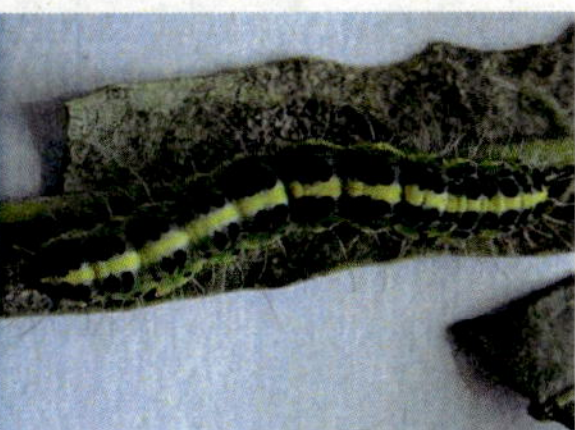

Adult and larva of *Xanthodes transversa*

Leaf caterpillar : *Spodoptera litura*

Family : Noctuidae

Order : Lepidoptera

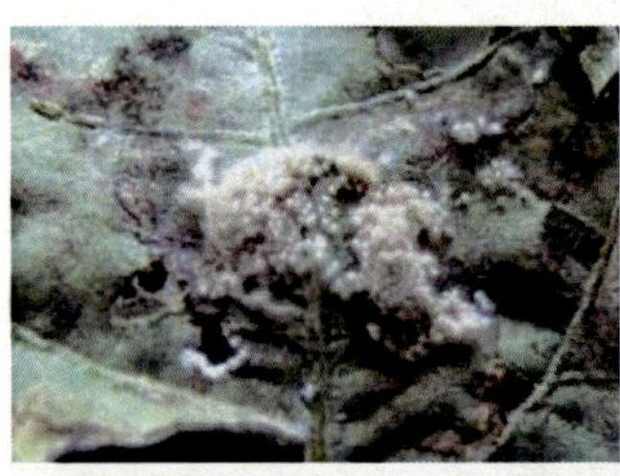
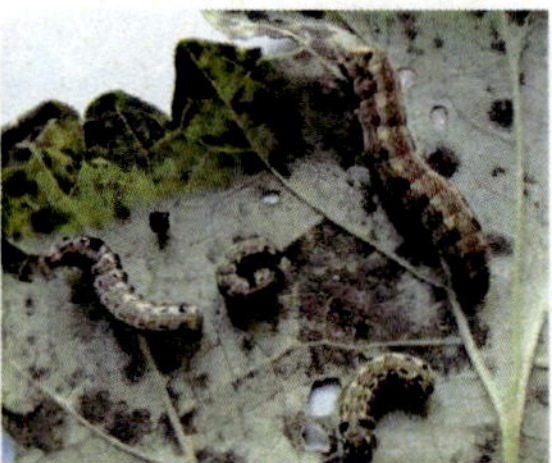
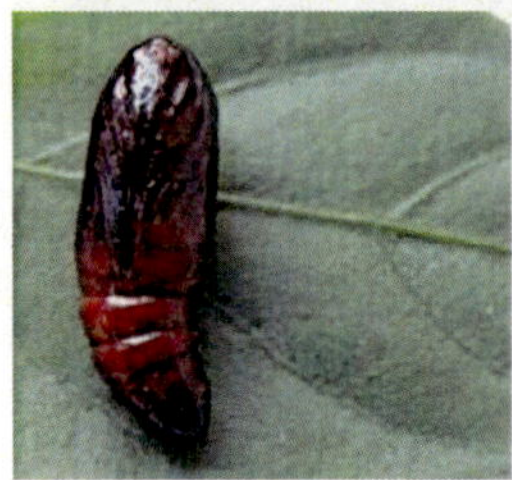
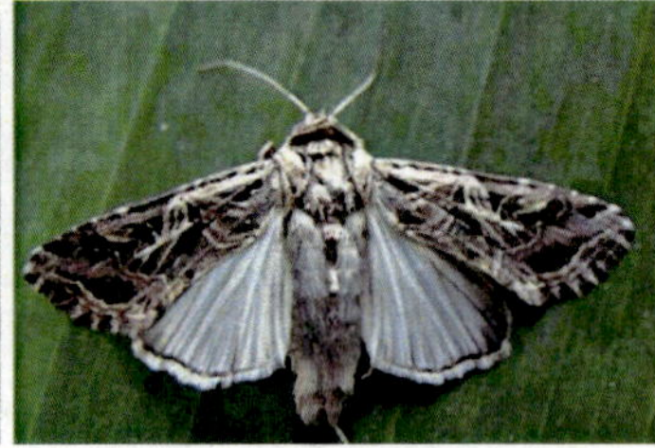

Eggs, larvae, pupa and adult of *Spodoptera litura*

Green semilooper : *Plusia/ Argyrogramma signata* F.

Family : Noctuidae

Order : Lepidoptera

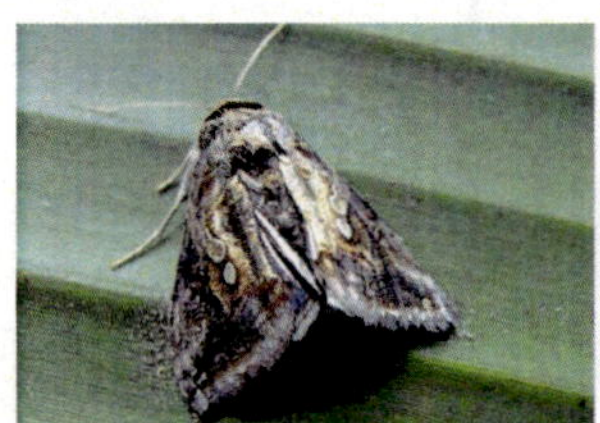
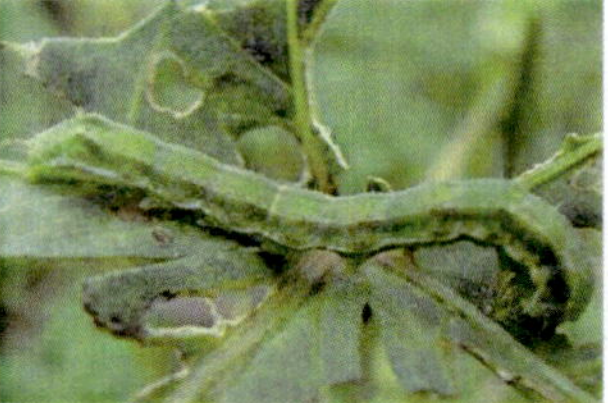

Adult and larva of *A. signata*

Management

- Spray any one of the insecticides starting from one month after planting at 15 days interval., NSKE 5%, Azadirachtin 1.0% 1.0-1.5mL/L
- In case of severe infestation spray any of the insecticides like flubendiamide 2ml in 10 l or emamectin benzoate 5 WG @ 4g/10L, or thiacloprid 240 Sc @ 1.5ml/10L or thiodicarb 75 WP@ 2g/L
- Avoid continuous use of synthetic pyrethroids as they cause resurgence of sucking pests
- Avoid using insecticide at the time of fruit maturation and harvest

Red Bug : *Dysdercus cingulatus*

Family : *Pyrrhocoridae*

Order : Hemiptera

Biology: Adults 12-15 mm long. Wings reddish and has a black spot or bar near the middle. The ventral side is red with white transverse stripes.

Eggs are laid in loose masses in moist soil or plant debris. Moisture is essential for development of the eggs. Egg period lasts for 1 week. Five nymphal instars with a duration of 4 weeks.

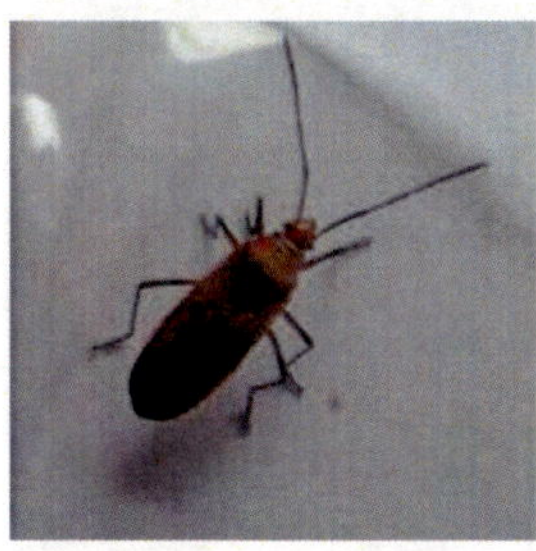

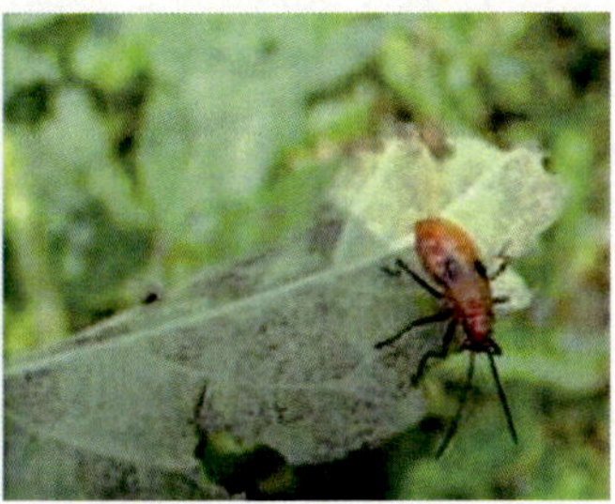

Adult and nymph of *Dysdercus cingulatus*

Nature of damage

Both nymphs and adults suck the sap from leaves shoots and developing seeds. All stages of the insect are seen on infested plants.

Leaf Hopper : *Amrasca biguttula biguttula*

Family : Cicadellidae

Order : Hemiptera

Biology: Adult hopper is green in colour and lays eggs singly within the leaf veins. Eggs are pear shaped, elongated and yellowish white in colour. Egg period is 4 to 6 days. Nymphs move diagonally when disturbed. Nymphs are yellowish and found in between the veins of the leaves.

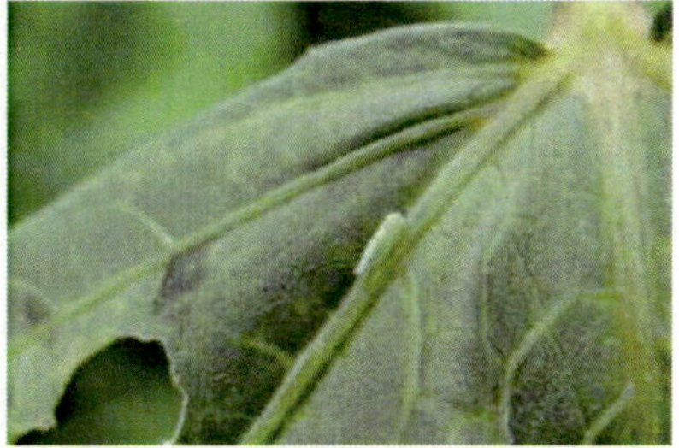

Adult of *Amrasca biguttula biguttula*

Nature of damage and symptoms

- The adult hoppers and nymphs suck sap from the leaves
- Injury is caused by the toxic material of the insect's saliva which is injected into the leaf during feeding
- The symptom is called 'hopper burn', characterised by marginal chlorosis, bronzing(browning), puckering (development of crinkles, curls and folds), and drying of leaves (Bindra *et al.*, 1981)
- The attacked plants are stunted and fail to grow and bear fruits.

Management

- Spray acetamiprid @ 2g/10L or thiamethoxam @ 2g/10L or imidacloprid @ 3mL/10L when attack is severe.

White fly : *Bemisia tabaci*

Family : *Aleyrodidae*

Order : Hemiptera

Biology: Adult with two pairs of pure white wings. The eggs are attached to the leaf surface. The young larvae move about in search of a suitable place where they settle down to feed for the rest of their life. Soon they moult and become legless, scale like, flattened and pressed to the leaf surface. Also their body gets covered with a kind of wax secreted by them. They further undergo two moults and then pupate, followed by the emergence of the adults.

Nature of damage

- Both adults and nymphs feed on leaves by sucking cell sap.
- They excrete honcy dcw which results in the development of sooty mould.
- Acts as vectors and transmit yellow vein mosaic virus.
- Chlorotic spots on the leaves which later coalesce forming irregular yellowing of leaves. Later dry and shed.

Management

- Grow resistant cultivars like Arka Abhay, Arka Anamika, Punjab Padmini and Parbhani Kranti.
- Foliar spray of imidacloprid 0.003% @ 3 mL/10L

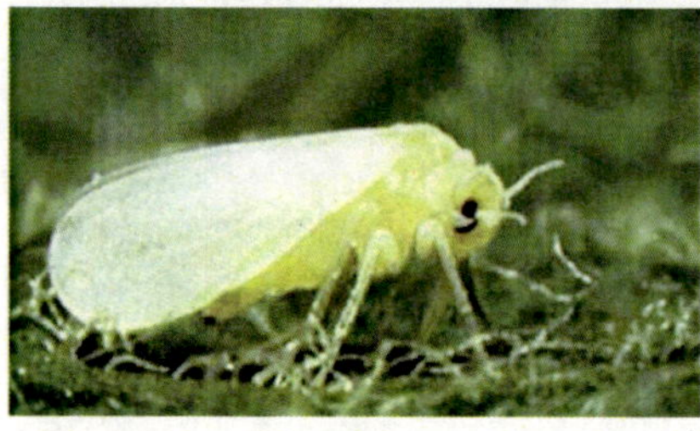
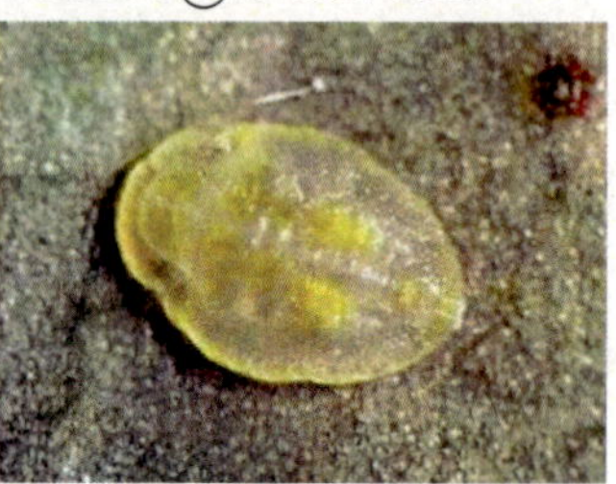

Adult and nymph of *Bemisia tabaci*

Aphids : *Aphis malvae, Aphis gossypii*

Family : Aphididae

Order : Hemiptera

They are gregarious in habit and completely cover the shoot tips, buds and lower surface of leaves.

Nature of damage

- Both nymphs and adults suck the sap and leaves curl
- The infestation causes the stunting of plants
- Sooty mould develops on the leaves due to the honey dew excretion

Management

- Clip off and destroy the infested parts
- Reduce application of nitrogenous fertilisers
- Encourage the activity of natural predators such as lady beetles, lacewings, and parasitic wasps (*Aphidius matricariae*, *Aphelinus semiflavus*) to reduce pest population
- Foliar spray with neem oil garlic emulsion 2% is effective during the initial stages
- Apply thiamethoxam @ 2g/10L or imidacloprid @ 3 mL/10L

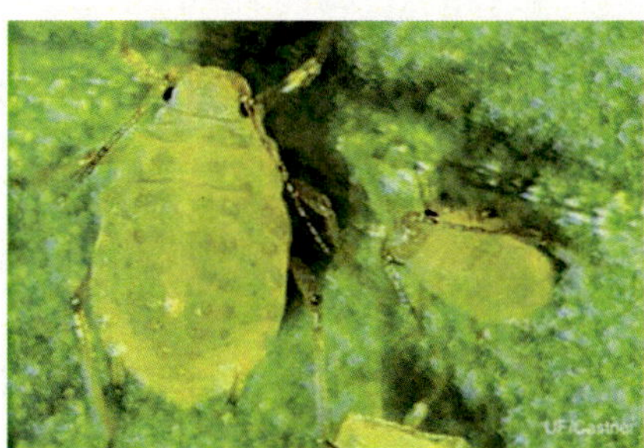

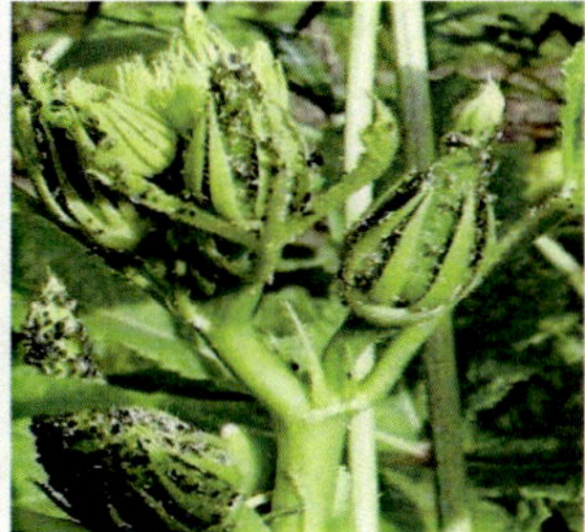

Adult of *Aphis gossypii* and its infestation on Bhindi

Dusky cotton bug : *Oxycarenus hyalinipennis*

Family : Lygaeidae

Order : Hemiptera

Nature od damage and symptoms

Grayish brown bug, with pointed head and white hyaline wings. Both nymphs and adults suck sap from developing seeds.

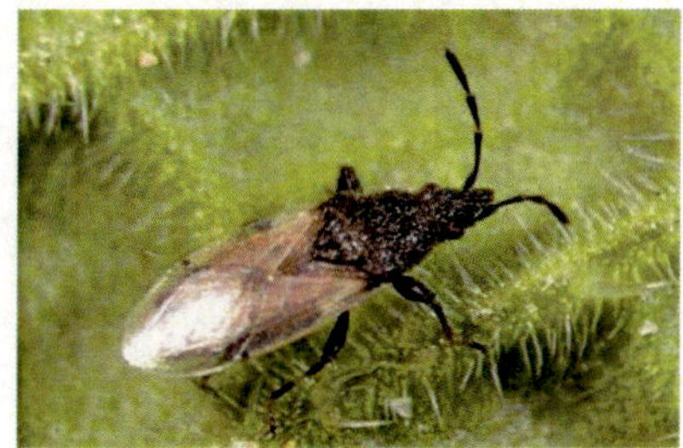

Adult of *Oxycarenus hyalinipennis*

Pink hibiscus mealybug : *Maconellicoccus hirsutus* Green

Family : Pseudococcidae

Order : Hemiptera

Nature of damage

- Crinkled or twisted leaves and shoots, bunched and unopened leaves, distorted or bushy shoots, called "Bunchy top".
- White fluffy mass on buds, stems, fruit, and roots.
- Presence of honeydew, black sooty mold, and ants. Unopened flowers which often shrivel and die. Small deformed fruits.

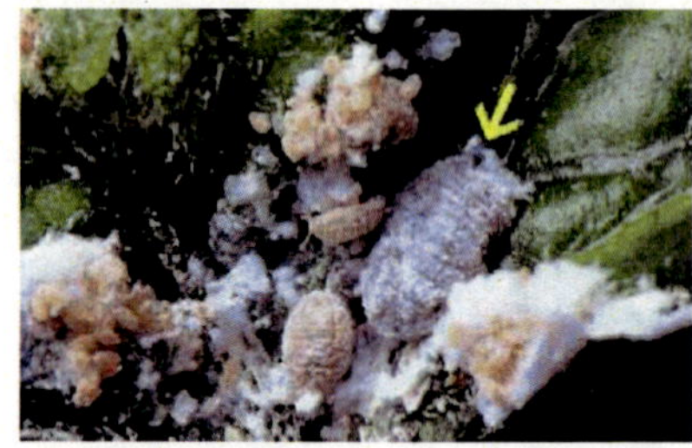

Adult & nymph of *Maconellicoccus hirsutus*

Petiole maggot : *Melanagromyza hibisci* Spencer

Family : Agromyzidae

Order : Diptera

Nature of damage and symptoms

- Maggot bores into tender stems and leaf petioles causing gall like swellings on them. Attack in the early stages results in the formation of nodulated galls and cracking of main stem.
- At later stages the maggots bores into the petioles and it results in the drying up of leaves.

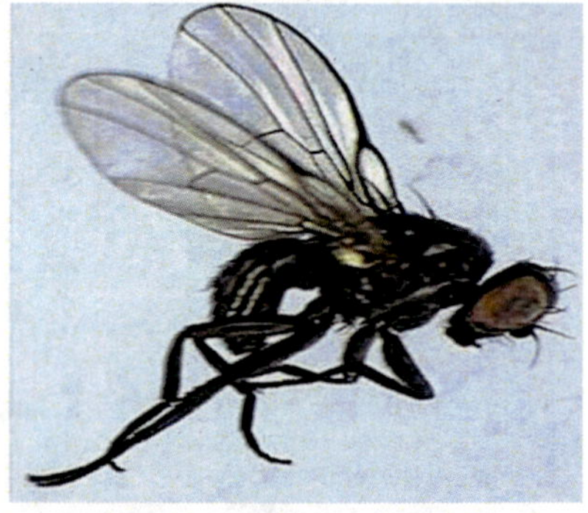

Adult of *Melanagromyza hibisci*

- Only one or two maggots can be observed on the main stem, as high as 20-25 maggots infest a single petiole. Affected leaves completely dry up.

Flower Beetles : *Oxycetonia* spp., *Popillio* spp.

Family : Scarabaeidae

Order : Coleoptera

Biology and nature of damage: Eggs are laid in soil. Egg period is 10 to 12 days. Larval period is 40 to 50 days. Pupation in soil for a period of 8 to 12 days. Injury is caused by the beetle feeding on the flowers and flower buds. Adults feed on flower and flower buds.

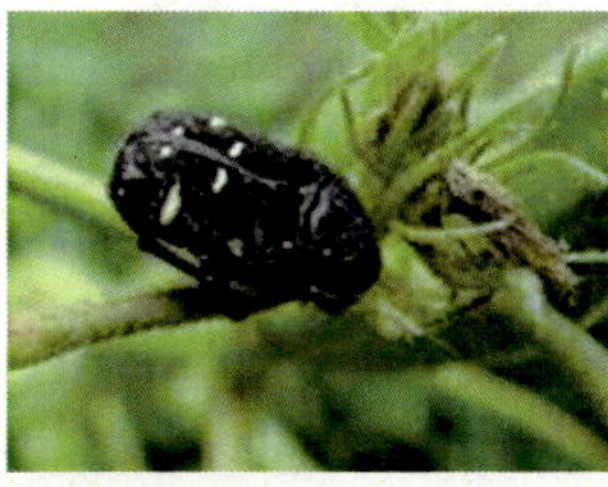
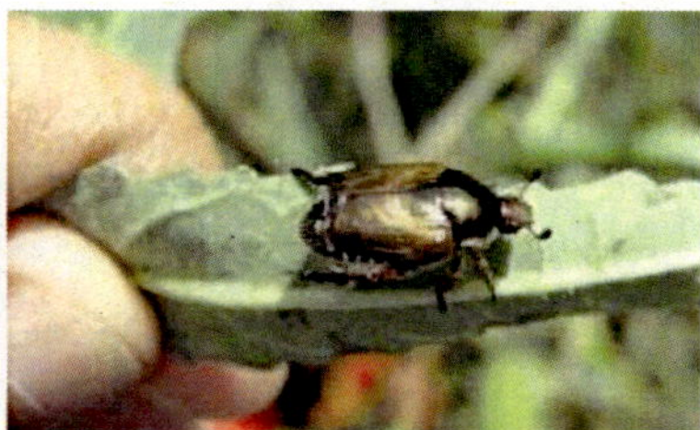

Adult of *Oxycetonia* sp.and *Popillio* sp.

Root knot nematode: *Meloidogyne incognita*

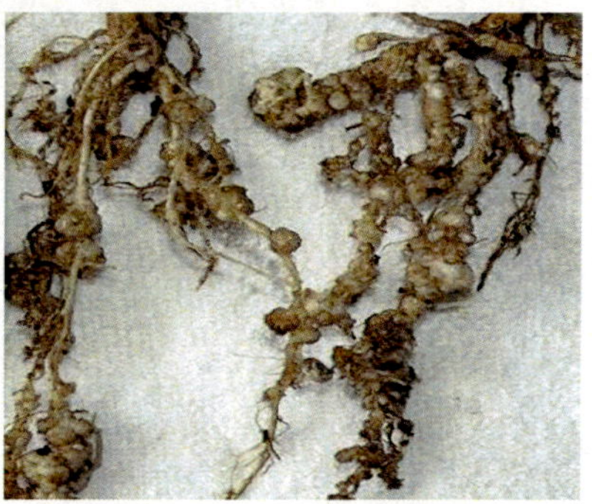

- On roots, galls are formed -affecting the translocation of food
- Foliar symptoms of nematode infestation generally involve stunting and general unthriftiness, premature wilting and leaf chlorosis.
- Damage more severe in seedlings
- Affected plants show development of galls on roots
- Affected plants become stunted with chlorotic symptoms

Management

- Seed treatment with *Pseudomonas flourescens* @ 10g/kg seeds
- *Trichoderma harzianum* application in the nursery beds (50g/m^2)
- Applicatiopn of *Trichoderma* enriched FYM @ 2 tonn/acre
- Neem cake @ 200 kg/acre
- Soil drenching with *Paecilomyces lilacinus* talc formulation@ 20g/L
- Trap cropping with marigold.

Red spider mite: *Tetranychus urticae* Koch.

Mite colonies infest the lower surface of leaves and during the initial stage of infestation, attacked leaves show chlorotic stippled appearance and later turn pale, yellow, dry up and fall off from the plant. In case of severe infestation, complete drying of leaves can be seen (Nirupa *et al.*, 2022).

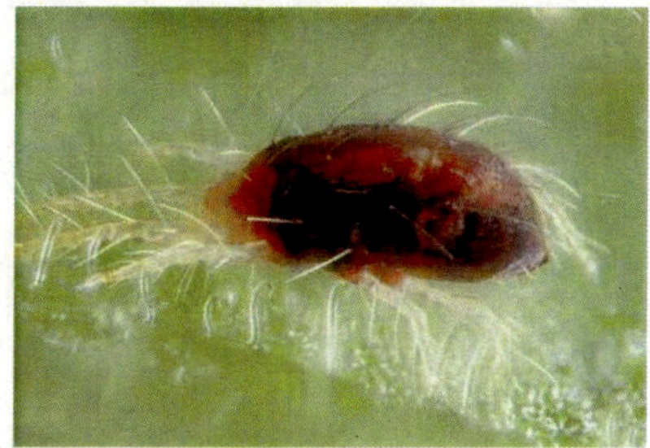

Tetranychus urticae

Management

- Azadirachtin 3000ppm @ 4mL/L is effective during the initial stags
- In case of severe infestation, foliar spraying with spiromesifen 25 EC @ 0.8 mL/L or propargite 57 EC @ 3mL/L is effective against mites

References

Bindra, O.; Mahal, M. Varietal resistance in eggplant (brinjal) (Solanum melongena) to the cotton jassid (Amrasca biguttula biguttula). Phytoparasitica 1981, 9, 119–131. [CrossRef]

Ewete, F.K. Insect species and description of damage caused on okra, Abelmoschus esculentus (L.) Moench. East Afr. Agric. For. J. 1978, 44, 152–163. [CrossRef]

Niruba, D., Chandrasekaran, M., Justin, C., & Kalyanasundaram, A. (2022). Bioefficacy of insecticides and plant based oils against red spider mite, Tetranychus urticae (Koch) (Acari: Tetranychidae) in okra. Pest Management in Horticultural Ecosystems, 28(2), 64-71.

Questions

1. What is the color pattern of the forewings of the moth?
   a) Brown with black spots
   b) White with a pea-green wedge-shaped band
   c) Yellow with red stripes
   d) Grey with white spots
2. Where does the female moth lay eggs?
   a) Only on fruits
   b) Only on leaves
   c) On tender parts of the plant, leaf axils, bracts, leaf veins, buds, flowers, and fruits
   d) Only on flowers
3. How do young *Anomis flava* larvae damage leaves?
   a) They eat entire leaves, leaving only the veins
   b) They tunnel into the roots
   c) They make small punctures on the leaf lamina
   d) They suck sap from the leaves
4. Which pest has a caterpillar with horse-shoe shaped black marks on each segment?
   a) *Sylepta derogata* b) *Xanthodes graellsi*
   c) *Anomis flava* d) *Spodoptera litura*
5. Which of the following insecticides is a systemic neonicotinoid recommended for managing leaf hopper infestations?
   a) Chlorpyrifos b) Thiamethoxam
   c) Fenvalerate d) *Bacillus thuringiensis*
6. What physiological effect does leaf hopper saliva have on plants?
   a) It blocks the xylem, causing wilting
   b) It introduces toxins that cause hopper burn symptoms
   c) It stimulates excessive leaf growth, leading to abnormal size
   d) It dissolves plant cell walls, creating feeding tunnels

7. What major deformity does *Maconellicoccus hirsutus* cause in plants?
   a) Root galls and nodules
   b) Formation of a bushy top with distorted and crinkled leaves
   c) Hollowed-out stems filled with frass
   d) Ring-like chlorotic patches on stems

8. Which of the following resistant cultivars is recommended for whitefly management?
   a) Arka Abhay
   b) Pusa Bold
   c) CO-2
   d) Sonalika

9. Which of the following is an effective cultural management practice against root-knot nematodes?
   a) Spraying neem oil on foliage
   b) Trap cropping with marigold
   c) Mulching with black plastic sheets
   d) Applying phosphatic fertilizers

10. What is a common symptom of severe spider mite infestation?
    a) The entire plant is covered in sooty mold
    b) Leaves become dry, discolored, and covered in webbing
    c) The plant stems develop deep cracks
    d) The roots produce excessive secondary shoots

11. Which of the following is a biological management practice for root-knot nematodes?
    a) Spraying synthetic pyrethroids
    b) Seed treatment with *Pseudomonas fluorescens*
    c) Foliar spray of imidacloprid
    d) Application of copper fungicides

12. **Assertion (A):** The leaf roller caterpillar (*Sylepta derogata*) rolls the leaf and feeds on it from within.

    Reason (R): This feeding habit protects the caterpillar from natural enemies and pesticide sprays.

    a) Both A and R are true, and R is the correct explanation of A.
    b) Both A and R are true, but R is not the correct explanation of A.

c) A is true, but R is false.

d) A is false, but R is true.

13. **Assertion (A):** Green semilooper larvae (*Anomis flava*) create small punctures in leaves during early infestation.

Reason (R): The larvae inject toxic saliva into the plant tissues, causing chlorosis.

a) Both A and R are true, and R is the correct explanation of A.

b) Both A and R are true, but R is not the correct explanation of A.

c) A is true, but R is false.

d) A is false, but R is true.

14. **Assertion (A):** Red bug (*Dysdercus cingulatus*) infestations are commonly observed on infested plants in all growth stages.

Reason (R): Both nymphs and adults of red bugs suck sap from leaves, shoots, and developing seeds.

a) Both A and R are true, and R is the correct explanation of A.

b) Both A and R are true, but R is not the correct explanation of A.

c) A is true, but R is false.

d) A is false, but R is true.

15. **Assertion (A):** Leaf hopper (*Amrasca biguttula biguttula*) infestations lead to leaf bronzing and puckering.

Reason (R): The injury is caused due to the toxic saliva injected by the insect while feeding.

a) Both A and R are true, and R is the correct explanation of A.

b) Both A and R are true, but R is not the correct explanation of A.

c) A is true, but R is false.

d) A is false, but R is true.

Answer Key

1	b	2	c	3	c	4	b	5	b	6	b	7	b
8	a	9	b	10	b	11	b	12	a	13	c	14	a
15	a												

6

Pests of Onion

Onions (*Allium cepa*) are a widely cultivated vegetable crop grown for their bulbs, which are used in cooking worldwide. However, onion crops are vulnerable to various pests that can significantly affect yield and quality.

Sl. No.	Common name	Scientific name	Family and Order	Site of oviposition	Site of pupation
			Sucking pests		
1	Onion thrips	*Thrips tabaci*	Thripidae Thysanoptera	Leaf tissues	Soil, usually near the base of the plant
2	Onion fly	*Delia antiqua*	Anthomyiidae Diptera	At the base of onion plants, on or just below the soil surface.	Soil
3	Cutworm	*Agrotis ipsilon*	Noctuidae Lepidoptera	Soil, often near the base of host plants	Soil

Onion thrips : *Thrips tabaci* L.

Family : Thripidae

Order : Thysanoptera

Distribution

Thrips tabaci is present in the central and southern regions of India, occupying about 36.4% of the land area under the current climate conditions. In central India, the states of Maharashtra, Karnataka, Madhya Pradesh, Gujarat, and parts of Rajasthan offer highly suitable habitats. In the northern region, areas such as Uttar Pradesh, Bihar, Jharkhand, Chhattisgarh, Delhi, Haryana, Punjab, Uttarakhand, & parts of the northeastern states are favorable. In southern India, Karnataka, Andhra Pradesh, Telangana, & Tamil Nadu are particularly suitable.

Biology Adults: Adult onion thrips overwinter in soil in onion, small grain, and hay fields. More mobile than immature stages, adults can fly and are attracted to white and yellow colours, often landing on clothing or skin. They are elongated, with body colour ranging from yellow to brown, and have pale, fringed wings. Adults measure 1.0–1.3 mm for females and 0.7 mm for males. Their lifespan is 16–42 days on garlic and 28–30 days on onion. Females lay eggs for up to three weeks after a one-week preoviposition period. In spring, adults emerge, colonize weed hosts, & can fly or be carried by wind to new plants.

Eggs

Females lay eggs individually in leaf tissue, with one end near the surface for immatures to emerge. The eggs are microscopic, kidney-shaped, and initially white or yellow, turning orange with reddish eye spots as they mature. On onion, eggs average 0.23 mm in length and 0.08 mm in width. The incubation period is 4–5 days on onion, with hatching occurring in 2–3 days in the lab, but 5–10 days in cooler field conditions.

Larvae

The first and second instars are the primary feeding stages. The first instar is small (0.35–0.38 mm in length), semi-transparent, and dull white, eventually transitioning to yellowish white. The second instar is larger, yellow, and measures 0.7–0.9 mm in length with red eyes. The abdomen consists of eight distinct segments, with a large conical posterior segment. The first instar lasts 2 to 3 days, while the second instar lasts 3 to 4 days (Gill *et al.*, 2015).

Pupae

The prepupa and pupa (1.0–1.2 mm) are inactive, non-feeding stages. Pupation occurs at the onion's apical meristem or in the soil. The prepupa is whitish-yellow, measuring 0.9 mm in length, and lasts 1–3 days. Fully formed pupae have folded antennae and developed wing pads. They are yellowish-white, turning yellow before adult emergence. The pupal stage lasts 3–10 days, depending on the region.

Symptoms

- Onion thrips puncture the leaf surface to extract sap, releasing substances that help predigest the tissue. They then consume the mesophyll cells, resulting in chlorophyll loss and reduced photosynthetic efficiency.
- The damage manifests as silvery streaks or patches on the leaves.
- Severe feeding damage by onion thrips is marked by small black "tar" spots, which are their excrement.
- Thrips are the primary vectors of tospoviruses, with onion thrips serving as the principal vector of the Iris yellow spot virus (IYSV tospovirus) in onions (Gill *et al.*, 2015).

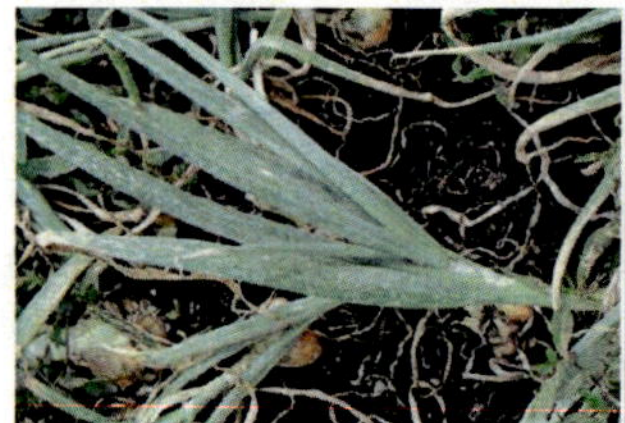

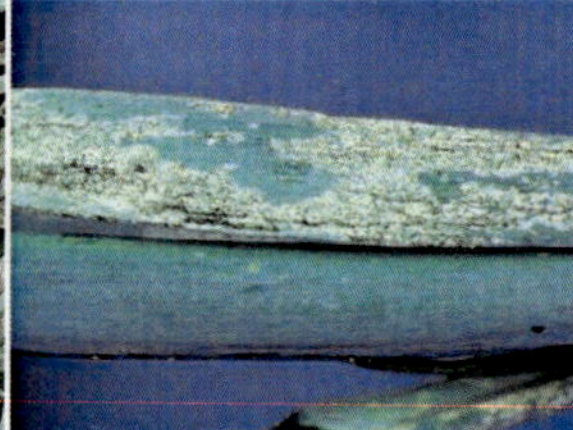

Feeding damage resulting from onion thrips (*T. tabaci*)

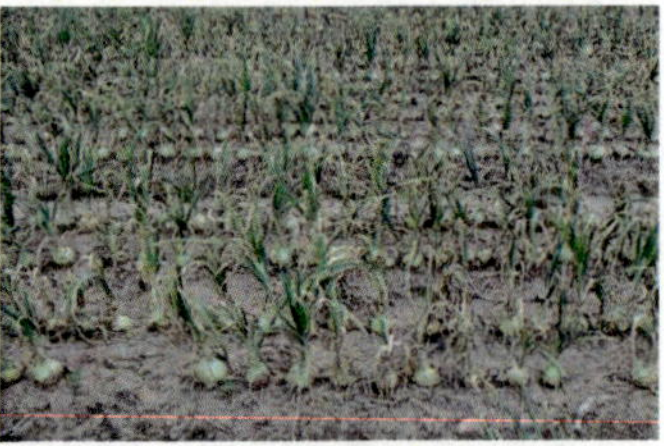

Onions affected by Iris yellow spot virus in the field

Management

- Adopt wider spacing
- Crop rotation with non-host crops like legumes should be followed
- Regular and adequate irrigation reduces thrips multiplication
- Avoid application of excess nitrogen which makes plants more succulent and attractive to thrips
- In case of severe infestation, apply imidacloprid 17.8% SL @ 0.3 ml/L or spinosad 45 SC @ 0.3 ml/L

Onion fly : *Delia antiqua* M.

Family : Anthomyiidae

Order : Diptera

Delia antiqua is distributed across various regions worldwide, including East Asia, North America, Western Europe, and Western Asia. However, comprehensive data on its distribution in India remains scarce in the existing literature (Ning *et al*., 2017).

Biology Eggs: Both mated and unmated onion flies deposit elongated white eggs, which darken to a deeper cream color as they incubate before hatching. The incubation period ranges from 1 to 2 days.

Maggot

The first instar maggot emerges through a transverse split at the anterior end of the egg shell. The legless maggots are cylindrical and creamy-white. Following hatching, the larvae pass through three instars over a period of approximately 5.4 to 5.7 days.

Pre-pupa and pupal period

Towards the end of the larval stage, the larvae became inactive, ceasing movement and feeding. They stayed in this state for a few days as they prepared for pupation, with their body color changing to a light reddish tint. The pre-pupa then developed into a dark reddish pupa, which remained motionless and non-feeding. The pupal stage lasts between 6.08 and 6.8 days.

Adults

The puparium has a cap-like lid that is dislodged when the fly emerges. Newly emerged flies are initially pale, soft, and have unexpanded wings. As they mature, their wings expand and their body turns ash-grey. Males generally emerge before females. The lifespan of the adult flies is influenced by mating status and environmental conditions. The entire life cycle spans from 15.29 to 16.73 days.

Symptoms

D. antiqua is a widespread pest of crops, with its maggots being a major pest of onions, as the onion fly is the primary pest for this species. Female adult onion flies lay significantly more eggs on older plants (4-8 times) compared to younger ones. Host plant odors are the main factor attracting and stimulating oviposition. The oviposition rate increases with the diameter of the onion stem. Females can lay approximately 200 eggs over their 30-day lifespan, with the eggs typically hatching into larvae after several days.

The first instar larva is particularly destructive, as it primarily infests young host seedlings, posing a considerable threat to agricultural systems. Its aggressive feeding often leads to the death of the plant before the maggot completes its development, after which it moves on to a new plant. Although the second and third instar maggots do not kill the plants, the damage caused to the onion bulbs makes them unfit for sale. The larvae feed on onion plant tissues using their hooked mouthparts (Nahar *et al.*, 2019)

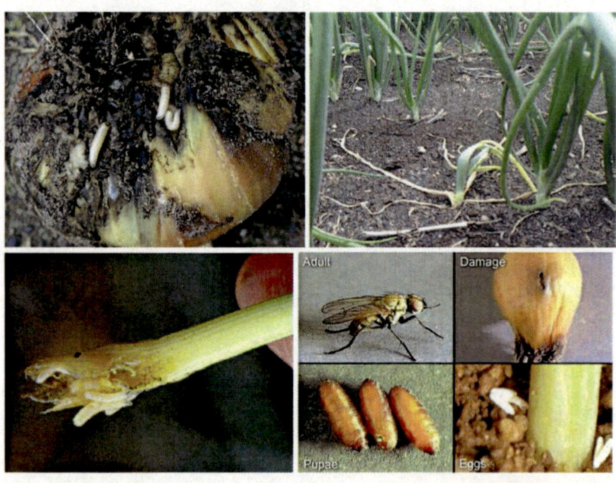

Management

- Field sanitation and crop rotation should be followed
- Soil solarization should be practiced during summer
- **Seed Treatment** with *thiamethoxam 70 WS* @ 3 g/kg of seed
- Foliar application of spinosad 45SC 3.3 mL/10L

Cutworm : *Agrotis ipsilon* H.

Family : Noctuidae

Order : Lepidoptera

Distribution

Agrotis ipsilon is a polyphagous pest found in potato-growing regions of northern India, from Punjab to Bengal and across Madhya Pradesh. With a host range of 41 plant species, it affects various vegetables, including cole crops, radish, turnip, peas, beans, okra, cucurbits, onion, brinjal, tomato, and fenugreek. In Telangana, it is a significant pest of cotton, while in northeastern India, it frequently infests cabbage, cauliflower, and knol khol. In Jammu and Kashmir, particularly in Srinagar, it dominates cole crops, and in Ladakh, it attacks nearly all vegetable crops.

Symptoms

Agrotis ipsilon is not classified as a climbing cutworm, as its feeding primarily occurs at soil level. The larvae feed above ground until reaching the fourth instar, during which time minimal foliage damage typically occurs. However, once the larvae reach the fourth instar, they can cause substantial harm by cutting young plants, with a single larva potentially damaging multiple plants in one night (Rodingpuia and Lalthanzara, 2021).

Biology Eggs: The eggs of *A. ipsilon* are small, slightly flattened spheres, ranging in size from 0.51 to 0.63 mm in width and 0.54 to 0.64 mm in height. They are initially pale yellow and feature narrow ridges radiating from the apex.

Larvae

Agrotis ipsilon larvae undergo six instars in total. After the fourth instar, they exhibit photonegative behavior, hiding in the soil during daylight hours. Older larvae generally cut plants at the soil surface and pull the plant tissues underground. Additionally, they display high levels of cannibalism. Larvae remain active throughout the night, with their peak activity occurring after midnight and about an hour before sunrise.

Pupae

Pupation occurs in the soil within earthen cells, and the pupal stage lasts for 12 to 14 days.

Adults

Adult moths are large, with a wingspan of 40–55 mm. Sexual differentiation is evident based on the antennae: males possess bipectinate antennae, while females have setaceous antennae. Females begin laying eggs 2 to 8 days after emergence, with egg-laying lasting for 4 to 8 days. The full life cycle of the species is completed within 39 to 53 days (Chandel *et al*., 2022) .

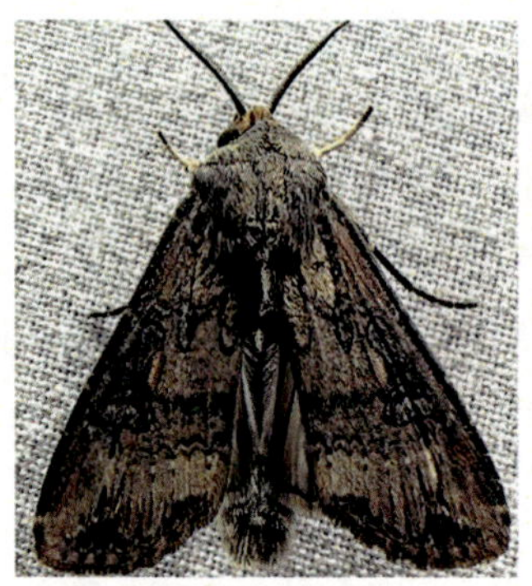

Adult

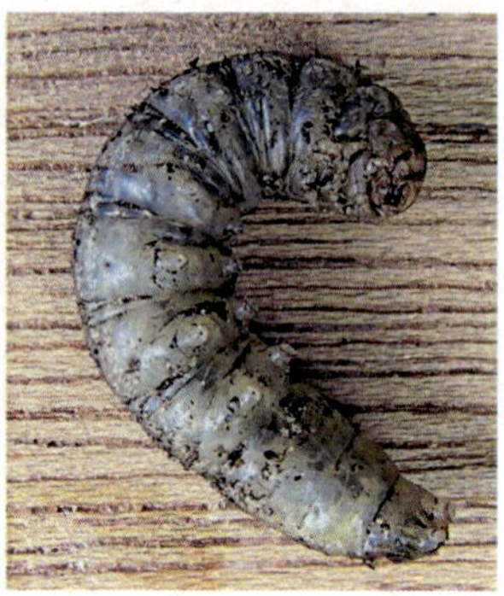

Larva

© Rodingpuia and Lalthanzara, 2021

Management

- Keep the field neat and clean by removing weeds and other plant debris that provide shelter to larvae
- Deep ploughing should be done during land preparation which exposes both larvae and pupae to hot sun and natural enemies including insectivorous birds
- Crop rotation should be practiced
- **Soil application** of insecticides before transplanting or during early seedling stage: **chlorpyrifos 20 EC** @ 2.5 mL/L water

References

Chandel, R.S., Verma, K.S., Rana, A., Sanjta, S., Badiyala, A., Vashisth, S., Kumar, R. and Baloda, A.S., 2022. The ecology and management of cutworms in India. Oriental Insects, 56(2), pp.245-270.

Gill, H.K., Garg, H., Gill, A.K., Gillett-Kaufman, J.L. and Nault, B.A., 2015. Onion thrips (Thysanoptera: Thripidae) biology, ecology, and management in onion production systems. Journal of Integrated Pest Management, 6(1), p.6.

Karuppaiah, V., Maruthadurai, R., Das, B., Soumia, P.S., Gadge, A.S., Thangasamy, A., Ramesh, S.V., Shirsat, D.V., Mahajan, V., Krishna, H. and Singh, M., 2023. Predicting the potential geographical distribution of onion thrips, Thrips tabaci in India based on climate change projections using MaxEnt. Scientific Reports, 13(1), p.7934

Nahar, K., Sultana, S., Akter, T., & Begum, S., 2019. Biological traits and susceptibility of Delia antiqua (Meigen, 1826) (Diptera: Anthomyiidae) in onion. Bangladesh Journal of Zoology, 47, pp. 325-332. https://doi.org/10.3329/bjz.v47i2.44343.

Ning, S., Wei, J., & Feng, J., 2017. Predicting the current potential and future world wide distribution of the onion maggot, Delia antiqua using maximum entropy ecological niche modeling. PLoS ONE, 12. https://doi.org/10.1371/journal.pone.0171190.

Rodingpuia,C. and Lalthanzara, H., 2021. An insight into black cutworm (Agrotis ipsilon): A glimpse on globally important crop pest. Science vision, 2, pp.36-42.

Questions

1. Which of the following is the most destructive pest of onion in India?
   a) Onion thrips b) Onion maggot
   c) Tobacco caterpillar d) Aphids
2. Thrips damage onion crops by:
   a) Boring into bulbs
   b) Feeding on leaves and sucking sap
   c) Laying eggs in roots
   d) Defoliating the entire plant
3. The scientific name of onion thrips is:
   a) *Thrips tabaci* b) *Spodoptera litura*
   c) *Delia antiqua* d) *Aphis gossypii*
4. Onion maggot (*Delia antiqua*) primarily damages which part of the plant?
   a) Roots b) Leaves
   c) Bulbs d) Flowers
5. The peak incidence of onion thrips occurs during:
   a) Rainy season b) Cold and dry weather
   c) Hot and humid weather d) Waterlogged conditions
6. Which natural enemy is effective against onion thrips?
   a) *Trichogramma chilonis* b) *Chrysoperla carnea*
   c) *Cotesia plutellae* d) *Bracon hebetor*
7. Which insecticide is commonly recommended against onion thrips?
   a) Imidacloprid b) Malathion
   c) Chlorpyrifos d) Fipronil
8. The typical damage symptom of thrips on onion is:
   a) Skeletonized leaves b) Silvery streaks and curling
   c) Black sooty mold d) White patches with holes
9. Cultural control of thrips includes:
   a) High nitrogen fertilization b) Wider spacing & crop rotation
   c) Water stress d) Continuous cropping

10. Which pest lays eggs at the base of the onion plant and the larvae bore into bulbs?
    a) Onion fly (*Delia antiqua*)
    b) Leaf miner
    c) Onion thrips
    d) Stem borer
11. **Assertion (A):** Onion thrips cause silvery patches and curling of onion leaves.
    Reason (R): Thrips suck the sap from the foliage, reducing photosynthesis
    a) Both A and R are true, and R is the correct explanation of A.
    b) Both A and R are true, but R is not the correct explanation of A.
    c) A is true, but R is false.
    d) A is false, but R is true.
12. **Assertion (A):** Onion maggots damage bulbs of onion crops.
    Reason (R): Adult flies feed on the leaves of the onion plant.
    a) Both A and R are true, and R is the correct explanation of A.
    b) Both A and R are true, but R is not the correct explanation of A.
    c) A is true, but R is false.
    d) A is false, but R is true.
13. **Assertion (A):** Cutworms damage onion seedlings by cutting them at the base.
    Reason (R): Cutworms feed on onion foliage during the day.
    a) Both A and R are true, and R is the correct explanation of A.
    b) Both A and R are true, but R is not the correct explanation of A.
    c) A is true, but R is false.
    d) A is false, but R is true.
14. **Tobacco Caterpillar (*Spodoptera litura*)**
    Assertion (A): *Spodoptera litura* causes defoliation in onion crops.
    Reason (R): The larvae feed voraciously on leaves during early stages.
    a) Both A and R are true, and R is the correct explanation of A.
    b) Both A and R are true, but R is not the correct explanation of A.
    c) A is true, but R is false.
    d) A is false, but R is true.

Answer Key

1	a	2	b	3	a	4	c	5	b	6	b	7	a
8	b	9	b	10	a	11	a	12	c	13	c	14	a

Pests of Solanaceous Vegetables

7

Pests of Brinjal

Brinjal (*Solanum melongena*), also known as eggplant or aubergine, is a major solanaceous vegetable crop grown in India and other parts of the world. It is affected by several insect pests throughout its growth period, significantly reducing both yield and quality.

Sl. No.	Common name	Scientific name	Family and Order	Site of oviposition	Site of pupation
			Borers		
1	Shoot and fruit borer	*Leucinodes orbonalis*	Crambidae, Lepidoptera	Under surface of leaves, tender shoots, flower buds & developing fruits	Plant parts
2	Stem borer	*Euzophera perticella*	Noctuidae, Lepidoptera	Basal portion of the stem	Inside stem/ soil
3	Epilachna beetle	*Henosepilachna vigintioctopunctata*	Coccinellidae Lepidoptera	On underside of leaves	Leaves
4	Leaf folder	*Antoba olivaceae*	Erebidae, Lepidoptera	On upper leaf surface	Within the leaf folds
5	Leaf webber	*Psara bipunctalis or Herpetogramma bipunctalis*	Crambidae, Lepidoptera	On leaf	Within the webbings
6	Ashweevil	*Myllocerus subfaciatus M. viridanus*	Curculionidae, Coleoptera	Soil	In soil
7	Ants	*Solenopsis geminata*	Formicidae, Hymenoptera	Soil	Soil
			Sucking pests		
8	Mealybugs	*Coccidohystrix insolitus*	Psuedococcidae, Hemiptera		
9	Leaf Hopper	*Amrasca biguttula biguttula Cestius phycitis*	Cicadellidae, Hemiptera	Within the leaf veins	
10	Lacewing bugs	*Urentius hystricellus*	Tingidae Hemiptera	On underside of leaves	
11	Aphids	*Myzus persicae, Aphis gossypii*	Aphididae, Hemiptera		

12	White fly	*Bemisia tabaci*	Aleyrodidae, Hemiptera	On leaf surface	
13	Mites	*Polyphago-tarsonemus latus*	Tarsonemidae Acarii Order: Trombidiformes	In plant tissues	

Shoot and fruit borer : *Leucinodes orbonalis* G.

Family : Crambidae

Order : Lepidoptera

Introduction

One of the major constraints in production and productivity of brinjal is the incidence of pests and diseases. The fruit and shoot borer is one of the most damaging pests of brinjal. Pest infestation starts from transplanting seedling stage and continues up to harvesting of the crop. Pest is active throughout the cropping season with peak infestation from last week of August to December

Distribution

China, India, Bangladesh, Malaysia, Thailand, Burma, Sri Lanka, Laos, Congo and South Africa

Host plants: *Solanum tuberosum* (potato), *Lycopersicon esculentum* (tomato), *Ipomoea batatas* (sweet potato), *Solanum indicum* and *Solanum torvum* (turkey berry). *Solanum gilo* (gilo) and *Solanum nigrum* (Black nightshade)

Biology: The grey delicate moth has white and hyaline wings with brown markings on the forewings. Eggs are laid on the under surface of leaves, tender shoots, flower buds and developing fruits. Egg period – 3 to 6 days. Adult female lay about 250 eggs and after hatching the larvae borne within shoots and fruits and feed on the internal tissues (Nair, 1999). Oviposition usually takes place on lower surfaces of leaves, shoots, flower buds and sometimes on the calyces of fruits.

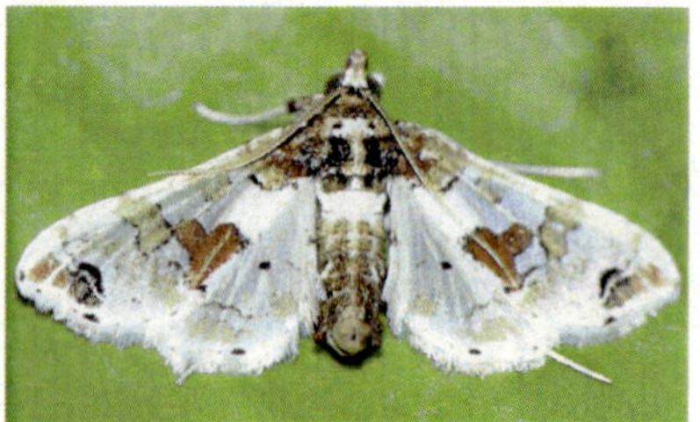

Adult moth

Source: Copyright @ Crop Pest Index NBAIR

The pinkish larva with sparsely distributed hairs or warts on the body and brownish head measuring about 1.6 cm when full grown. Larval period from 12 to 15 days during summer and extends up to 28 days during winter. The mature larvae come out of their feeding tunnels and pupate in tough silken cocoons on the plant. Pre pupal and pupal periods are 3-4 days and 7-10 days respectively. In winter season pupation prolongs for 15 days (Srivastava and

Butani, 2009). Total life cycle lasts for 21-45 days with five overlapping generations in an year (Srivastava and Kunjwal, 2018).

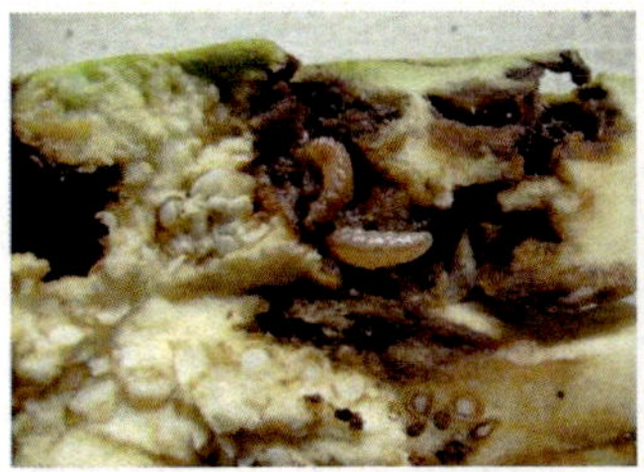
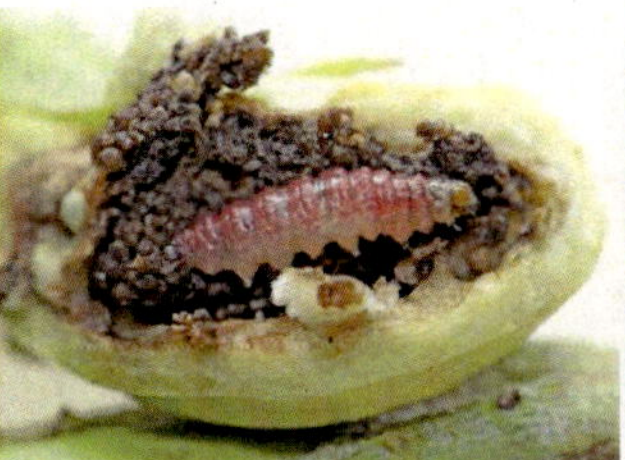
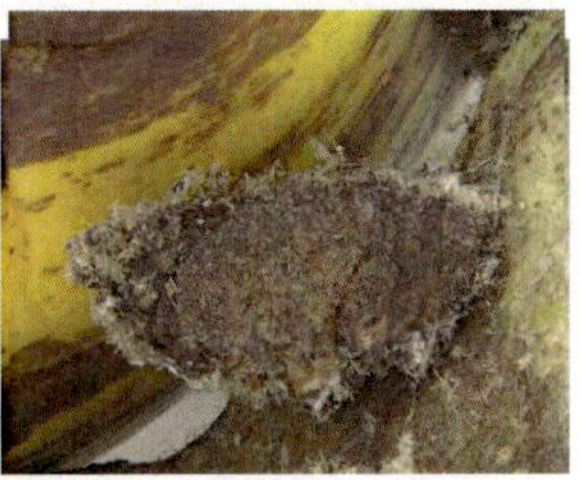

Tunneling made by the larva Pupa

Source: Copyright @ Crop Pest Index NBAIR

Nature of damage

- Young plants are more prone to attack
- Initially the caterpillar bores into the petiole and midribs of large leaves and young tender shoots situated very close to the entry point
- The caterpillars bore into the shoots and fruits and feed on the internal tissues

Symptoms

- Appearance of wilted and droopy shoots and leaves
- Damaged fruits have holes on them, plugged with excreta
- Premature flower shedding
- Reduction in fruit number and size

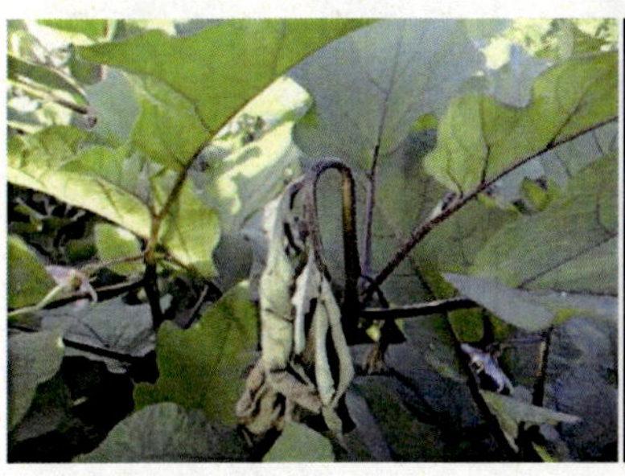
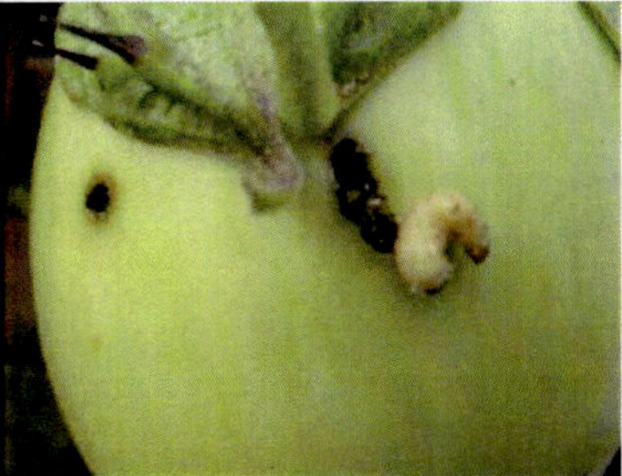

Integrated pest management

- Use of resistant varieties viz., Pusa purple long, Pusa purple round, Annamalai, Arka Kusumakar, Doli-5, Chaklasi Doli, Pusa Purple Long, SM 6, SM 68 and Pant Samrat for cultivation
- Avoid continuous cropping of brinjal and ratooning
- Crop rotation with nonhost plants should be practiced

- Crops like maize, cowpea and coriander can be used for inter cropping and this will help to enhances the natural habitat for natural enemies of this pest
- Uproot and burn old plants before planting new plants since they harbour pest and carry over infestation
- Collect and destroy the damaged tender shoots, fallen fruits and fruits with bore holes to prevent population build up
- Use light traps @ 1/ha to attract and kill the moths
- Predatory coccinellids viz., *Cheilomenes sexmaculata*, *Coccinella septempunctata*, *Brumoides suturalis*, predatory mirid bug *Campyloneura* sp and parasitoids (*Trichogramma chilonis*, *Pseudoperichaeta* sp., *Phanerotoma* sp., *Itamoplex* sp., *Eriborus argenteopilosus*, *Diadegma apostate*) can be used for pest management
- Release egg parasitoids *Trichogramma chilonis* @ 50000 /ha
- Spray Bt formulations of *B. thuringiensis* var. *kurstaki* such as Dipel @ 1.5 to 2 ml /L of water at weekly intervals starting from flowering
- Spray any one of the insecticides starting from one month after planting at 15 days interval., NSKE 5%, Azadirachtin 1.0% 1.0-1.5 ml/l
- In case of severe infestation spray any of the insecticides like Flubendiamide 2 ml in 10 l or Emamectin benzoate 5 WG @ 4g/10l, or Thiacloprid 240 Sc @ 1.5 ml/10l or Thiodicarb 75 WP@ 2g/l
- Avoid continuous use of synthetic pyrethroids as they cause resurgence of sucking pests
- Avoid using insecticides at the time of fruit maturation and harvest

Stem Borer	:	***Euzophera perticella*** Ragonot (Snout moths)
Family	:	Pyralidae
Order	:	Lepidoptera

Distribution: Indian sub-continent

Host plants : Brinjal, chilly, tomato and potato

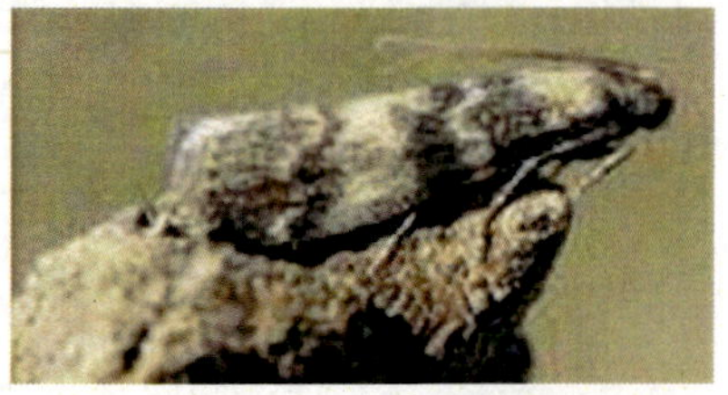
Euzophera perticella Ragonot

Biology: Female moths prefer young leaves, petioles and tender shoots for oviposition. Eggs are laid singly or in clusters. Incubation period lasts for about 3 to 10 days. Immediately after hatching the neonate make a hole on the stem and bores into it and move downwards making tunnels inside the stem. The larval stages lasts for 26 to 58 days and the pupal duration is about 9-16 days (Srivastava and Butani, 2009). Total life cycle will be completed within 35-76 days. Usually 3-4 generations occur within an year sometimes extending upto eight overlapping generations (Srivastava, 1961 and Prem Chand, 1995).

- Moths are medium sized
- Fore wings pale or greyish brown with vertical black lines beyond middle of the wing
- Hind wings are whitish
- Eggs are laid singly or in clusters on young leaves, petioles or tender shoots.
- Full grown caterpillars are whitish. Pupation is in stem. Life cycle is completed in 30-60 days.

Nature of damage

Matured plants are more prone to attack

- Pencil-thick and woody stem is usually preferred by the larvae
- Soon after hatching the caterpillar bores into stem near the ground level
- Make tunnels inside the stem and attacked plants wither and wilt

Symptoms

Larva bore the main stem and feeds the internal contents. Due to continuous feeding and tunnelling made by the larva, drooping and wilting of infested plant occurs. At the entry point there is a distinct thickening of stem. Fruit bearing capacity is also adversely affected.

Management

- Avoid continuous cropping of brinjal and practice crop rotation with nonhost plants
- Crop sanitation should be practiced and severely infested plants should be destroyed
- Installation of light traps @1/ha to attract and kill the moths
- Larval paarsitoids - *Pristomerus testaceus* and *P. euzopherae* are to be conserved
- Pupal parasitoids like *Xanthopimpla* sp., *Apanteles* sp. *Goryphus* sp. Are also effective in reducing the pest population
- Spray neem seed kernel extract 5%
- Spray flubendiamide @ 2 ml/10L if infestation is severe

Epilachna beetle : *Henosepilachna vigintioctopunctata*
Family : Coccinellidae
Order : Coleoptera

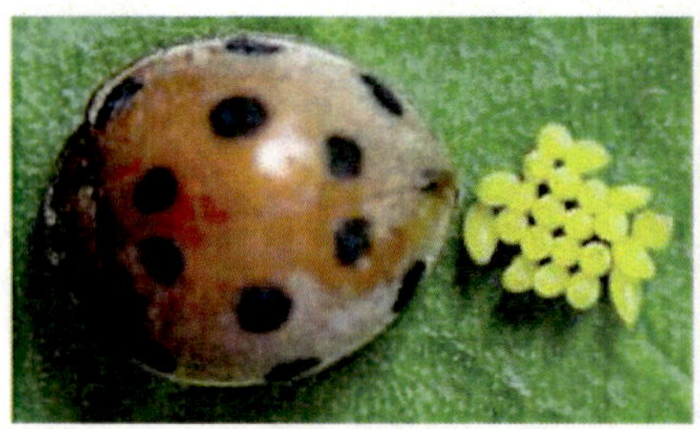
Adult beetle and egg mass

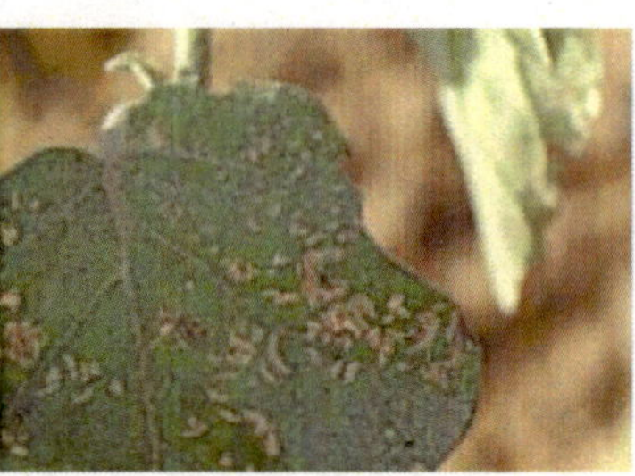
Damage symptom on leaf

Adult beetle is hemispherical, reddish brown with 12 to 28 black spots dorsally.

Distribution

Native to southeastern Asia, mainly India, and has been accidentally introduced to other regions of the world, including Australia and New Zealand. Occurrence of this pest has also been documented in Brazil and Argentina since 1996.

Host plants

Brinjal, potato, chillies, tomato and other plants belonging to Solanaceae Family

Biology: The females lay cigar shaped and yellowish eggs in erect clusters on the lower side of leaves.

Egg period: 2-4 days: Eggs cigar shaped, laid in clusters on leaf surface, yellow; 120-460 eggs/female and the grub period have a duration of 10-35 days. The grubs are yellow, fleshy and covered with hairs and six rows of longitudinal spines. Total duration of life cycle varies between 20-50 days depending upon the weather parameters (Kunjwal and Srivastava, 2018).

- *E. dodecastigma*: Copper-coloured, 6 spots / elytra
- *E. demurille*: Dull appearance, light copper coloured and six black spots surrounded by yellowish area on each elytra
- *E. vigintioctopunctata*: 14 spots on each elytra, deep red. Total life period: 20-50 days 7 generations / year.

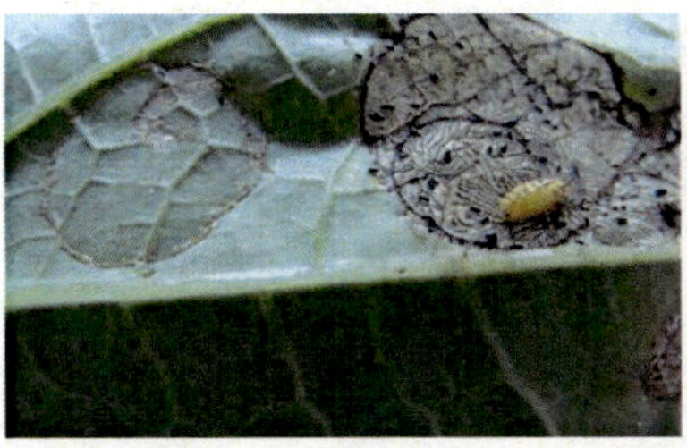
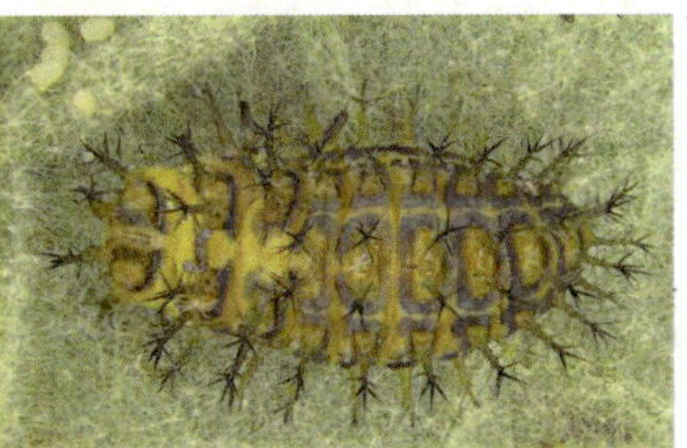

Grub feeding on leaf Grub

Source: Copyright @ Crop Pest Index NBAIR

- Pupation is on the leaf surface/ stem, Pupal period: 5-6 days.
- Yellowish pupa with spines on posterior part; anterior portion being devoid of spines
- Life cycle is completed in 3 to 5 weeks.

Nature of damage and symptoms

- Both the adults and grubs scrape surface tissues of the leaves causing irregular holes on the leaves.
- They eat up regular areas of leaf tissues leaving parallel bands of uneaten tissue in between
- The leaves, thus present a lace like appearance. They turn brown & dry up
- In case of severe infestation, skeletonization occurs

Natural enemies

Egg parasitoid	:	*Tetrastichus ovulorum.*
Larval parasitoid	:	*Pleurotropis epilachnae, P. faveloatus.*
Pupal parasitoid	:	*Pediobius epilachnae, Tetrastichus* sp., *Chrysocharis johnsoni*

Management

- Collect and destroy egg masses, grubs and adults of the pest.
- Neem based formulations 4 ml/l
- Spray NSKE 5%
- Spray neem oil garlic emulsion 2%
- Spray *Beauveria bassiana* @ 20g/l at weekly intervals
- Foliar spray of quinalphos @ 2 ml/l is also effective in reducing the pest

Leaf folder / leaf roller : *Antoba olevaceae* (Walker)

Family : Erebidae

Order : Lepidoptera

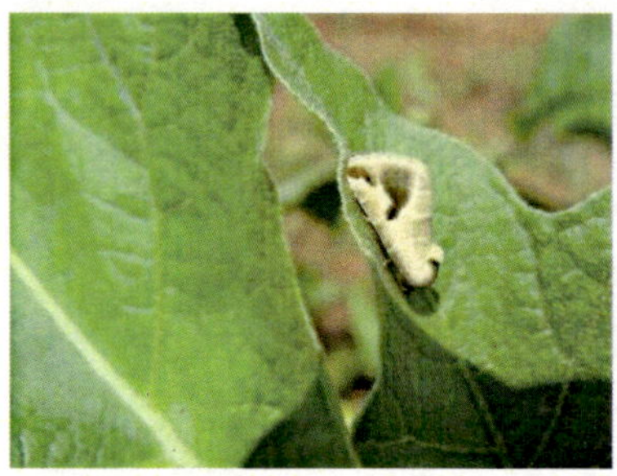
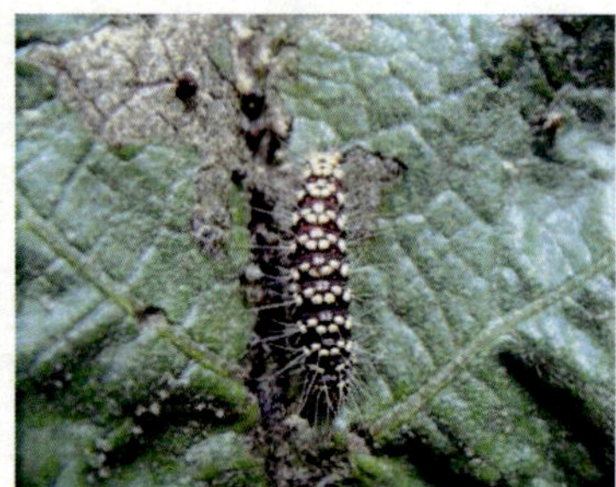

Distribution

Botswana, Eritrea, Madagascar, Malawi, Mozambique, Nigeria, South Africa,Tanzania, Uganda and Zimbabwe. It is also found in Sri Lanka and India.

Host plants : Brinjal, and wild solanaceous crops

Biology: Adult is a stout moth, the wings have olive green colouration. The larva is hairy and purple brown with yellow spots. Eggs are laid (30-40 eggs) on upper leaf surface in an irregular manner. Larvae cause damage by folding the leaves and feeding the chlorophyll from within. Pupation also occurs inside the leaf fold.

Nature of damage and symptoms

Larva folds the tender leaf and feed on surface tissues, infested leaves later dry up. Larvae sometimes bore the tender shoots and feed the internal tissues resulting in withering and wilting of the affected plants.

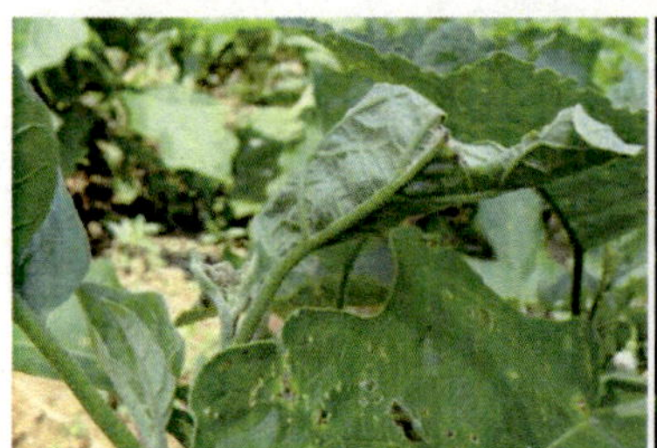
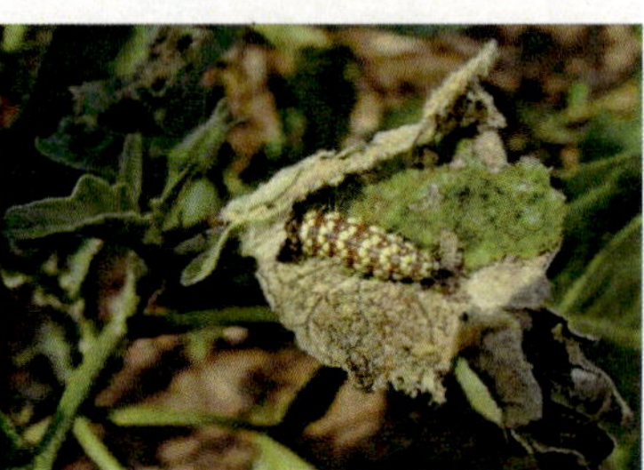

Leaf fold Larva inside the leaf fold

Source: Copyright @ Crop Pest Index NBAIR

Leaf Webber	:	*Psara bipunctalis/ Herpetogramma bipunctalis* F.
Family	:	Pyralidae
Order	:	Lepidoptera
Host plants	:	Brinjal, *Codiaeum* sp., *Solanum torvum, S. indicum, Alternanthera sessilis*.

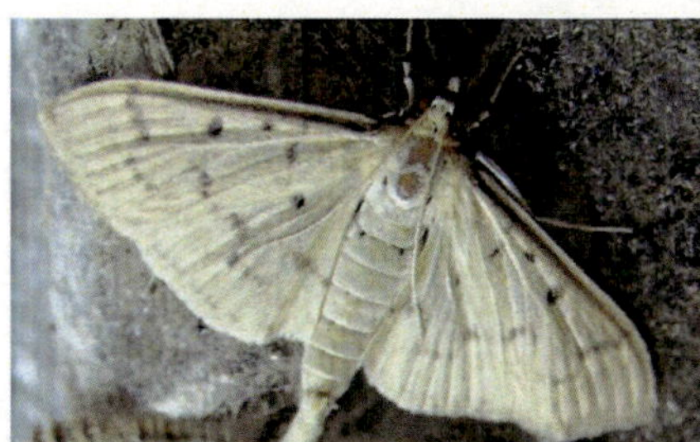
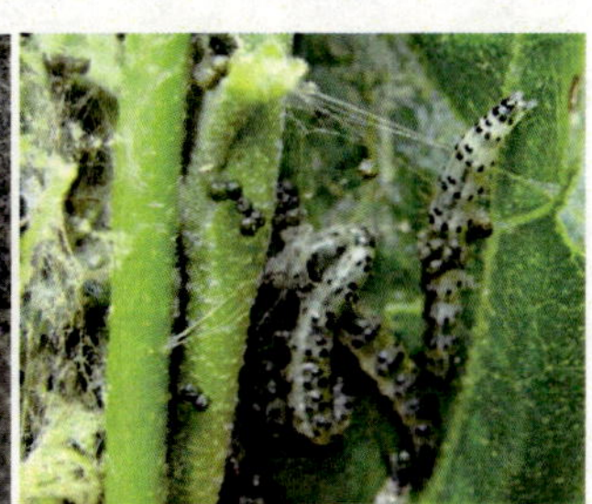

Biology: Straw coloured moth with black dots and lines on the wings. Caterpillar is green in colour with black spots.

Nature of damage and symptoms

Caterpillar webs together the leaves and feed from within. The leaves are totally eaten up leaving only the veins and webbings. Pupation is inside these webbings.

Management

- Collection and destruction of affected plant parts along with insects
- NSKE 5% spray
- In case of severe infestation foliar spray of flubendiamide @ 2 mL/10L or chlorantraniliprole @ 3 mL/10L

Ash weevil	:	*Myllocerus viridanus* F., *M.subfasciatus*
Family	:	Curculionidae
Order	:	Coleoptera

Biology: Ash weevil is an important pest of brinjal and other vegetables. It primarily damages the crop by feeding on leaves and roots. Eggs are creamy white and oval shaped and laid in soil near the plant base or in soil cracks. Hatch in 3-5 days. Grub is white in color. Legless, cylindrical in shape, completes development in 1-2 months. Pupation in soil inside earthen cocoon, pupa creamy white in colour. Pupal period is about 1 week.

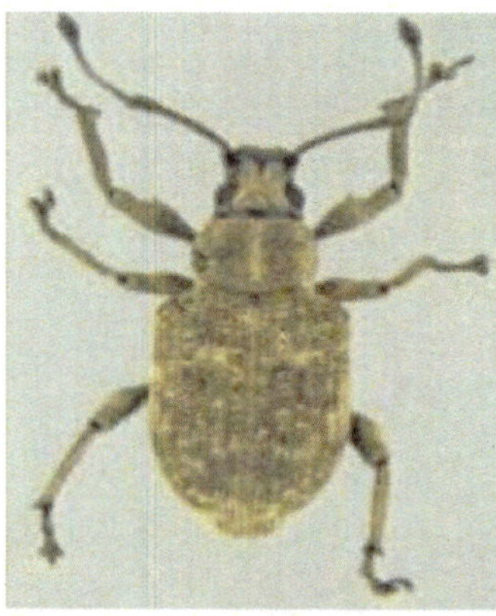

Myllocerus subfasciatus

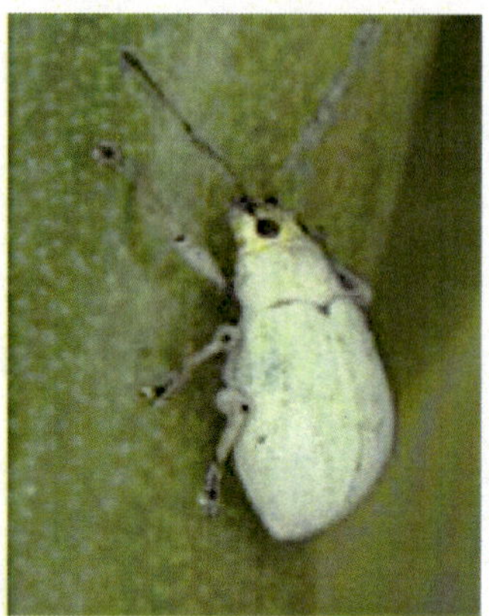

M. viridanus

Nature of damage and symptoms

Both adult weevils and grubs cause damage to the plant. Adult feeds on leaves and cause notching symptoms on the leaf. Grubs feed on the roots and cause wilting of plants in patches.

Management

- Collect and destroy adults
- Deep summer ploughing to expose grubs and pupae to natural enemies and hot sun
- Apply Neem cake @ 500 kg / ha at the time of last ploughing
- Spray NSKE 5%
- In case of severe infestation spray Cyantraniliprole @ 2mL/L
- For destroying grubs and pupae soil drenching with chlorpyrifos @ 2.5 mL/L should be done

Ants : *Solenopsis geminata*
Family : Formicidae
Order : Hymenoptera

Minute brown ants make tunnels around the roots and nibble at them. It also bores into the buds and terminal shoots. Destroy the anthills with insecticides, keep a sugar trap; smear jaggery on the inner surface of a coconut shell and sprinkle some insecticidal granules. Place it near the anthill.

Mealy Bug : *Coccidohystrix insolitus* G.
Family : Pseudococcidae
Order : Hemiptera

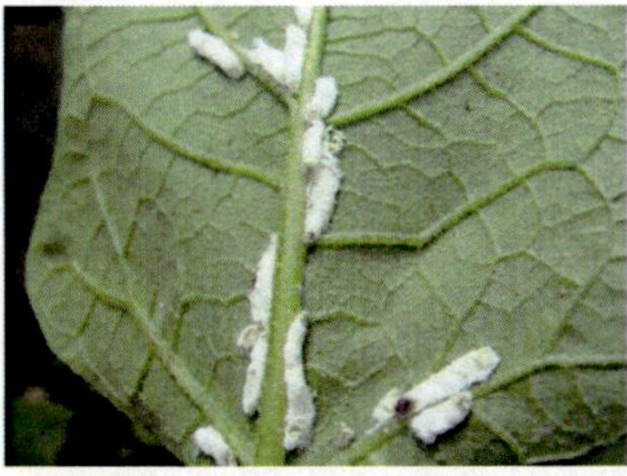
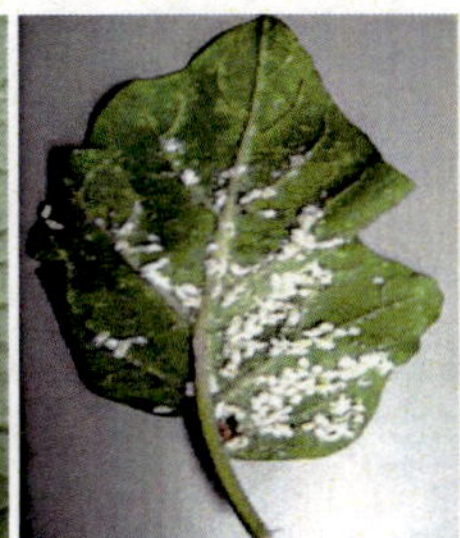

Mealybug population on the leaf

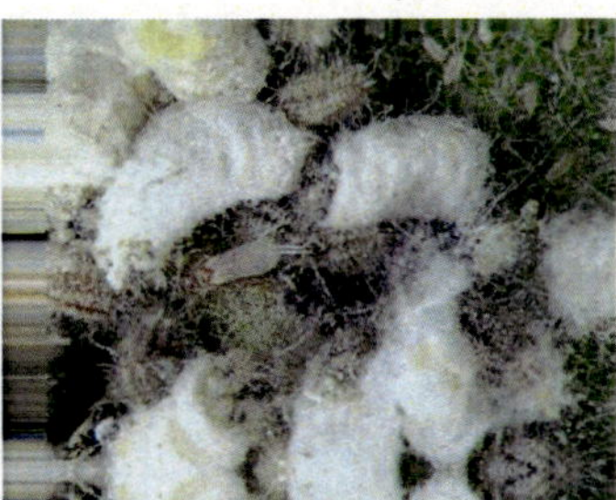

Mealybug adults

Distribution

It is a highly polyphagous pest with its origin in India and is widely distributed to all over the world.

Host plants : Brinjal, pigeon pea and other Solanum spp. Also infests members of Malvaceae Family.

Biology: Parthenogenesis is not recorded in this species. Ovisac of the adult female is seen protruded out from the posterior end of the abdomen. A fertilised adult female will lay upto 100-200 eggs in an ovisac. Hatching period is about 3-8 days. All the developmental stages (3 nymphal instars) will be completed within 22-25 days (Srivastava and Butani, 2009).

Nature of damage and symptoms

- Both nymphs and adults congregate on the tender plant parts viz., leaves. tender shoots, flower buds and fruits and suck sap from these plant parts
- Continuous desapping will devitalise the plant
- Mealybugs Infest leaves, tender shoots and fruits
- Leaves turn yellow and crinkle resulting in the drying of leaves. Infestation on flower blooms affect fruit set
- Fruits become dried and shrivelled and premature fruit drop occurs
- Numerous mealy bugs can be seen on all the tender parts and fruits
- Due to honeydew excretion, a wet surface is formed facilitating the growth of black coloured sooty mould (*Capnodium* sp.)

Management

- Pruning and destruction of severely infested plant parts
- Conservation of predatory coccinellids like *Scymnus* sp., *Coccinella septumpunctata* etc.
- In case of severe infestation spraying of imidacloprid @ 3 ml/10 litre or thiamethoxam @ 2g/10 litres is effective in reducing the infestation

Leaf hoppers – *Amrasca bigutula bigutula* (Ishida), *Cestius phycitis* (Distant), *Empoasca binotata* Pruthi, *E. parathea* Pruthi and *E. punjabensis* Pruthi

Among the different leaf hoppers infesting brinjal, *A. bigutula bigutula* is the most common and destructive one.

Host plants : Brinjal (*Solanum melongenum*), cotton (*Gossypium* spp.) and okra (*Abelmoschus esculentus*). Other alternate host plants are Sunflower *Helianthus annus* L., Cowpea *Vigna unguiculata* L., China Rose (*Hibiscus rosasinensis* L.), Pigeon pea (*Cajanus cajan* Millsp.) and several grasses including durva lawns (*Cynodon dactylon* L.).

Biology: A single female lay about 15-30 eggs and are inserted to the plant tissues. The eggs will be hatched within a period of 4-10 days. The nymphs are white to light green in colour and go through a 7–21 day nymphal cycle. Usually, they traverse leaves in a diagonal manner. Adults live for around two weeks (Srivastava and Butani, 1998).

Nature of damage and symptoms

Nymphs and adults suck sap from the ventral surface of leaves especially near the vein region. They are phloem feeders. Apart from sucking sap, these insects inject toxic saliva to the plant tissues leading to hypertrophy and thus resulting in the rupturing of phloem tubes. They also act as vectors for the viral disease, little leaf of brinjal.

- Yellowing starts from the leaf margins and progress towards the centre
- Crinkling of leaves
- In severe cases, hopper burn symptoms appear giving a burnt appearance of the plant

Management

- Leafhoppers are repelled by the length and density of the trichomes (hairs) in tolerant or resistant cultivars with hairy leaves
- It is said that Bangladeshi cultivar Bagun 6 and Indian cultivars Manjari Gota, Vaishali, Mukta Kesi, Round Green, and Kalyanipur T3, Purple Long, Nepali, and Neelum are tolerant (Ghosh and Karmakar, 2021)
- Intercropping with pigeon pea and other non-host plants will reduce the pest infestation
- Installation of yellow sticky traps will help to monitor the pest at the same time will help to reduce the pest population

- Release of green lacewings *Chrysoperla zastrowii* Zillemi @ 100000 eggs / ha if effective in reducing leaf hopper population thrice at fortnightly intervals reduce all sucking pests including hoppers
- Application of two per cent neem oil emulsion will reduce the infestation
- Foliar spray with spinosad @ 3.3 mL/10L is effective to manage the pest population
- In severe cases, imidacloprid 3 mL/ 10L or thiamethoxam @ 2g/ 10L will manage the pest

Lace Wing Bug: *Urentius hystricellus* Tingidae ; Hemiptera

It is a small bug, body covered with spines and the wings show a distinct lace-like appearance. Nymphs resemble adults, but are initially wingless, developing wings as they grow. Both adults and nymphs are usually found in groups on the underside of leaves. It is a specific pest of brinjal

Host plants : Brinjal

Biology: Eggs are laid singly in the leaf tissues. A total of 35-40 eggs are laid by a single female. Hatching period lasts for about 3-12 days and the nymphal period lasts for 10-23 days.

Nature of damage and symptoms

Both nymphs and adults suck sap from the leaves causing whitish to yellowish mottled patches on the leaves. In case of serious infestation the leaves turn entirely yellow, then dry and drop off. Attacked leaves are speckled with black shiny spots, which are the faeces of the bugs.

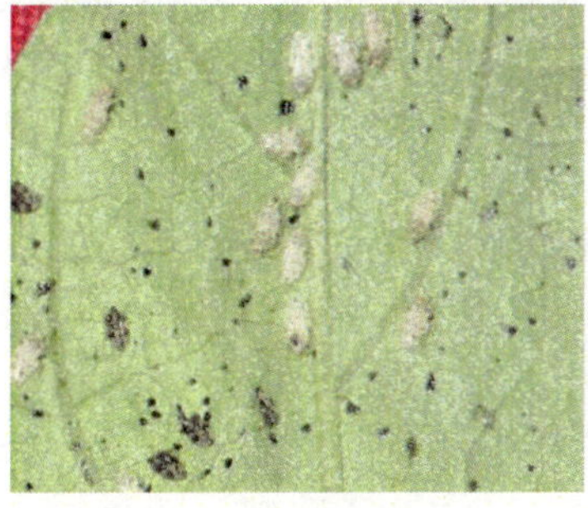

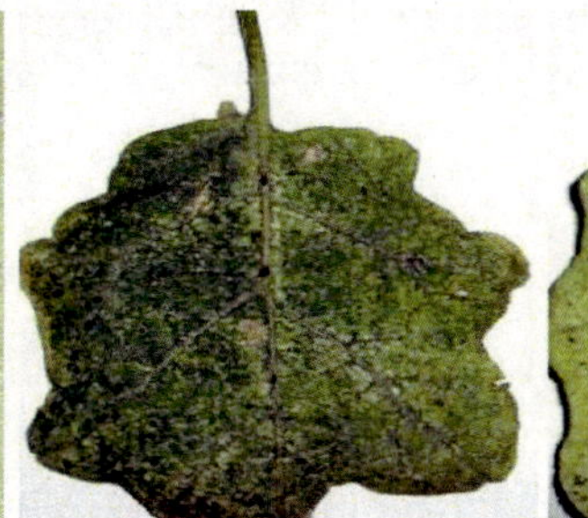

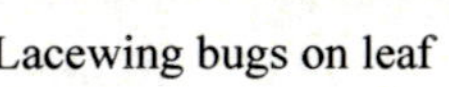

Lacewing bugs on leaf

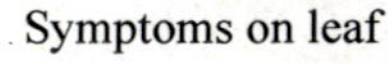

Symptoms on leaf

Aphids : Cotton aphid, *Aphis gossypii* Glover, and green peach aphid, *Myzus persicae* Sulzer.

Family : Aphididae

Order : Hemiptera

Greenish brown aphid, Occurrence of aphids can be identified by the presence of ants that feed on honeydew. Plant becomes weak and leaves curled and crinkled. Congregation of both nymphs and adults can be seen on all the tender plant parts.

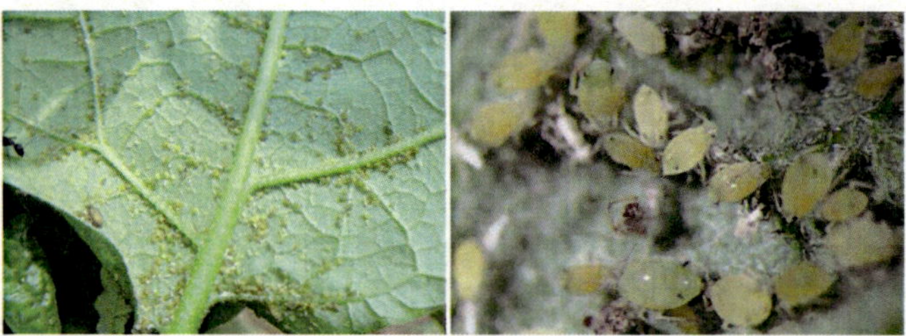

Nymphs and adults-lower leaf surface-Adults

Distribution: Worldwide distribution except the colder parts of Asia and Canada

Biology: Parthenogenetic viviparity is the mode of reproduction in *A. gossypii*. Fecundity of the adult female ranges from Usually the nymphs are greenish brown or yellowish in colour while the adults are yellowish green in colour. The total nymphal period (4 instars) is 5.09 $^{+}$ 0.30 days in brinjal. Incubation period lasts for 0.96 to 1.10 days. Total life cycle will be completed within 13.55 to 15.35 days (Shah *et al.*, 2009). Adults of *Myzus persicae* are greenish in colour. Overwintering and migration are common in aphids. Usually *A. gossypii* prefers brinjal and other vegetables for breeding during winter season and during summer they migrate to cucurbits and by the end of June these aphids will return to cotton. In case of green peach aphid, parthenogenetic viviparity dominates during Summer, Monsoon and Autumn seasons and sexual reproduction prevails in cooler regions during winter (Srivastava and Butani, 2009).

Nature of damage and symptoms

Both nymphs and adults colonise on almost all the tender plant parts and suck sap. More population can be seen on the under surface of leaves. Honey dew excretion and associated *Capnodium* (sooty mold) growth which make black colouration to the severely infested plants. Ants are always seen associating with the aphid colonies for the nutrient rich honey dew. Due to continuous desapping the following symptoms are observed in plants

- Loss of plant vigour
- Curling, crinkling and deformation of affected plant parts
- Shedding of flowers and malformation of fruits
- In case of severe infestation, stunted growth occurs

White fly : *Bemesia tabacii*

Family : Aleyrodidae

Order : Hemiptera

White flies are one of the most common and destructive sucking pest of vegetables and ornamentals. Population of white flies can be seen on all the tender plant parts especially lower surface of leaves.

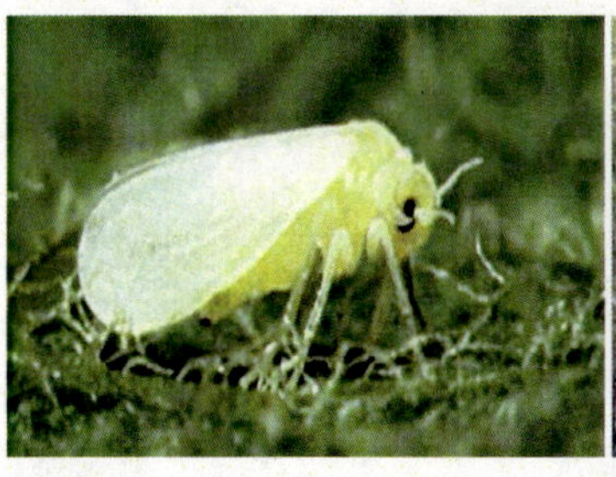

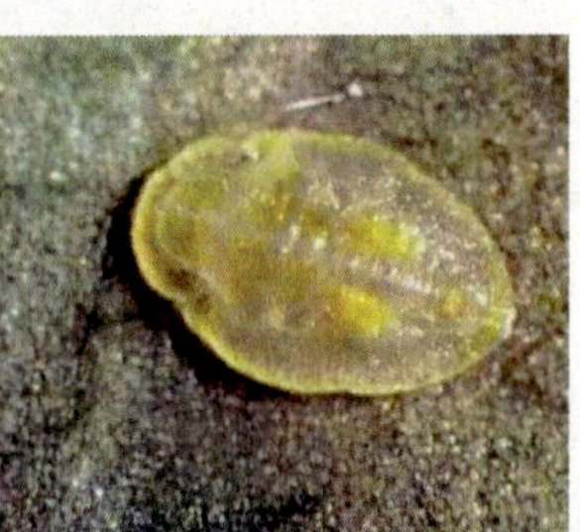

Yellow mite : *Polyphagotarsonemus latus*

Family : Tarsonemidae

Order : Trombidiformes

Nature of damage and symptoms

Both adults and nymphs suck sap from the lower leaf surface and also from the tender plant parts resulting in characteristic bleaching, and stunted growth.

Management

- Encourage the activity of predatory mite: *Amblyseius ovalis*
- Application of azadirachtin @ 5 ml/l (in initial stages), neemoil garlic emulsion 2% is effective to reduce the infestation
- In case of severe infestation, spray wettable sulfur 80 WP @ 3g/L Propargite 57% EC 3 mL/L or spiromesifen 22.9 SC (Oberon) @ 8 mL/10L or fenazaquin 10 EC @ 2.5 mL/L or fenpyroximate 5 EC @ 1 mL/L

References

Ghosh, S. K., & Karmakar, R. (2021). Sustainable management of leaf hopper (Amrasca biguttula biguttula) on eggplant/brinjal (Solanum melongena (Linn.) and related crops. Hi-Tech Crop Production and Pest Management.-Biotech Books. Daryaganj, New Delhi, 231-255.

Kunjwal, N., & Srivastava, R. M. (2018). Insect Pests of Vegetables. Pests and Their Management, 163–221. doi:10.1007/978-981-10-8687-8_7

Shah, M. A. S., Singh, T. K., & Radhakrishore, R. K. (2009). Comparative biology of cotton aphid, Aphis gossypii Glover (Homoptera-Aphididae) on okra and brinjal.

Srivastava K., P. and Butani, D., K. Pest management in vegetables Vol I. Studium Press (India) Publishers p. 381.

Questions

1. Which of the following is the most serious pest of brinjal?
   a) Fruit borer (*Leucinodes orbonalis*)
   b) Aphids (*Aphis gossypii*)
   c) Whitefly (*Bemisia tabaci*)
   d) Jassids (*Amrasca biguttula biguttula*)
2. Leucinodes orbonalis damages brinjal by:
   a) Sucking sap from leaves
   b) Boring into flowers & fruits
   c) Defoliating the plant
   d) Feeding on roots
3. The egg-laying habit of *Leucinodes orbonalis* is:
   a) Eggs laid in the soil
   b) Eggs laid singly on tender parts
   c) Eggs laid in clusters on mature leaves
   d) Eggs inserted into fruits
4. Characteristic symptom of brinjal fruit and shoot borer infestation is:
   a) Yellowing of lower leaves
   b) Curling of leaves
   c) Drooping of shoots and holes in fruits
   d) Webbing of leaves
5. Which of the following pest causes 'hopper burn' in brinjal?
   a) Aphid
   b) Whitefly
   c) Jassid
   d) Thrips
6. Which pest is known to transmit little leaf disease in brinjal?
   a) Whitefly
   b) Aphid
   c) Thrips
   d) Jassid
7. Which insecticide is commonly recommended for managing fruit and shoot borer in brinjal?
   a) Imidacloprid
   b) Malathion
   c) Emamectin benzoate
   d) Acephate
8. Biological control agent for *Leucinodes orbonalis* includes:
   a) *Trichogramma chilonis*
   b) *Coccinella septempunctata*
   c) *Cryptolaemus montrouzieri*
   d) *Aphidius colemani*

9. Which brinjal pest is responsible for transmitting viruses?

   a) Aphid
   b) Thrips
   c) Whitefly
   d) Leafhopper

10. Eggs of *Leucinodes orbonalis* are laid on:

   a) Soil near plant base
   b) Underside of leaves
   c) Tender shoots and flower buds
   d) Fruits only

11. **Assertion (A):** Fruit and shoot borer causes extensive economic losses in brinjal production.

    Reason (R): The larvae bore into the fruits and shoots, causing internal feeding and damage.

    a) Both A and R are true, and R is the correct explanation of A
    b) Both A and R are true, but R is not the correct explanation of A
    c) A is true, but R is false
    d) A is false, but R is true

12. **Assertion (A):** Jassids cause curling and yellowing of brinjal leaves.

    Reason (R): Jassids inject toxins during feeding that result in 'hopper burn'.

    a) Both A and R are true, and R is the correct explanation of A
    b) Both A and R are true, but R is not the correct explanation of A
    c) A is true, but R is false
    d) A is false, but R is true

13. **Assertion (A):** Whitefly infestation in brinjal leads to sooty mold development.

    Reason (R): Whiteflies excrete honeydew which promotes fungal growth.

    a) Both A and R are true, and R is the correct explanation of A
    b) Both A and R are true, but R is not the correct explanation of A
    c) A is true, but R is false
    d) A is false, but R is true

14. **Assertion (A):** *Leucinodes orbonalis* is difficult to control once it enters the fruit.

    Reason (R): Internal feeding makes contact insecticides ineffective.

    a) Both A and R are true, and R is the correct explanation of A
    b) Both A and R are true, but R is not the correct explanation of A
    c) A is true, but R is false
    d) A is false, but R is true

15. **Assertion (A):** Brinjal fruit and shoot borer (*Leucinodes orbonalis*) is the most destructive pest of brinjal.

    Reason (R): The larvae feed externally on brinjal leaves and stems.

    a) Both A and R are true, and R is the correct explanation of A
    b) Both A and R are true, but R is not the correct explanation of A
    c) A is true, but R is false
    d) A is false, but R is true

16. **Assertion (A):** Severe infestation by ash weevil (*Myllocerus viridanus*) leads to wilting and yellowing of brinjal.

    Reason (R): Ash weevil grubs feed on the roots resulting in yellowing and wilting

    a) Both A and R are true, and R is the correct explanation of A
    b) Both A and R are true, but R is not the correct explanation of A
    c) A is true, but R is false
    d) A is false, but R is true

17. **Assertion (A):** Whitefly (*Bemisia tabaci*) infestation leads to the development of sooty mold on brinjal leaves.

    Reason (R): Whiteflies secrete honeydew that promotes fungal growth.

    a) Both A and R are true, and R is the correct explanation of A
    b) Both A and R are true, but R is not the correct explanation of A
    c) A is true, but R is false
    d) A is false, but R is true

18. **Assertion (A):** *Leucinodes orbonalis* is difficult to manage with contact insecticides.

    Reason (R): The larvae feed internally within shoots and fruits, making them inaccessible.

    a) Both A and R are true, and R is the correct explanation of A

    b) Both A and R are true, but R is not the correct explanation of A

    c) A is true, but R is false

    d) A is false, but R is true

19. **Assertion (A):** Jassid infestation in brinjal is usually higher during hot and dry weather.

    Reason (R): Dry conditions favour population build up of sucking pests.

    a) Both A and R are true, and R is the correct explanation of A

    b) Both A and R are true, but R is not the correct explanation of A

    c) A is true, but R is false

    d) A is false, but R is true

20. **Assertion (A):** Biological control using *Trichogramma chilonis* can help manage fruit and shoot borer in brinjal.

    Reason (R): *Trichogramma chilonis* parasitizes the eggs of *Leucinodes orbonalis*.

    a) Both A and R are true, and R is the correct explanation of A

    b) Both A and R are true, but R is not the correct explanation of A

    c) A is true, but R is false

    d) A is false, but R is true

21. **Assertion (A):** Use of neem-based biopesticides is effective against sucking pests in brinjal.

    Reason (R): Neem compounds act as antifeedants, repellents, and growth regulators.

    a) Both A and R are true, and R is the correct explanation of A

    b) Both A and R are true, but R is not the correct explanation of A

    c) A is true, but R is false

    d) A is false, but R is true

Answer Key

1		2		3		4		5		6		7	
8		9		10		11		12		13		14	
15		16		17		18		19		20		21	

8

Pests of Chilli

Chilli (*Capsicum annuum* L.), a member of the Solanaceae, is a significant spice and vegetable crop in India, extensively cultivated over warm temperate, tropical, and subtropical regions. Approximately 51 insect pests and two mite species from 27 families and 9 orders were discovered to be infesting chillies (Reddy and Puttaswamy, 1983). The yield losses range from 50-90 per cent due to insect pests in chilli (Nelson and Natrajan, 1994)

Sl No.	Common name	Scientific name	Family and Order
1	Chilli thrips	*Scirtothrips dorsalis* *Thrips parvispinus*	Thripidae, Thysanoptera
2	Green peach aphid	*Myzus persicae*	Aphididae, Hemiptera
3	Yellow mite	*Polyphagotarsonemus latus*	Tarsonemidae, Acarina
4	White fly	*Bemisia tabaci*	Aleurodidae, Hemiptera
5	Tobacco cutworm	*Spodoptera litura*	Noctuidae, Lepidoptera
6	Gram caterpillar	*Helicoverpa armigera*	Noctuidae, Lepidoptera

Chilli thrips: *Scirtothrips dorsalis*, Thripidae, Thysanoptera Biology

The adults are slender, yellowish brown in colour, with long, narrow, and heavily fringed wings. The adult female inserts eggs into the tissues of the leaves and shoots. The nymphs are similar to adults, except they are smaller and wingless. With the exception of the rainy season, the pest is present all year round. The life cycle is completed over a period of two weeks. Over the course of a year, multiple generations overlap.

Recently introduced invasive thrips in chilly is *Thrips parvispinus* Karny. It causes premature flower drop, shedding of fruits and malformations resulting in severe yield loss. The average fecundity is about 56 eggs with a mean developmental period of 18.8 days (Muray *et al*., 2009).

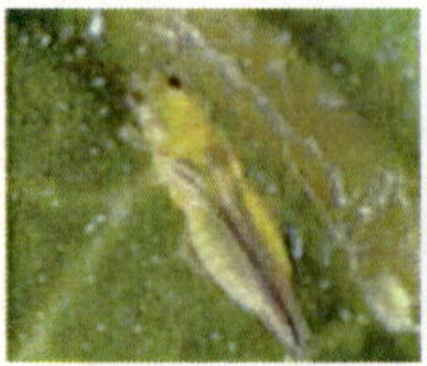
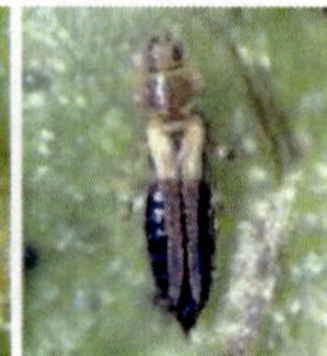
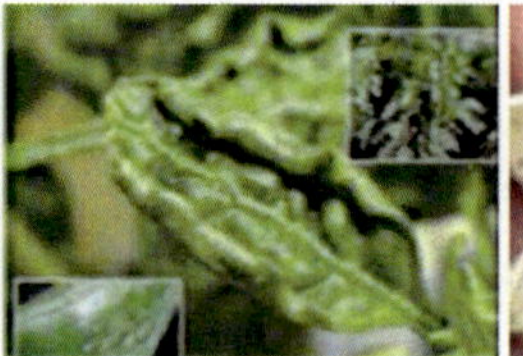
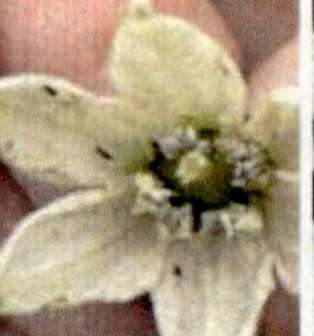
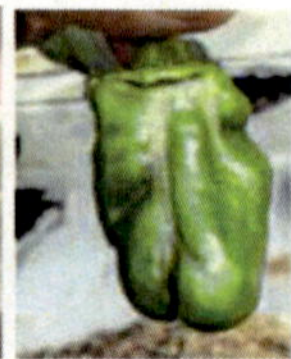

S. dorsalis *T.parvispinus* Symptoms on leaf, flower and fruit

Nature of damage and symptoms

- The attacked leaves get crinkled, curled upward, and shed
- In case of severe infestation leaves, flower buds, flowers and fruits are malformed
- Upward curling of leaves
- Shedding of flowers and fruits
- The attacked plants are stunted and may dry up

Management

- Provide shade plants that regulate the thrips population
- Sprinkle water over the seedlings
- Setting up of bright blue sticky traps
- Place plastic/paper mulch to suppress the emergence of pupae
- Thrips are preyed upon by predacious thrips like *Franklinothrips vespiformis, Erythrothrips* spp., and *Scolothrips* spp.
- In case of severe incidence spray imidacloprid 17.8 SL @ 3 ml/10l or acetamiprid 20 SP @ 2g/10l or emamectin benzoate 5 SG @ 4g/10l or spinosad 45 Sc @3-3.3 ml/l or Thiacloprid 21.7 SC @ 4.5 ml/10l or Cyantraniliprole @ 1.2 ml/l (Tatagar *et al.*, 2014)

Green peach aphid: Myzus persicae, Aphididae, Hemiptera

Adults are yellowish-green in colour. Nymphs initially are greenish, but soon turn yellowish. The infested plants turn pale with sickly appearance.

Nature of damage and symptoms

- The affected leaves become curled and crinkled
- Honeydew excretion leads to the development of sooty mould
- In case of severe infestation plants show stunted growth

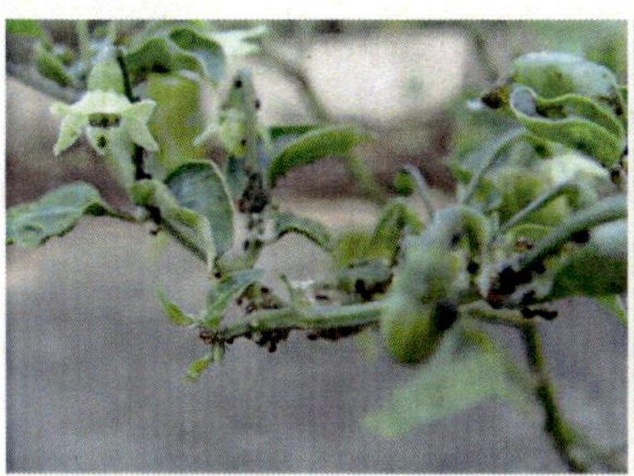

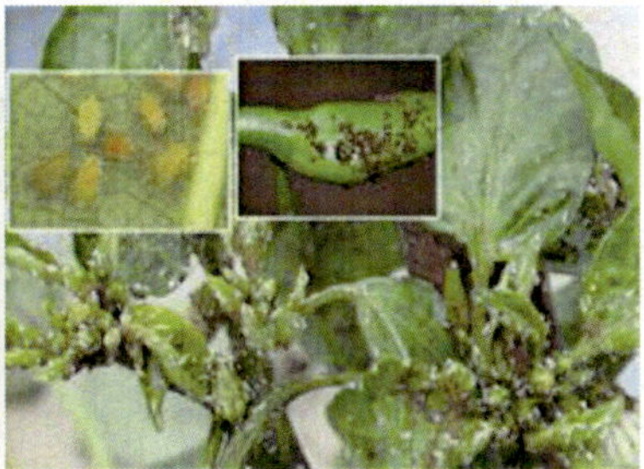

Management

- Severely affected plant parts should be clipped off and destroyed
- Spray *Verticillium/Lecanicillium lecanii* @ 20g/l, and repeat application at 10-12 days interval
- 80–90% of chillies in field are known to be parasitized by *Aphidius* and *Aphelinus* species (Mani & Krishnamoorthy, 1994)
- Apply insecticides like imidacloprid @ 3 mL/10L or acetamiprid @ 2g/10L or thiamethoxam @ 2g/10L

1. Yellow mite or muranai mite: *Polyphagotarsonemus latus*, Tarsonemidae, Acarii

Biology: The adult mites are yellowish green colour with four pairs of legs. They lay tiny, oval-shaped eggs on the ventral side of immature leaves or on leaf buds. The larva moves slowly and has three pairs of legs. The durations of the egg, larval, nymphal, and adult phases are 1.5–2, 1.5, 1, and 8–10 days, respectively.

Nature of damage and symptoms

- Infected leaves show downward curling and crinkling
- Leaves with elongated petiole
- In case of severe infestation plants show stunted growth

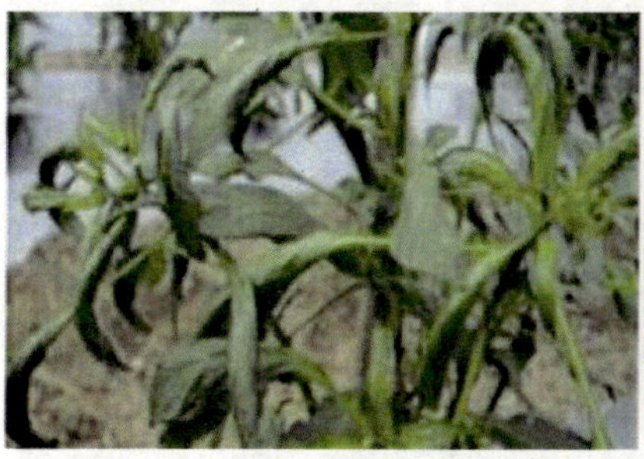

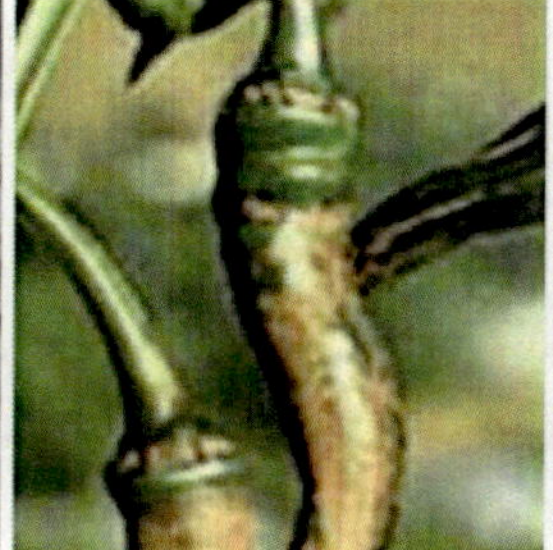

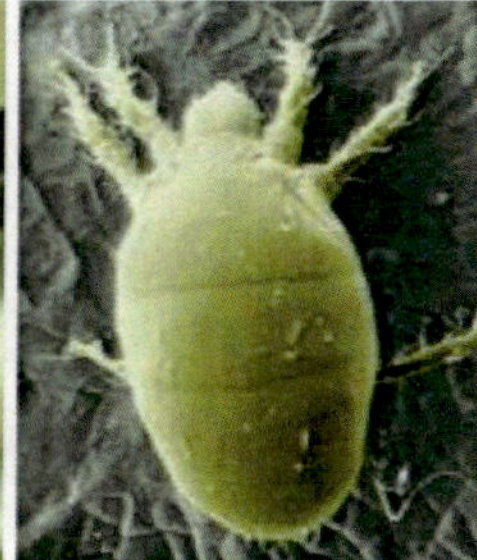

Downward curling of leaves Malformation and bronzing of fruits *P.latus* adult

Management

- Encourage the activity of predatory mite: *Amblyseius ovalis*
- Application of azadirachtin @ 5 ml/l (in initial stages), neemoil garlic emulsion 2%
- In case of severe infestation, spray wettable sulfur 80 WP @ 3g/L Propargite 57% EC 3 mL/L or spiromesifen 22.9 SC (Oberon) @ 8 mL/10L or fenazaquin 10 EC @ 2.5 mL/L or fenpyroximate 5 EC @ 1 mL/L

2. White fly: *Bemisia tabaci*, Aleurodidae, Hemiptera

Biology: The adults are winged and their yellowish bodies are dusted with white waxy powder. The adult females insert their light-yellow eggs singly on the underside of the leaves. The nymphs are yellowish, louse-like and sluggish and are seen clustering on the undersurface of the leaves. Pupation occurs on the leaves.

Nature of damage and symptoms

- The nymphs and adults suck sap from the leaves, lowering the vitality of the plant
- The growth and yield of the plant is adversely affected during severe infestation

Management

- Severely affected plant parts should be clipped off and destroyed
- Place yellow sticky traps @ 12/ha
- In case of severe infestation use thiamethoxam (Actara) @ 4g/10l

3. Tobacco cutworm: *Spodoptera litura,* Noctuidae, Lepidoptera

Biology: The adults are brown in colour—brown forewings with white wavy markings and white hindwings with brown patch along margin. The golden yellow coloured eggs are laid in mass and covered with silky hairs. The caterpillars are light green with black heads or black spots; they can be seen in groups feeding on the plant.

Nature of damage and symptoms

- Newly hatched larvae scrap the green matter in the leaf
- Affected leaf looks like a papery white structure
- The larvae bore within the fruit during the fruiting period, filling the boreholes with excrement and harming the crop financially (Meena *et al.*, 2012)

- Affected fruits decay and fall off
- In severe infestations, they feed voraciously on the entire lamina, petiole, and sometimes even the tender twigs or the terminal shoots of plants, also feed on the floral parts and bore into the fruits

Management

- Plough the soil to expose and kill pupae
- Collect and destroy the egg masses, gregarious larvae and grownup caterpillars
- Application of *Beauveria bassiana* @ 20g /L
- Spray SlNPV @ $1.5x10^{12}$ POB/ha in the evening hour
- In case of severe infestation apply Chlorantraniliprole @ 3 mL/10L or spinosad 3.2 mL/10L or flubendiamide 2 mL/10L or cyantraniliprole @ 1.2 mL/l or emamectin benzoate 5 SG@ 4g/10L or indoxacarb 14.5 SC (Avaunth) @ 7 mL/10L

4. Gram caterpillar: *Helicoverpa armigera,* Noctuidae, Lepidoptera

Biology: The adult females are stout brownish-yellow moths, while the males are light greenish with characteristic V-shaped markings. The creamy white eggs are laid singly. Pupation occurs in soil, leaf, pod and crop debris.

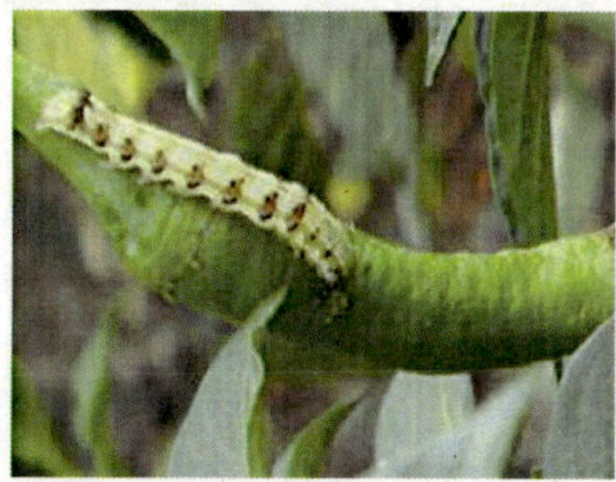

Larva feeding on fruit

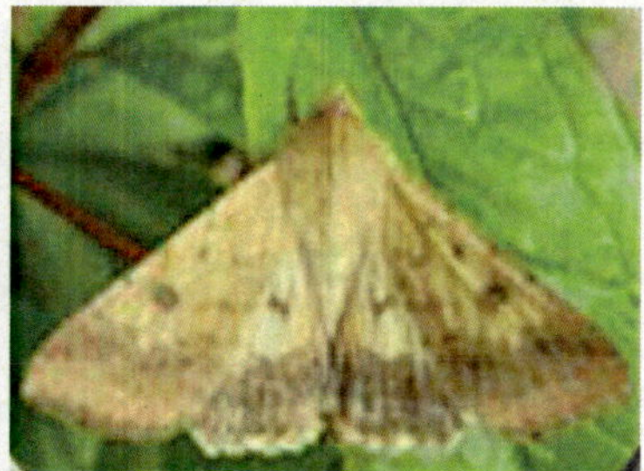

H. armigera - adult

Nature of damage and symptoms

- Early instar feeds on foliage
- Grown up larvae mainly bore into the fruits

Management

- Plough the soil to expose and kill pupae
- Collect and destroy the infected fruits and grownup larvae
- Chilli intercropped with marigold (trap crop) in the row proportion of 20:1, 18:1 or 16:1 was found effective (Shivarmu., 1999)

- Fruit borer populations can be effectively reduced by using organic amendments, such as vermicompost (2500 kg/ha) and neemcake (500 kg/ha) (Varma & Supare, 1997).
- Application of *Beauveria bassiana* @ 20g /L
- Spray HaNPV @ 1.5x10^{12} POB/ha in evening hour
- In case of severe infestation apply Chlorantraniliprole @ 3 mL/10L or spinosad 3.2 mL/10L or flubendiamide 2 mL/10L or cyantraniliprole @ 1.2 mL/L or emamectin benzoate 5SG @ 4 g/10L or indoxacarb 14.5 SC (Avaunth) @ 7 mL/10L

References

Mani, M., & Krishnamoorthy, A. (1994). Impact of the parasitoids on the suppression of greenpeach aphid, Myzus persicae (Sulz.) on chillies and sweet pepper in India. Journal of Biological Control, 8,81–84

Meena, U. P., Kulkarni, A. V., & Gavkare, O. (2012). Bioefficacy of flubendiamide 39.35% SC against chilli fruit borer (Spodoptera litura). Indian Journal of Plant Protection, 40(3),214–220

Murai T, Watanabe H, Foriumi W, Adati T, Okajima S (2009) Damage to vegetable crops by Thrips parvispinus Karny (Thysanoptera: Thripidae) and preliminary studies on biology and control. J Insect Sci 10 : 166

Nelson SJ and Natarajan S. Economic threshold level of thrips in semi-dry chilli. South Indian Horticulture. 1994; 42(5):336-338.

Reddy DNR, Puttaswamy. Pest infesting chilli (Capsicum annuum L.) in the nursery. Mysore. Journal of Agriculture Science. 1983; 17(3):122-125.

Shivarmu, K., 1999. Investigation on fruit borer, Helicoverpa armigera (Hubner) in chilli. Ph.D. Thesis, Univ.Agric.Sci., Dharwad, Karnataka, India (Cross ref.)

Tatagar, M. H., Kumar, H. D., Mesta, R. K., & Shivaprasad, M. (2014). Bioefficacy of newmolecule, Flubendiamide 24% + Thiacloprid 24%–48% SC against Chilli thrips, Scirtothrips dorsalis. Karnataka. Journal of Agricultural Sciences, 27(1), 25–27

Varma, N. R. G., & Supare, N. R. (1997). Effect of vermicompost in combination with FYM and chemical fertilizers against sucking pests of chilli. Andhra Agricultural Journal, 44, 186–187

Questions

1. _________feed on chili flowers resulting in pre-mature dropping of flowers and also cause bud necrosis

   a) *Scirtothrips dorsalis* b) *Helicoverpa armigera*

   c) *Spodoptera litura*

2. Muranai disease is caused by_________on chillies

   a) *Bemisia tabaci* b) *Polyphagotarsonemus latus*

   c) *Myzus persicae*

3. Name the predatory mite feeding on *Polyphagotarsonemus latus*

   a) *Aceria cajani* b) *Aceria sorghi*

   c) *Amblyseius ovalis*

4. Vectors of leaf curl disease of chilli

   a) *Bemisia tabaci* b) *Scirtothrips dorsalis*

   c) *Myzus persicae*

5. Upward leaf curl symptom in chilli is caused by

   a) *Polyphagotarsonemus latus* b) *Scirtothrips dorsalis*

   c) *Myzus persicae*

6. Downward leaf curl symptom in chilli is caused by

   a) *Polyphagotarsonemus latus* b) *Scirtothrips dorsalis*

   c) *Myzus persicae*

Answer Key

1	a	2	b	3	c	4	b	5	b	6	a		

9

Pests of Tomato

Sl No.	Common name	Scientific name	Family and Order
1	Fruit borer	*Helicoverpa armigera*	Noctuidae, Lepidoptera
2	Tomato pin worm	*Tuta absoluta*	Gelechidae, Lepidoptera
3	Serpentine leaf miner	*Liriomyza trifolii*	Agromyzidae, Diptera
4	Tobacco cutworm	*Spodoptera litura*	Noctuidae, Lepidoptera
5	Whitefly	*Bemisia tabaci*	Aleyrodidae, Hemiptera
6	Thrips	*Thrips tabaci*	Thripidae, Thysanoptera
7	Striped mealybug	*Ferrisia virgata*	Pseudococcidae, Hemiptera
8	Red spider mite	*Tetranychus* spp	Tetranychidae, Acarina

Fruit borer: *Helicoverpa armigera*, Noctuidae, Lepidoptera

Biology: The adult females are light pale brownish-yellow stout moths while the male moths are pale greenish with V-shaped speck. The eggs are creamy white and sculptured type. They are laid singly. The larva shows colour variation from greenish to brown. It has dark brown grey lines on the body with lateral white lines and also has a dark band. Pupation occurs in soil, leaf, fruit, and crop debris.

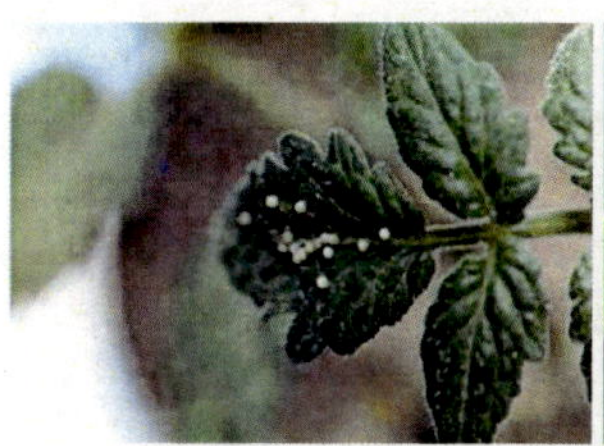
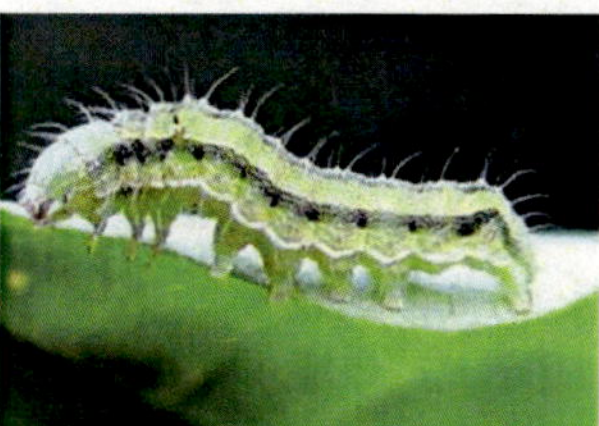
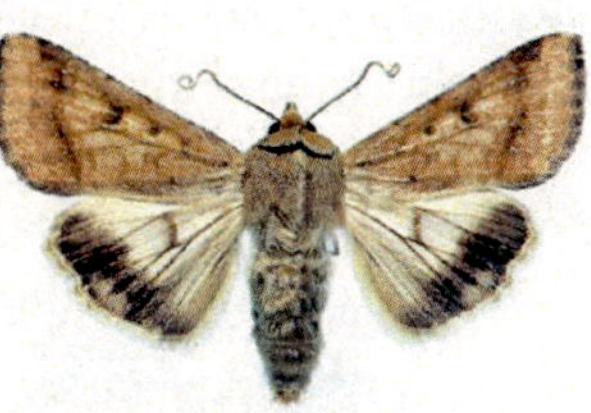

Nature of damage and symptoms

- The young larvae feed on tender foliage
- Mature larvae bore into fruit through circular holes
- Larva thrust only a part of its body into fruit and eat the inner content

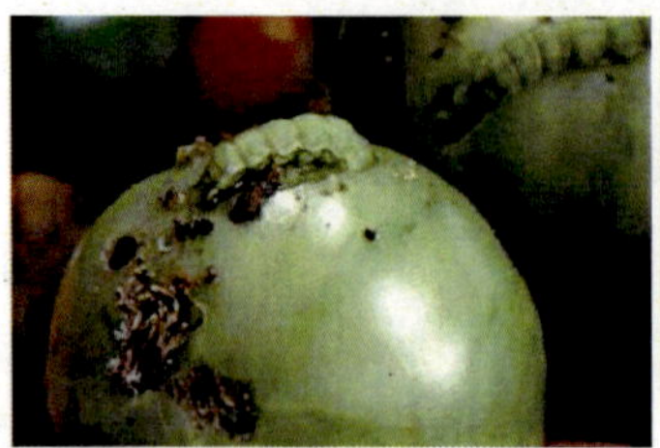
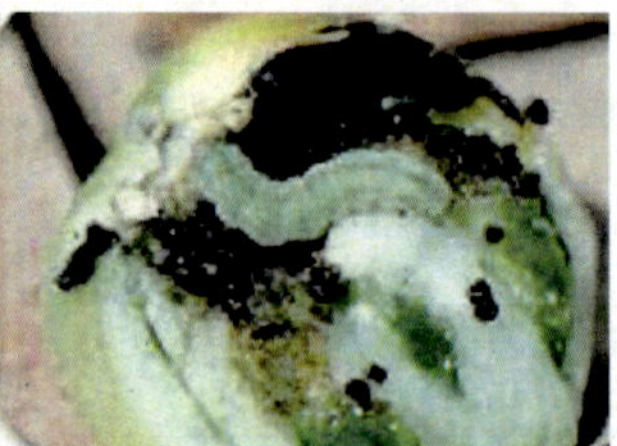

Symptoms on the fruit

Management

- Collect and destroy the infested fruits and grown up larvae
- Setup pheromone trap with Helilure at 12/ha
- Release *Trichogramma pretiosum* @ 1 lakh /ha/release at an interval of 7 days starting from flower initiation
- Spray HaNPV @ 1.5 x 10^{12} POBs/ha (Mohan *et al.*, 1996)
- Spray *Bacillus thuringiensis* 2g/L
- In case of severe infestation apply flubendiamide 2 mL/10L, chlorantraniliprole 3mL/10L, novaluron 10 EC 1.5mL/L

Tomato pin worm: *Tuta absoluta*, Gelechidae, Lepidoptera

Biology: Adult moths are 5-7 mm long and with a wingspan of 8-10 mm, with silverish- grey scales. Eggs are Small, cylindrical, creamy white to yellow, 0.35 mm long, and laid on the underside of leaves or stems. Hatching takes place after 4-6 days. The first-instar larvae are whitish soon after eclosion, becoming greenish or light pink in the second to fourth instars according to food. There are usually four instars. Larval period lasts 10–15 days. Pupation occurs inside mines or fruit. Pupae are obtect, with greenish coloration at first, turning chestnut brown and dark brown near adult emergence. Pupation takes place within 10 days. The total life cycle is completed in 30–40 days. There are up to 12 generations per year (Nayana & Kalleshwaraswamy, 2015).

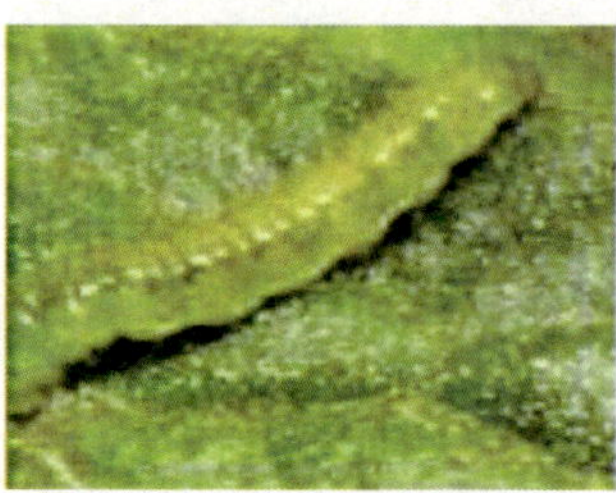
Larva

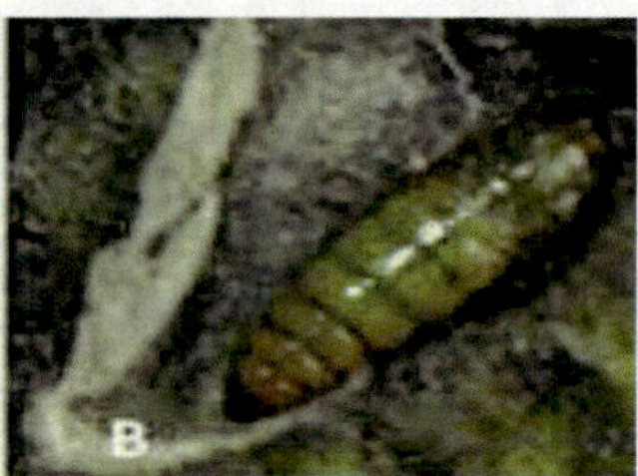

Pupa

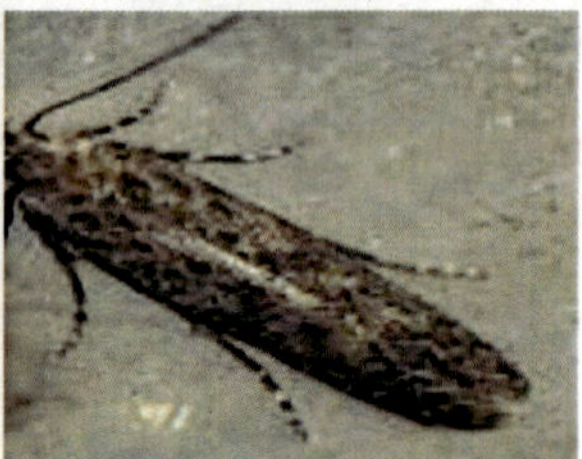
Adult

Nature of damage and symptoms

- Tomato plants can be attacked from seedlings to mature plants. This pest damage occurs throughout the entire growing cycle of tomatoes
- The larvae of *T. absoluta* mine the leaves producing large galleries and burrow into the fruit
- The larvae feed on mesophyll tissues and make irregular mines on the leaf surface
- Damage fruits by making pin holes and feeding within them
- Infestation found on apical buds, leaves, stems, flowers, and fruits also on which the black frass is visible

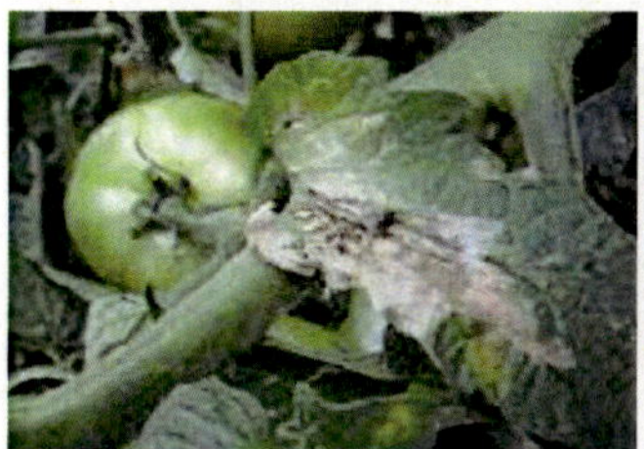 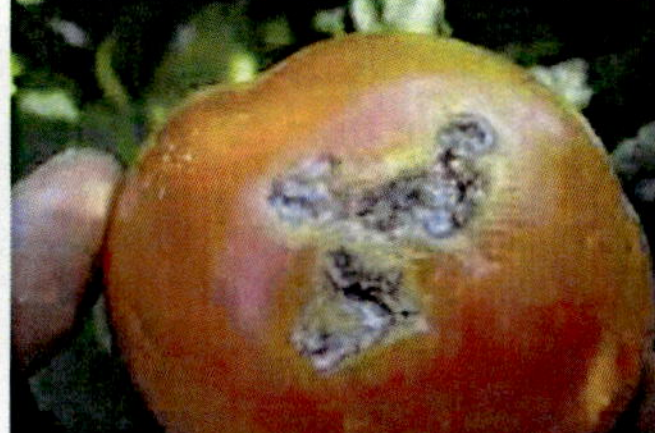 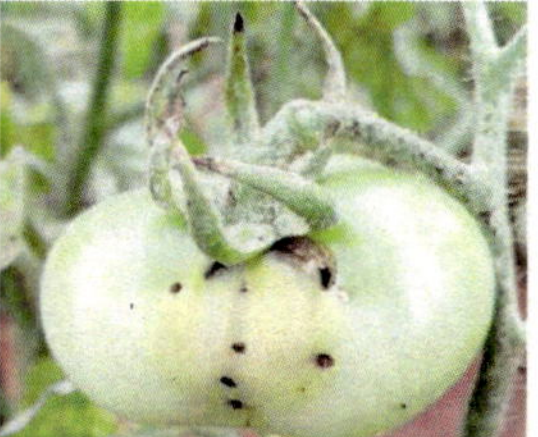

Symptoms on the leaf and fruit

Management

- Collection and destruction of affected plants and plant parts
- Apply NSKE 5% or neem oil 3%
- In case of severe infestation apply any of the insecticides *viz.* chlorantraniliprole 18.5% SC at 3 mL/10L or cyantraniliprole 10% OD at 1.2 mL/L or flubendiamide 480SC 2mL/10L or indoxacarb 14.5% SC at 1mL/L and Spinosad 45SC 3.3mL/L

Serpentine leaf miner: *Liriomyza trifolii,* Agromyzidae, Diptera

Biology: The adult insects are pale yellow in colour. Eggs are inserted into the epidermis of the under surface of the leaf. The egg period is two to three days. Maggots are minute orange, yellowish, and apodous. Pupation occurs within mines. The life cycle is completed within a period of 20-25 days.

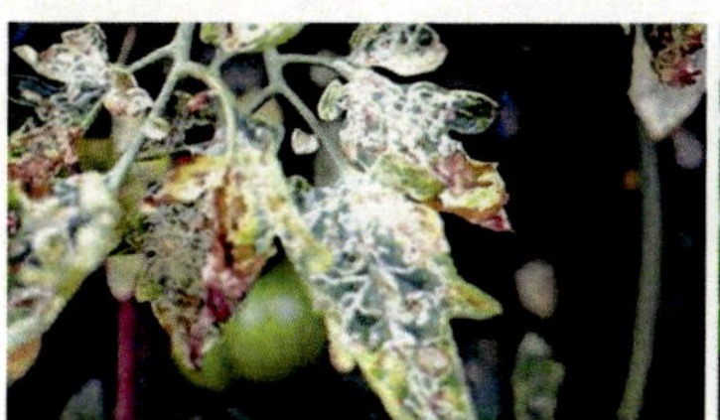 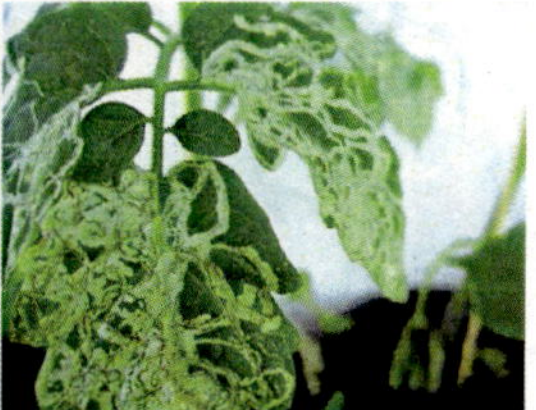

Symptoms on leaves

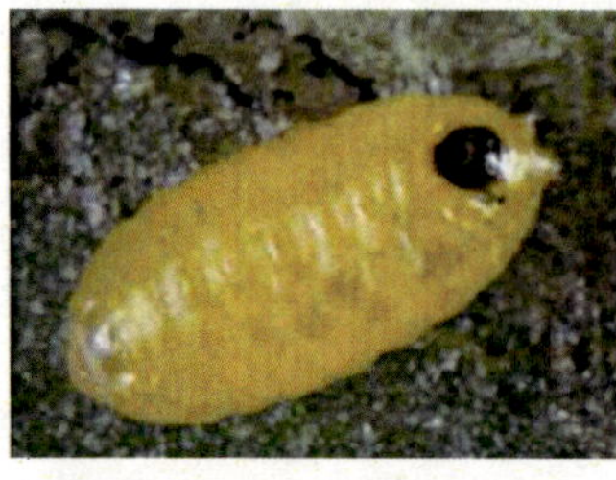
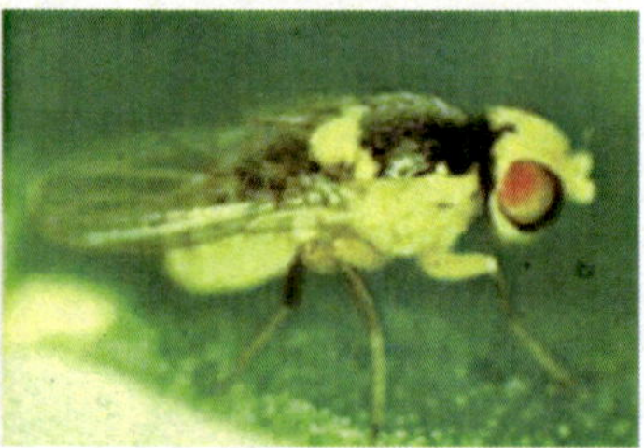

Pupa and adult *L.trifolii*

Nature of damage and symptoms

- Larva feeds on the mesophyll cells leading to the formation of serpentine mines
- Serpentine like mines on the leaves
- Continuous feeding leads to drying and drooping of leaves
- Severe infestation leads to drying of leaves

Management

- Collect and destroy mined leaves
- Spray NSKE 5% or neem formulations, azadirachtin 3000ppm@5mL/L
- Parasitism by the indigenous natural enemies goes upto 40% in India-*Hemiptarsenus varicornis* (Girault) (Shivalingaswamy *et al*., 2022)
- In case of severe infestation, apply fipronil 5SC 2mL/L or spinosad 45SC 3.3mL/10L

Tobacco cutworm: *Spodoptera litura,* Noctuidae, Lepidoptera

Biology: The adults are brown in colour, brown forewings with white wavy markings and white hindwings with brown patches along the margin. The golden yellow coloured eggs are laid in mass and covered with silky hairs. The caterpillars are light green with blackheads or black spots; they can be seen in groups feeding on the plant.

Nature of damage and symptoms

- The early instar caterpillars are gregarious and give the leaf lamina a papery white look by scraping out the chlorophyll content
- Later instars are voracious feeders and make irregular holes in leaves
- Severe feeding causes skeletonization until only veins and petioles remain
- Cause severe defoliation and irregularly shaped, bored fruits

Management

- Plough the soil to expose and kill pupae
- Collect and destroy the egg masses, gregarious larvae and grownup caterpillars
- Application of *Beauveria bassiana* @ 20g /l
- Spray SlNPV @ $1.5x10^{12}$ POB/ha in the evening hour
- In case of severe infestation apply Chlorantraniliprole @ 3 mL/10L or spinosad 3.3 mL/10L or flubendiamide 2 mL/10L or cyantraniliprole @ 1.2 mL/L or emamectin benzoate 5SG @ 4g/10L or indoxacarb 14.5 SC @ 1 mL/L

Whitefly: *Bemisia tabaci*, Aleyrodidae, Hemiptera

Biology: Adults are tiny, whitish moth-like covered with white waxy bloom. The eggs are pear shaped, light yellowish in colour. The egg period lasts for 5-8 days. The emerging nymphs are oval, scale-like, and greenish-white in colour. The life cycle is completed within 18-30 days.

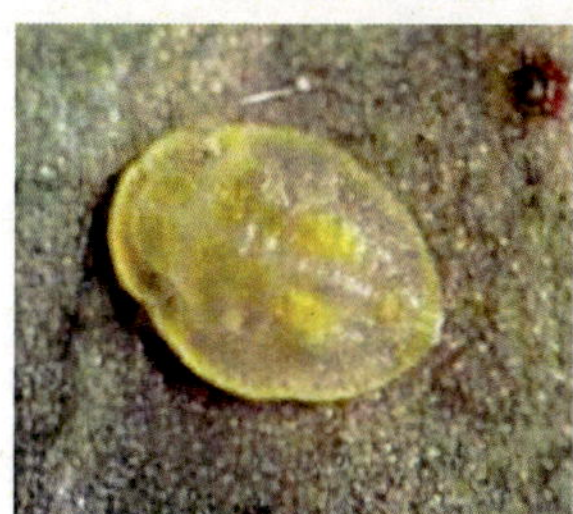

Nymph

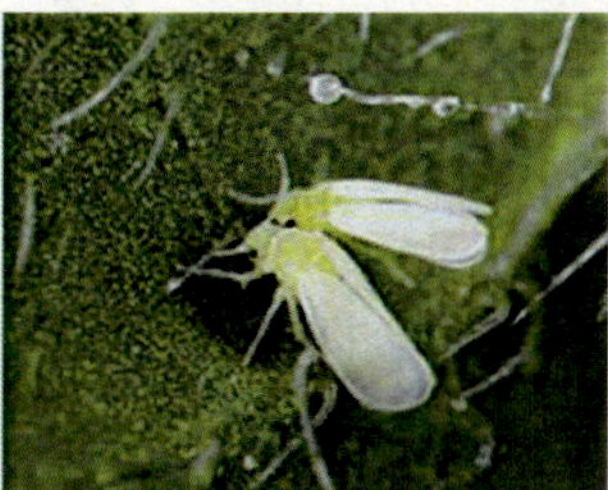

Adult

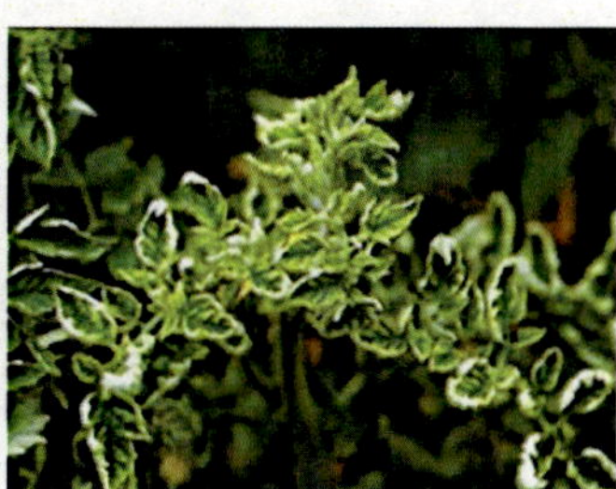

Tomato leaf curl virus infested plant

Nature of damage and symptoms

- The nymphs and adults suck sap from plants resulting in reduced vigour
- The honeydew excretion leads to the formation of sooty mould disease
- They are vectors of the leaf curl virus
- Affected plants will not form flowers

Management

- Uproot and destroy the diseased leaf curl plants
- Avoid excess application of nitrogen
- Remove alternate weed host *Abutilon indicum*
- Use yellow sticky traps at 12/ha to attract and kill insects
- In case of severe infestation apply imidacloprid17.8SL @ 3mL/10L or thiamethoxam 25WG@ 4g/10L

Thrips: *Thrips tabaci,* Thripidae, Thysanoptera

Biology: The adults are tiny dark coloured with fringed wings. The nymphs are yellowish.

Nature of damage and symptoms

- Feeding leads to silvery streaks on the leaf surface
- Cause pre-mature dropping of flowers
- Bud necrosis
- They are also vector of the tomato spotted wilt virus

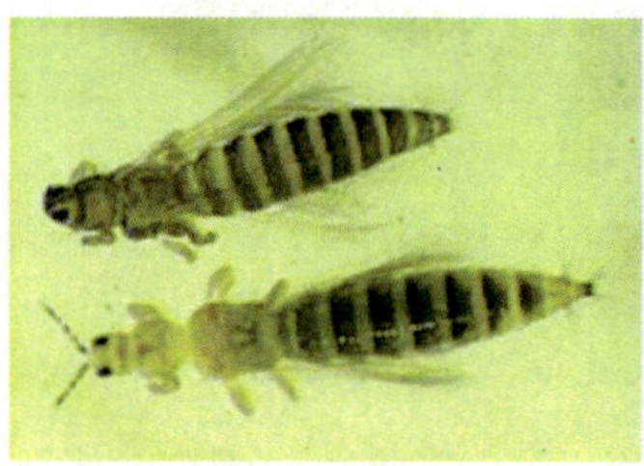

T.tabaci – adults

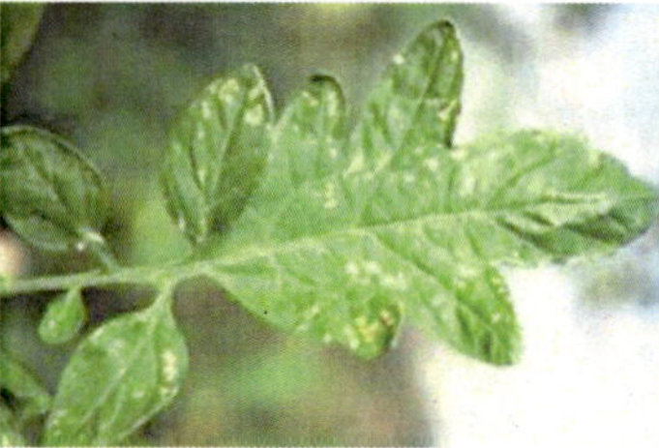

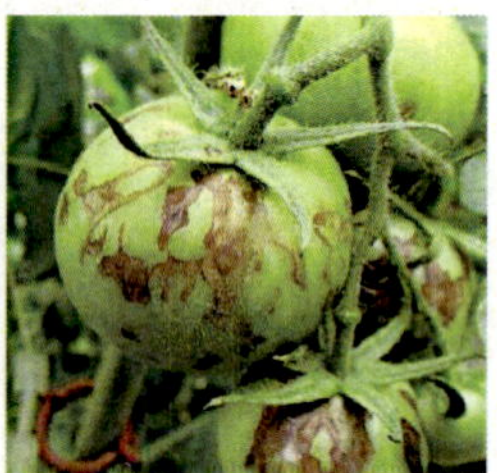

Symptoms on leaf and fruit

Management

- Release larvae of *Chrysoperla zastrowii* @ 10,000/ ha
- Spray dimethoate 30 EC @ 1.5 mL/L or spinosad @ 3.2 mL/10L or spiromesifen @ 8 mL/10L or fipronil 5 SC @ 2 mL/L

1. Striped mealybug: *Ferrisia virgata,* Pseudococcidae, Hemiptera

Biology: Females are apterous, long, slender, and covered with white waxy secretion, while the crawlers are yellowish to pale white.

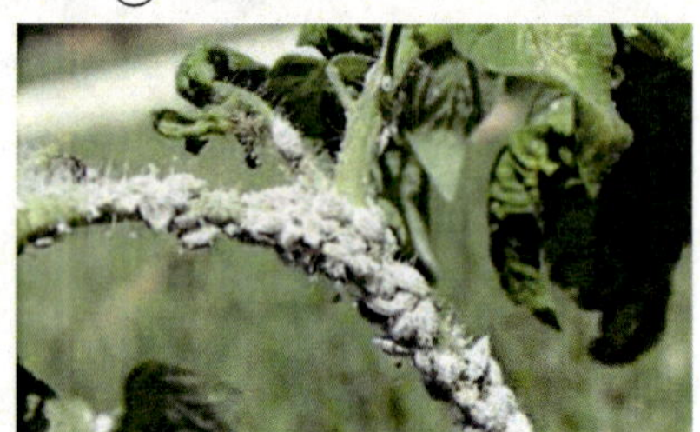

Mealybugs on tomato plant

Nature of damage and symptoms

- Presence of white, cottony mealy bugs on the leaves and twigs
- Continuous feeding leads to stunted growth
- Honeydew excretion favours growth of sooty mould fungus

Management

- Spray neem oil emulsion 2%
- Spray *Lecanicillium lecanii* @ 20g/L and repeat the application at 15 days interval
- Spray imidacloprid 0.005% @ 3 mL/10Lor thiamethoxam @ 2g/10L

2. Red spider mite, *Tetranychus* spp, Tetranychidae, Acarina

Biology: The adult mites are tiny red coloured ones. The globular eggs are laid in mass. The emerging nymphs are yellowish in colour. Nymphs seen in silken webbing on the leaves

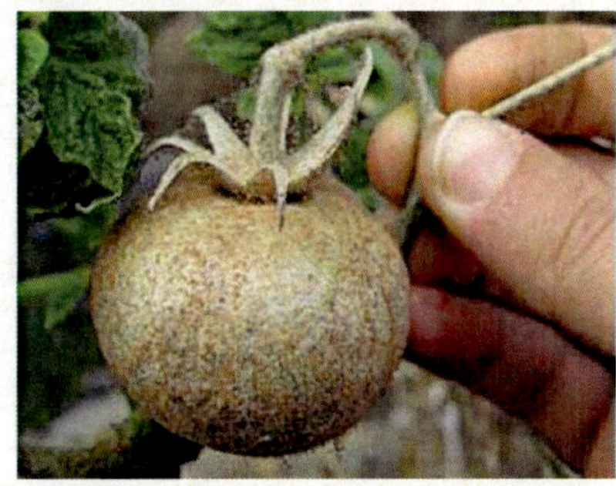
Mite infested fruit

Nature of damage and symptoms

- Affected leaves become reddish brown and bronzy
- Later affected leaves wither and dry
- Flower and fruit formation are affected

Management

Spray dicofol 18.5 EC 2.5 mL/L or wettable sulphur 50 WP 3g/L or Fenazaquin 2.5 mL/L

References

Shivalingaswamy, T.M., Udayakumar, A. and Mani, M., 2022. Pests and their management in chillies and bell pepper. Trends in Horticultural Entomology, pp.971-982.

Mohan, K. S., Asokan, R., & Gopalkrishnan, C. (1996). Isolation and field application of a nuclearpolyhedrosis virus for the control of fruit borer, Helicoverpa armigera (Hub.) on tomato. Pest Management in Horticultural Ecosystems, 2,1–8.

Nayana, B. P., & Kalleshwaraswamy, C. M. (2015). Biology and external morphology of invasivetomato leaf miner, Tuta absoluta (Meyrick) (Lepidoptera: Gelechiidae). Pest Management in Horticultural Ecosystems, 21(2), 169–174

Questions

1. Presence of circular holes and larva feeding by thrusting only a part of its body into tomato fruit is symptom of

   a) *Helicoverpa armigera* b) *Tuta absoluta*

   c) *Spodoptera litura*

2. Vector of tomato leaf curl virus

   a) *Bemisia tabaci* b) *Thrips tabaci*

   c) *Liriomyza trifolii*

3. Vector of tomato spotted wilt virus

   a) *Bemisia tabaci* b) *Thrips tabaci*

   c) *Liriomyza trifolii*

Answer Key

1	a	2	a	3	b

10

Pests of Potato

Introduction

Potato is a tuber crop belonging to the Family solanaceae. In India large number of insects are attacking potato both in field as well as storage thereby causing both direct and indirect losses to farmers.

Distribution

Potatoes are cultivated in almost all states of India, but the majority of the crop is grown in the Indo-Gangetic plains of North India. The major potato growing states are Uttar Pradesh, West Bengal, Punjab, Bihar, and Karnataka (Rana and Anwer, 2018).

Major pest

S. No.	Common name	Scientific name	Family	Order
1.	Green peach aphid	*Myzus persicae*	Aphididae	Hemiptera
2.	Potato aphid	*Macrosiphum euphorbiae*	Aphididae	Hemiptera
3.	Colorado potato beetle	*Leptinotarsa decemlineata*	Chrysomelidae	Coleoptera
4.	Potato tuber moth	*Gnorimoschema (Phthorimaea) operculella*	Gelechidae	Lepidoptera
5.	Cutworms	*Agrotis ipsilon* *A. segetum, A. nigrum*	Noctuidae	Lepidoptera
6.	White grubs	*Holotrichia* spp. *Melolontha* spp. *Brahmina* spp.	Scarabaeidae	Coleoptera
7.	Leaf hopper	*Empoasca kerri E. fabae* *Amrasca biguttula biguttula*	Cicadellidae	Hemiptera

Aphids

Green peach aphid - *Myzus persicae* (Hemiptera: Aphididae)

Potato aphid - *Macrosiphum euphorbiae* (Hemiptera: Aphididae)

Distribution

Most potato cultivating fields of North India

Host plants: Carrot, broccoli, cabbage, mustard, radish, cucumber, pepper, wheat, rice (Holman, 2009).

Symptoms of damage

- Nymphs and adults suck sap causing reduction in photosynthetic area (Ali *et al.*, 2023)
- Malformation of infested plant parts
- Leaf curling and stunted growth
- Honeydew secretion and development of sooty mould on leaves (Heuvel and peters, 1990)
- Chlorosis and necrosis seen in infested plants
- Wilting and defoliation of plants
- Vector of Potato Leafroll Virus and Potato Virus Y (Eigenbrode *et al.*, 2002).

Biology: Green peach aphid - *Myzus persicae*

Egg: Yellowish to green, elliptical in shape and laid on leaves

Nymph: Initially greenish but turn yellowish green with 4 nymphal instars (Ali *et al.*, 2023)

Adult: Black head and thorax with yellowish green abdomen (Alate forms) Pale green abdomen is seen in wingless forms

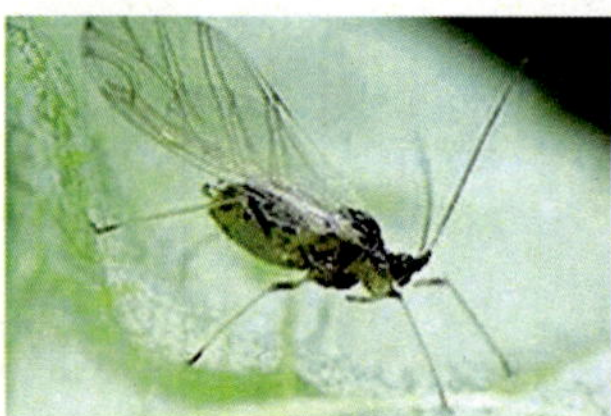

Winged adult - *M.persicae*

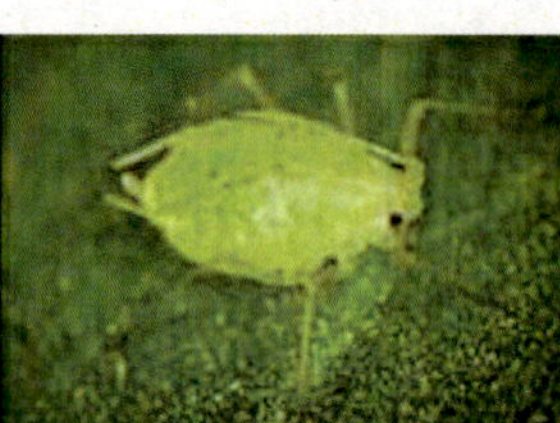

Wingless adult - *M.persicae*

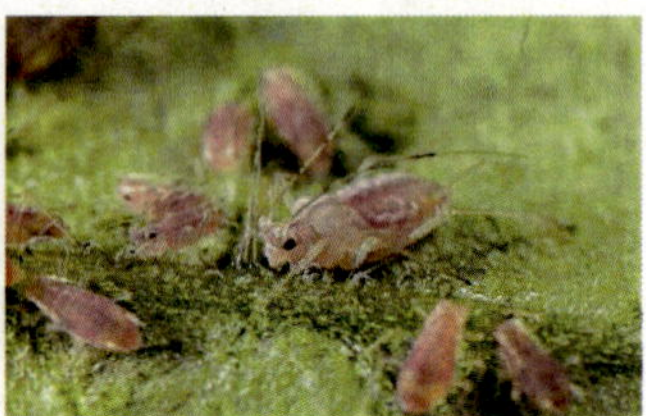

M.euphorbiae - Nymphs

Potato aphid: *Macrosiphum euphorbiae*

Egg: Overwintering of eggs is seen (Cloutier *et al.*, 1981) Nymphs: Longitudinal black stripe is seen in greenish abdomen

Adult: Greenish or occasionally pinkish coloured abdomen with pear shaped body in wingless forms. Winged forms are pinkish in colour

Management

- Removal of alternate host plants like nightshade
- Avoid monocropping of potato especially during winter season
- Conservation of predators and parasitoids
- Application of neem leaf extract or azadirachtin 1%

Colorado potato beetle: *Leptinotarsa decemlineata* (Coleoptera: Chrysomelidae).

There are currently no reports of the Colorado potato beetle, *L.decemlineata*, being introduced in India. However, because of its destructive tendency, particularly on potatoes (*Solanum tuberosum*) and other solanaceous crops like tomato and brinjal, it is regarded as a high-risk quarantine pest in India. Although it originated in North America, it has since expanded to Asia and Europe. Indian officials are careful to prevent its entry due to its strong potential for invasion and resistance to numerous pesticides.

Distribution: Europe, Central Asia, Asia minor, Iran, Western China, North America, and Africa (Vincent *et al.*, 2013)

Host plants: Tomato, brinjal, and other wild solanaceous Family members (Vincent *et al.*, 2013)

Symptoms of damage

- Larva and adult feed on leaves and causes complete defoliation of plants
- Reduced tuber yield due to defoliation
- Adult beetles also feed on exposed tubers and stem which result in yield loss (Balasko *et al.,* 2020)

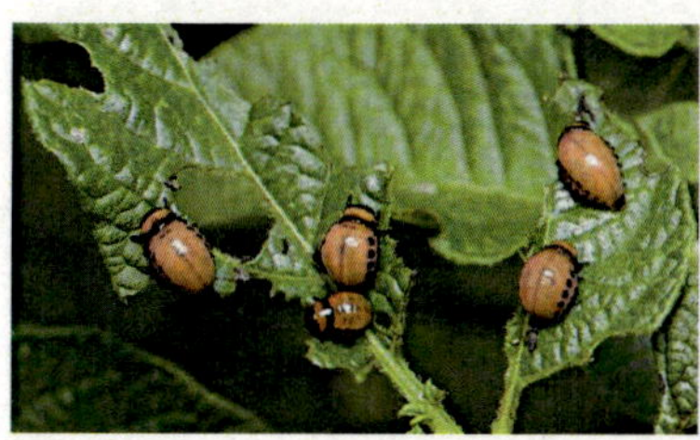

Adults feeding on leaves

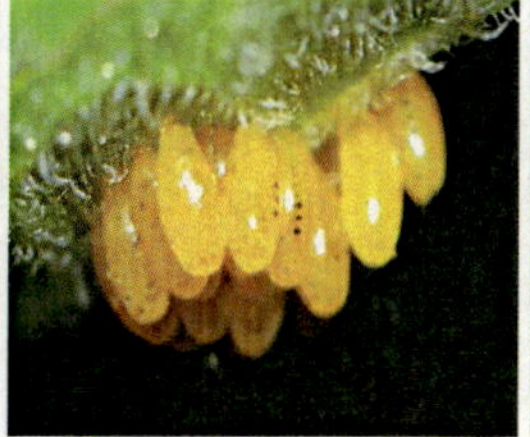

Eggs

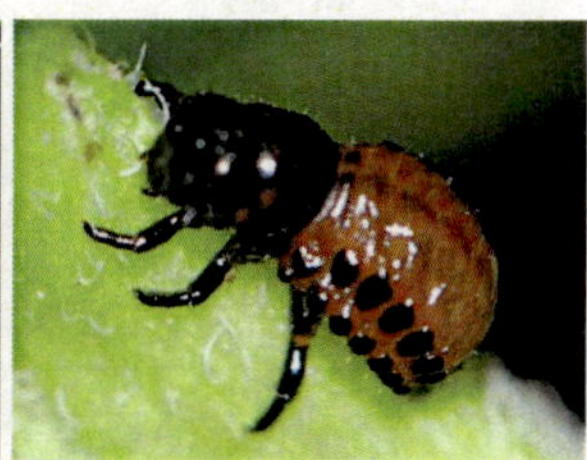

Grub

Biology: Eggs are bright orange in colour and ovalshaped laid in clusters on the undersurface of leaves.

Larva: Eruciform larva, reddish orange colour with 2 rows of black spots on either side. Four grub stages are seen

Pupa: Pupation takes place in soil at a depth of 5-8 cm (Aloykhin *et al.*, 2013)

Adult: Adults are pale yellow in colour, oval shaped with black stripes on elytra and, head and pronotum with black spots. Adults undergo diapause during winter season

Management

- Crop rotation with non-host plants reduces pest incidence
- Collection and destruction of early instar larvae
- Digging trenches between field to reduce population immigration
- Mulching with straw reduces population of larva in small fields

Potato tuber moth – *Gnorimoschema (Phthorimaea) operculella* (Lepidoptera: Gelechidae)

Distribution: Africa, Asia, Europe, North and South America.

Host range: Potato, tomato, eggplant, pepper, tobacco and wild solanaceous plants including Jimson weed and datura (Adhikari *et al.,* 2022).

Symptoms of damage

Damage is caused in both field and storage

- Larva mines the leaf and feed within (Adhikari *et al.,* 2022)
- Tunneling of stem and petiole is also seen which results in wilting and death of plants (Adhikari *et al.,* 2022)

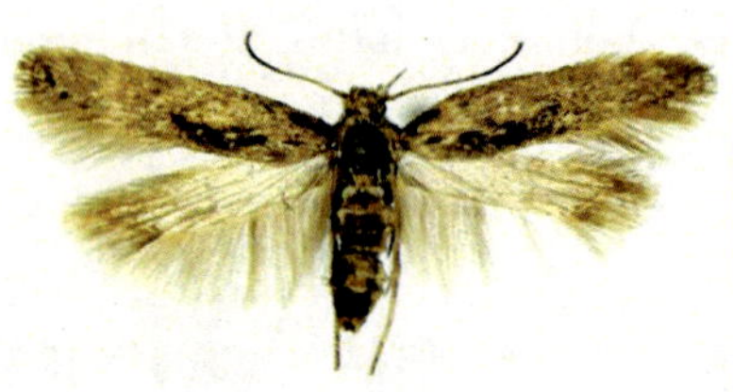

Adult – moth

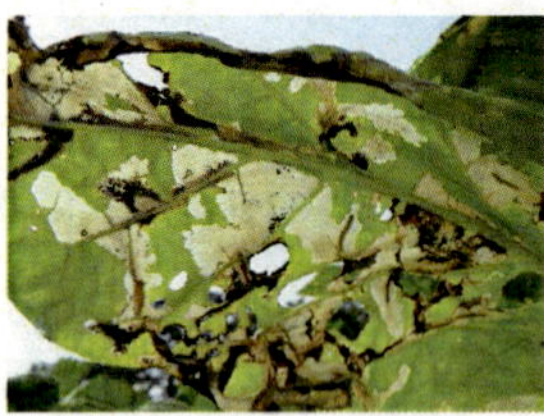

Mining in leaves

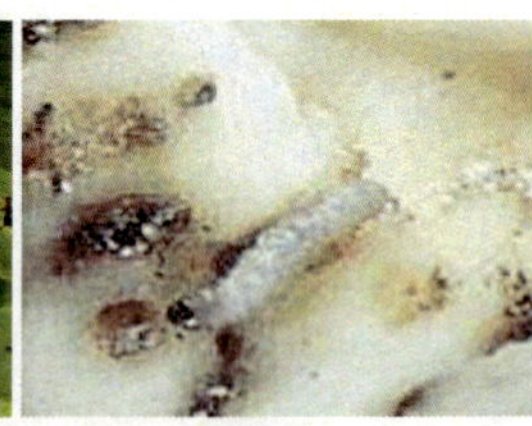

Galleries in tubers

- In storage, larva bore into the tubers causing galleries and tunnels which results in losses both qualitatively and quantitatively (Adhikari *et al.,* 2022).
- The injuries also cause secondary infections of fungus like *Erwinia* sp. (Adhikari *et al.,* 2022).

Biology

Egg: Adults lay eggs in lower side of leaves, exposed tubers or soil near tubers Eggs are transparent, round, white to yellowish brown in colour (Adhikari *et al.,* 2022)

Larva: Larvae are pale white with brownish head

Pupa: Pupation occurs in silken cocoon in dead potato leaves or soil or tubers

Adult: Tiny moth with both pair of wings having fringed borders and black markings on forewings. Male moths with 2-3 black spots on forewings and females with X shaped marking on forewings (Adhikari *et al.,* 2022)

Management

- Use healthy tubers for sowing
- Avoid shallow planting of tubers
- Crop rotation with non-host crops
- Harvest potatoes as soon as crop reaches maturity
- Avoid leaving harvested potatoes in field over night as they serve as potential egg laying site
- Cover the potato tubers with dried and crushed leaves of *Eupatorium* to repel ovipositing moths (Adhikari *et al.,* 2022)
- Release egg larval parasitoid *Chelonus blackburnii* @ 30000/ ha twice at 40 and 70 days after planting
- Spray NSKE 5% or quinalphos 20 EC 2 ml/l to control the foliar damage

Cutworms: *Agrotis ipsilon, A. segetum, A. nigrum* (Lepidoptera: Noctuidae)
Distribution: India, China, Northern Europe, Canada, Japan, New Zealand.

Host range: Most vegetable crops along with other species like alfalfa, clover, cotton, rice, sorghum, tobacco and strawberry (Joshi *et al*., 2020).

Symptoms of damage

- Early stage larva feeds on leaves causing small holes
- Larva cut germinating seedlings which result in gaps in field
- Matured larvae entirely cut plants or tunnel into the stem of the plants
- Infested fields have grazed appearance (Joshi *et al*., 2020)

Biology

Egg: Eggs are spherical shaped, whitish brown colour and laid on foliage in clusters

Larva: Grayish black colour larva with brown head and dark spots over the body. Larva are nocturnal and feed during night time (Joshi *et al*., 2020).

Pupa: Pupation occurs below the soil

Adult: Adult moths are large in size with wingspan of 40 to 55 mm. Forewings are uniformly dark brown with distal area having bean-shaped spot

Hind wings are whitish gray in colour (Joshi *et al*., 2020)

Management

- Deep summer ploughing to expose pupa to hot sun and natural enemies
- Avoid growing tomato or okra in nearby fields
- Early sowing in last week of October
- Handpicking and destruction of larvae
- Conserve *Braconids, Microgaster sp., Bracon kitcheneri,* parasitoids in the field
- Broadcast chlorpyrifos 20% EC treated sand (3 L / 10 kg sand) @ 10 kg treated sand per ha in field before planting
- Spray quinalphos 25 EC @ 1000 mL / ha (Joshi *et al*., 2020)

White grubs: *Holotrichia* spp., *Melolontha* spp., *Brahmina* Spp. (Coleoptera: Scarabaeidae)

Distribution: Cosmopolitan in distribution all over the world

Host range: Ground nut, pearl millet, sorghum, cowpea, soybean, cluster bean, ginger *etc*. (Chandel *et al.,* 2017).

Symptoms of damage

- Young grubs feed on mother tubers and roots of developing plants causing wilting and dying of young seedlings
- Later stage grubs feed on tubers making large, shallow and irregular holes making them unfit for marketing
- Tuber damage often exceeds 50% in endemic areas (Chandel *et al.,* 2017)

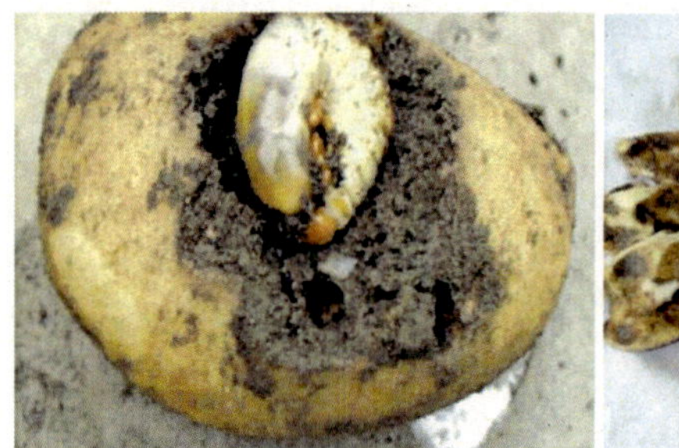

Grub of *Melolontha indica*

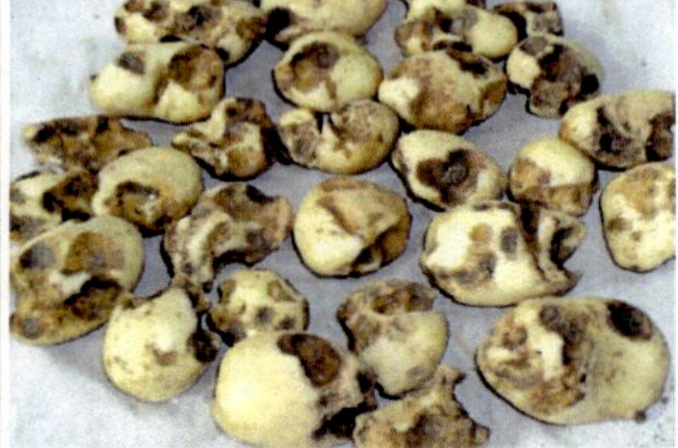

Tuber damage

Biology

Egg: Egg period 9-11 days. 20 to 30 eggs are laid by a single female in soil.

Grub: 3 larval instars with a grub period of 9-10 months. Characteristic C shaped larva which are creamy white in colour

Pupa: Pupates inside soil in cocoon with a pupal period of 15 – 21 days

Adult: Adult emergence in first week of July. Adults are shiny brown beetles (Chandel *et al.,* 2017)

Management

- Summer ploughing for exposing larva and pupa to sunlight
- Application of well decomposed organic manure reduces the incidence of pest
- Combining *Beauveria bassiana / Metarhizium anisoplae* in farm yard manure can effectively reduce infestation
- Cadavers of *Galleria mellonella* infected with *Heterorhabditis indica* can be applied at a ratio of 1: 7 (Cadaver: Plant).
- Soil drenching with chlorpyriphos causes mortality of eggs and grubs in endemic regions
- earthing up provides effective control (Chandel *et al.,* 2017)

Leaf hopper: *Empoasca kerri, E. fabae, Amrasca biguttula biguttula* (Hemiptera: Cicadellidae)

Distribution: North America, Egypt, Central Asia, Southern Europe, India.

Host range: Alfalfa, Soybean, Clover, Apple, Beans, Ground nut, and most pulse crops (Chasen *et al.,* 2014)

Symptoms of damage

- Adults and nymphs suck sap from underside of leaves
- Brown triangular lesions are seen on the leaves (Hopper burn system)
- Late instar nymphs cause more yield loss than adults
- Yield loss is more severe when the plants are in early tuber bulking stage
- Stunted growth and crinkling of leaves is seen
- Vector of Potato Yellow Dwarf Virus and Beet Curly Top Virus (Munyaneza and Henne, 2013)

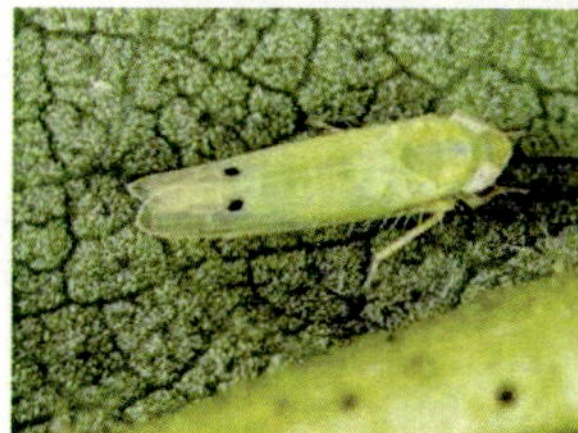

A. biguttula biguttula

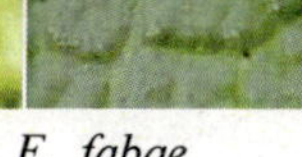

E. fabae

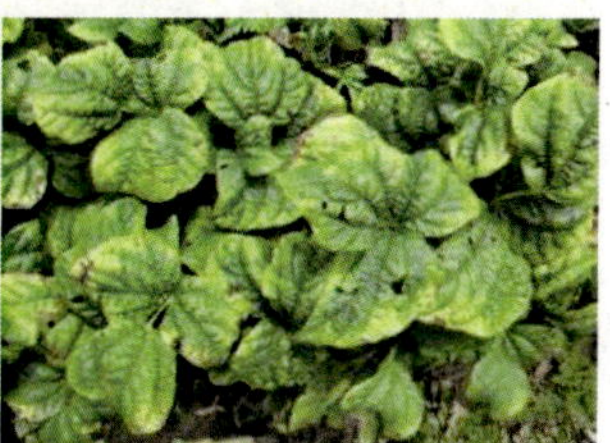

Marginal yellowin crinkling of leaves

Biology

Eggs: Pear shaped yellowish white in colour and laid on leaves at 15 to 30 eggs per female. Egg period is 4-10 days

Nymphs: 7 to 21 days of nymphal period with whitish green nymphs.

Adults are pale green in colour with black dot on posterior portion of forewing. Adults live for about 2 weeks (Munyaneza and Henne, 2013)

Eggs: Transparent to pale yellow in colour and laid on veins and petioles of leaves at 200 to 300 eggs per female. Egg period is around 10 days

Nymphs: 15 days of nymphal period with whitish green nymphs

Adults are pale green in colour and live for about 30 – 60 days (Munyaneza and Henne, 2013)

Management

- Crop rotation with non-host plants
- Maintain proper plant spacing
- Avoid use of excessive fertilisers especially nitrogenous fertilisers
- Application of insecticides, imidacloprid 17.8SL@3mL/10L or thiame thoxam 25WG@2g/10L at the appearance of insects

References

Adhikari, A., Oli, D., Pokhrel, A., Dhungana, B., Paudel, B., Pandit, S., and Dhakal, A. 2022. A review on the biology and management of potato tuber moth. Agriculture (pol'nohospodarstvo), 68(3): 97-109.

Ali, J., Bayram, A., Mukarram, M., Zhou, F., Karim, M. F., Hafez, M. M. A., ... and Shamsi, I. H. 2023. Peach–Potato Aphid Myzus persicae: Current Management Strategies, Challenges, and Proposed Solutions. Sustainability, 15(14): 11150.

Alyokhin, A., Udalov, M., and Benkovskaya, G. 2013. Potatoes and their Pests Setting the Stage In: Giordanengo, P., Alyokhin, A., and Vincent, C. (eds.). Insect Pests of Potato Global Perspectives on Biology and Management Academic Publishers Oxford UK. 11-29.

Balasko, M. K., Mikac, K. M., Bazok, R., and Lemic, D. 2020. Modern techniques in Colorado po[ta]to beetle (Leptinotarsa decemlineata Say) control and resistance management: History review and future perspectives. Insects, 11(9): 581.

Chandel, R. S., Vashisth, S., and Verm, K. S. 2017. Whitegrubs in Potato and their control. In: Handbook of Agriculture (6th Ed.). ICAR, New Delhi, pp: 40 – 43

Chasen, M. E., Dietrich, C., Backus, E. A., and Cullen, E. M. 2014. Potato leafhopper (Hemiptera: Cicadellidae) ecology and integrated pest management focused on alfalfa. Journal of integrated pest management, 5(1).

Cloutier, C., McNeil, J. N., and Regniere, J. 1981. Fecundity, longevity, and sex ratio of Aphidius nigripes (Hymenoptera: Aphididae) parasitizing different stages of its host, Macrosiphum euphorbiae (Homoptera: Aphididae). The Canadian Entomologist, 113(3): 193-198.

Eigenbrode, S. D., Ding, H., Shiel, P., and Berger, P. H. 2002. Volatiles from potato plants infected with potato leafroll virus attract and arrest the virus vector, Myzus persicae (Homoptera: Aphididae). Proceedings of the Royal Society of London. Series B: Biological Sciences, 269(1490): 455-460.

Heuvel, J. V. D., and Peters, D. 1990. Transmission of potato leafroll virus in relation to the honeydew excretion of Myzus persicae. Annals of applied biology, 116(3): 493-502.

Joshi, M. J., V, P. R., Solanki, C. B., and V, B. V. 2020. Potato cutworm, Agrotis ipsilon: An overview and their management. Agriculture and food, 2(5): 188 – 191

Munyaneza, J. E. and Henne, D. C. 2013. Leafhopper and Psyllid Pests of Potato. In: Giordanengo, P., Vincent, C., and Alyokhin, A. (eds.), Insect Pests of Potato (1st Ed.). Elsevier, Amsterdam, pp. 11-30

Rana, R. K., and Anwer, M. D. 2018. Potato production scenario and analysis of its total factor productivity in India. Indian Journal of Agricultural Sciences, 88(9): 1354-61.

Vincent, C., Alyokhin, A., and Giordanengo, P. 2013. Potatoes and their Pests Setting the Stage In: Giordanengo, P., Alyokhin, A., and Vincent, C. (eds.). Insect Pests of Potato Global Perspectives on Biology and Management Academic Publishers Oxford UK. 5-8.

Questions

1. Which of the following is a major defoliating pest of potato in temperate regions?
   a) *Leptinotarsa decemlineata* b) *Helicoverpa armigera*
   c) *Phthorimaea operculella* d) *Myzus persicae*
2. The scientific name of the potato tuber moth is:
   a) *Phthorimaea operculella* b) *Agrotis ipsilon*
   c) *Tuta absoluta* d) *Leucinodes orbonalis*
3. Which pest causes mining of potato leaves and damage to tubers in storage?
   a) *Spodoptera litura* b) *Phthorimaea operculella*
   c) *Myzus persicae* d) *Bemisia tabaci*
4. Which insect pest of potato acts as a vector of Potato leafroll virus?
   a) *Empoasca kerri* b) *Phthorimaea operculella*
   c) *Myzus persicae* d) *Leptinotarsa decemlineata*
5. Which of the following pests is not directly associated with potato?
   a) *Leptinotarsa decemlineata* b) *Phthorimaea operculella*
   c) *Bactrocera cucurbitae* d) *Myzus persicae*
6. **Assertion (A):** *Phthorimaea operculella* is a major pest of potato in both field and storage.

   Reason (R): The larvae of *Phthorimaea operculella* mine into the tubers and foliage.

   a) Both A and R are true, and R is the correct explanation of A.
   b) Both A and R are true, but R is not the correct explanation of A.
   c) A is true, but R is false.
   d) A is false, but R is true.
7. **Assertion (A):** *Myzus persicae* transmits potato viruses like PLRV and PVY.

   Reason (R): *Myzus persicae* has chewing mouthparts.

   a) Both A and R are true, and R is the correct explanation of A.
   b) Both A and R are true, but R is not the correct explanation of A.
   c) A is true, but R is false.
   d) A is false, but R is true.

8. **Assertion (A):** *Leptinotarsa decemlineata* is a major threat to Indian potato crops.

   Reason (R): It is an endemic pest in Indian potato fields.

   a) Both A and R are true, and R is the correct explanation of A.

   b) Both A and R are true, but R is not the correct explanation of A.

   c) A is true, but R is false.

   d) A is false, but R is true.

9. **Assertion (A):** Aphids infest potato plants mainly during early stages of crop growth.

   Reason (R): Young potato leaves are soft and rich in nutrients.

   a) Both A and R are true, and R is the correct explanation of A.

   b) Both A and R are true, but R is not the correct explanation of A.

   c) A is true, but R is false.

   d) A is false, but R is true.

Answer Key

1	a	2	a	3	b	4	c	5	c	6	a	7	c
8	c	9	a										

Pests of Spices

11

Pests of Black Pepper

Black pepper, popularly known as the "King of spices", is the most popular spice crop in the world, and the crop originated in the Western Ghats and Malabar coast of India. India was the centre of pepper trade from time immemorial. Recently, black pepper production in the country remained stagnant at around 90000 tonnes in the last few years. Hence, India is losing its status as a leading producer and exporter of black pepper. Kerala accounts for 75 per cent of total black pepper production in the country. It has been noted that the increase in area under cultivation is not in tune with the increase in production. Low productivity is mainly due to the incidence of pests and diseases.

Black pepper is infested by 56 species of insects in India; among these, pollu beetle, (*Lanka ramakrishnae* Prathapan & Viraktamath), top shoot borer (*Cydia hemidoxa* Meyr), scale insects (*Lepidosaphes piperis* and *Aspidiotus destructor*) are considered as major pests (Devasahayam, 2000).

Sl. No.	Common name	Scientific name	Family and Order	Site of oviposition	Site of pupation
		Borers			
1	Pollu beetle	*Lanka ramakrishnae*	Chrysomelidae Coleoptera	tender berries and shoots	Soil
2	Topshoot borer	*Cydia hemidoxa/ Laspeyresia hemidoxa*	Eucosmidae, Lepidoptera	tender terminal shoots	Inside shoot
		Sucking pests			
3	Scales	Mussel scale (*Lepidosaphes piperis* and coconut scale *Aspidiotus destructor* Soft scale *Marsipococcus marsupial and Lecanium* sp	Diaspididae, Hemiptera Coccidae, Hemiptera		
4	Marginal gall thrips	*Liothrips karnyii*	Thripidae Thysanoptera		

Major pests

Pollu beetle : *Lanka ramakrishnae* Pratapan & Viraktamath

Family : Chrysomelidae

Order : Coleoptera

It is one of the most destructive pests of black pepper and the infestation is severe in plains of Malabar region (20-30 %) and low in hilly tracts (Wayanad and Idukki) and South Kerala.

Distribution: Tamil Nadu, Karnataka and Kerala.

Host plants: Castor, turmeric, guava, mulberry, *etc.*

Biology: The adult flea beetle is bluish yellow with stout hind legs. On the delicate berries or the developing shoots, the female beetle scoopes out tiny holes, depositing one or two eggs in each. Egg period lasts for 5-8 days and the larval phase completes within 30-32 days. Pupation takes place in soil in an earthen shell. Period of pupation lasts for 6-7 days.

Nature of damage and symptoms

Damage is caused by both adults and grubs. Adult beetles feed on the tender plant parts such as shoots, leaves and spikes. Beetles scrape the plant tissues and feed on them, resulting in sunken black patches. Besides feeding injuries, adult females are also causing indirect damage by laying eggs on the rind of berries in shallow elliptical holes made by scraping the tissues. The feeding activity of adults results in small, irregular, circular holes on leaves. Grubs also cause severe damage by boring into the tender berries and feeding on the internal contents (Verma *et al.*, 2023).

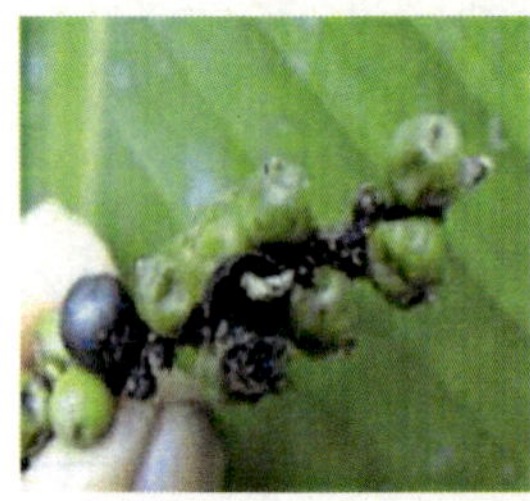

Grubs feeding on berries

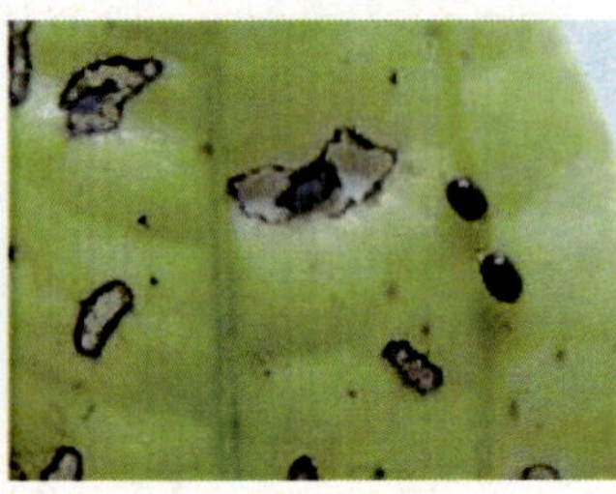

Symptoms on leaf -adult

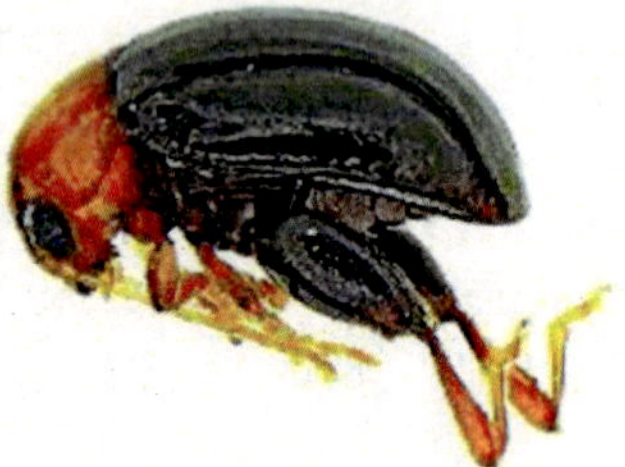

L. ramakrishnae

Appearance of holes and black patches on leaves and shoots of new flushes. Drying of tender spikes, partially or wholly and later turn dark coloured. Dropping of dried spikes also occurs.

On emergence, the grubs bore into the berries, feed on their internal contents, and hollow them. The infested berries turn yellow initially and later black and crumble when pressed, hence the name pollu beetle. Usually, the entire distal portion of the spike dries up. The infested shoots and spikes turn black and drop (Prathapan, 2015).

The pest population is more severe in shaded areas. Vines trailed on standards producing heavy shade result in more severe infestation. The adult population was higher during July – January and May—September, coinciding with the monsoon showers.

Management

- Shade regulation should be practiced in plantations with heavy shade
- Entomopathogenic fungus, *Beauveria bassiana* spraying should be done @ 20g/L at 15day intervals, starting from the onset of monsoon
- Spray neem garlic emulsion 2% as three sprays at spike emergence, berry formation and berry maturation stage
- Spraying quinalphos @.05% during July and October will reduce the infestation
- Spraying with cypermethrin 10 EC @ 1 mL/L twice, once at berry formation stage and the second at one month after the first spray
- Thorough coverage should be ensured while spraying, under surface of leaves as well as the spikes are to be sprayed thoroughly

Top shoot borer : *Cydia hemidoxa* Mayrick/ *Laspeyresia hemidoxa*

Family : Eucosmidae

Order : Lepidoptera

Young plantations (up to 2 to 3 years old) are more susceptible to the infestation of the top shoot borer. It is widely distributed in plains and higher altitudes in Kerala. In case of severe infestation, cent per cent infestation of young shoots has been recorded in some places.

Nature of damage and symptoms

The caterpillars infest young, tender orthotropic shoots, especially those that adhere to the standards. The neonates scrape and feed on the epidermis of the tender terminal shoots and sometimes on tender leaves. The matured larvae bore into the tender shoots and feed on their internal contents, resulting in decay and drying of the infested shoots.

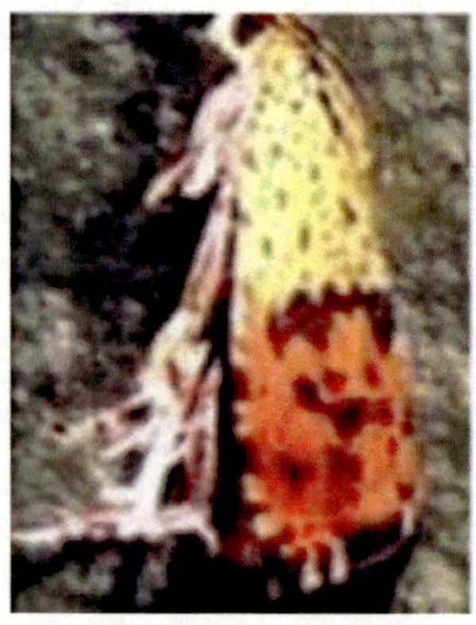

C. hemidoxa

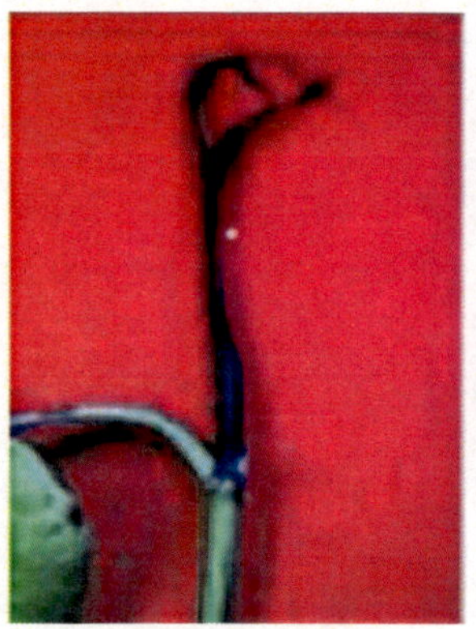

Infested terminal shoot

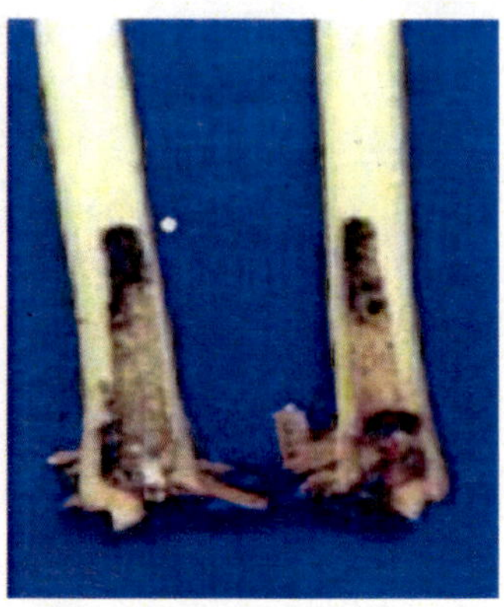

Tunneling made by larva

Decaying the terminal shots followed by drying will induce auxiliary bud formation, and the pest will also infest those shoots. Repeated infestation of the tender terminal shoots affects the growth and establishment of the vine, resulting in stunted growth (Devasahayam, 2000).

Pest infestation is observed in the field throughout the year and the peak infestation is observed during the monsoon period (August-December) coinciding with the active growth of vines and new succulent shoots formed.

Management

- NSKE 5% spray during the initial periods
- *Beauveria bassiana* spray @ 20g/mL at 15 day intervals starting from the monsoon period onwards
- In case of severe infestation, dimethoate 30 EC (@ 1.5 mL/L should be sprayed on the tender shoots and new flushes

Scale insects – Mussel scale (*Lepidosaphes piperis* Gr.) and coconut scale (*Aspidiotus destructor*) belongs to the family Diapididae and soft scales (*Marsipococcus marsupial* and *Lecanium* sp.) belonging to Coccidae family.

Incidence of scale insects are more severe in higher altitudes. Three different species of scale insects are more common in Idukki district, the black pepper mussel scale infest all parts of vines, coconut scale suck sap from the under surface of leaves and soft scale *Marsipococcus marsupiale* confine to the upper leaf surface. Another soft scale, *Lecanium* sp. is, occasionally observed to infest both the foliage and vines at higher altitudes. Among all these, infestation by mussel scales causes significant yield loss as it infests all parts of the plants, including berries (Devasahayam and Koya, 1994).

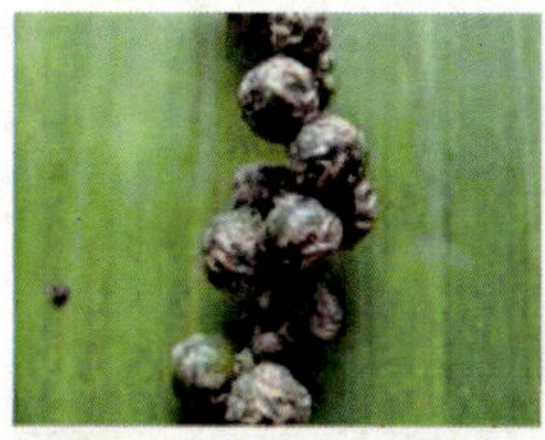
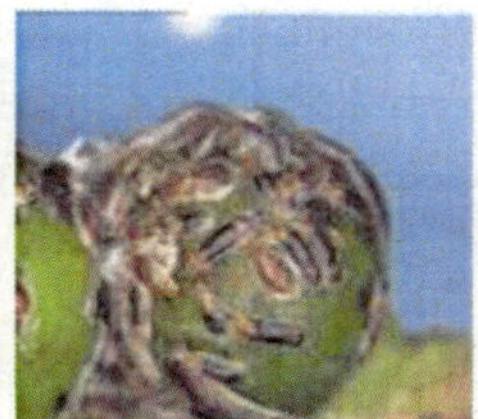
L. piperis infesting berries

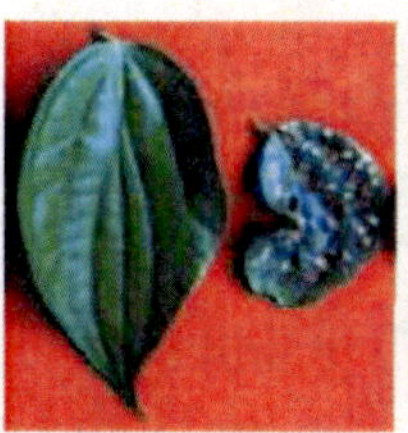
M. marsupiale

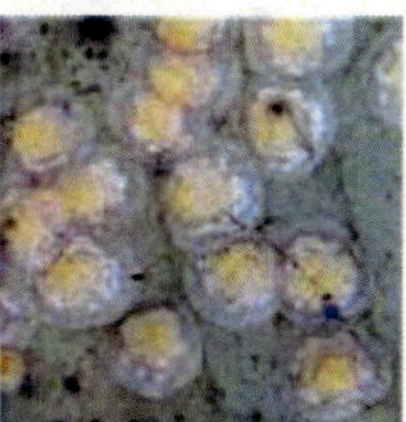
A. destructor

Nature of damage and symptoms

- Mussel scales encrust the main stem of young vines and lateral branches, mature leaves, spikes and berries.
- The infestation results in chlorotic spots / patches, yellowing and necrosis of leaves due to desapping
- Young vines succumb to the infestation where as older infested lateral branches wilt and dry in patches
- Infestation by mussel which is specific to black pepper causes significant loss in production as it affects all parts of the plant including berries
- Coconut scales infest on undersurface of leaves and very rarely on other parts.
- The pest infestation leads to chlorotic streaks on the upper surface of leaves.
- Soft scales are confined on the upper leaf surface and vines at high altitudes.
- Vines become sick and drying of vines occurs in case of severe infestation

Management

- Prune the infested plant parts and destroy them to reduce the population
- During the initial period of infestation, two sprays of azadirachtin 5000 ppm @ 1 mL/L at fortnightly intervals reduce the scale attack
- Black pepper mussel scale can be effectively controlled by two sprays of dimethoate 0.05% @ 1.5 mL/L at fortnightly intervals
- Thiamethoxam 25WG @ 2g/10L- two sprays at an interval of 15 days, was also found to reduce the infestation
- Soft scale, *Lecanium* sp. can be controlled by spraying 0.05% quinalphos @ 2 mL/L

Leaf gall thrips : *Liothrips karnyi* Bagn.

Family : Thripidae

Order : Thysanoptera

Leaf gall thrips are persistent pests of black pepper, more severe on younger vines at high range situations. In plains, this pest is very common in nurseries. Severe infestations of this pest have been reported from the South Wayanad region.

Nature of damage and symptoms

Leaf gall thrips initially infest the tender leaves and make the leaf margins curl downwards and inwards, forming tubular galls. Both nymphs and adults lacerate the plant tissues and suck the exuding sap. As the infested vines grow, the infested parts become crinkled, malformed and reduced in size. Pest infestation is more severe on younger vines (Dhanush and Patil, 2021).

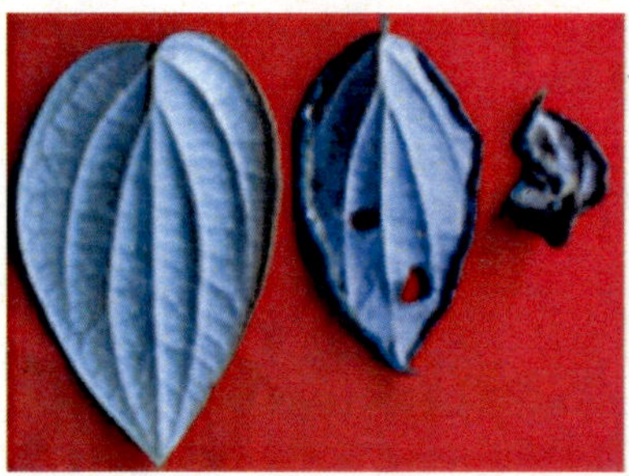

Healthy leaf and thrips infested leaves

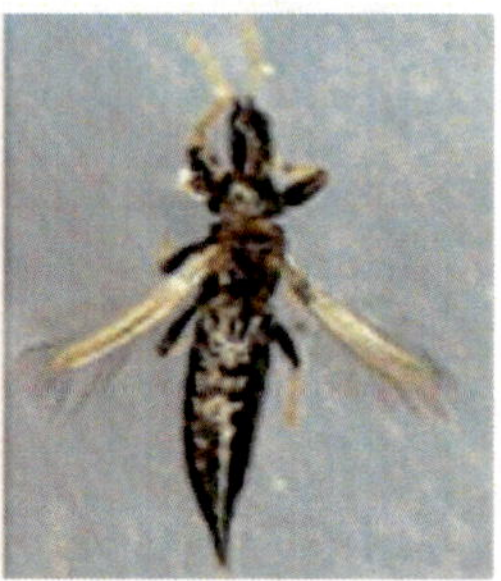

L. karnyi

A number of predators have been reported against this pest. Among the different predators, *Montandonia moraguesi* (Puton) (Anthocoridae) and *Andothrips flavipes* Schmutz (Phleothripidae) play an important role in regulating the pest. In case of severe infestation dimethoate 0.05% @ 1.5 mL/L can be sprayed to reduce the infestation.

Mealy bugs

Several species of mealy bugs have been identified in black pepper.

Against foliage infesting mealy bugs, *viz.*, *Ferrisia virgata, Planococcus* spp., application of the Entomopathogenic fungus (EPF), *Lecanicillium lecanii* @ 20 g/L is found to be effective. If the infestation is severe, the insecticides imidacloprid @ 3 mL/10L or thiamethoxam @ 2g/10L can be sprayed to reduce the infestation. Root mealy bugs such as *Planococcus* sp., *Dysmicoccus brevipes* , *Formicoccus polysperes, Xenococcus annandalei* and *Pseudococcus* sp. are causing more severe yield loss since they attack the roots, resulting in wilting, yellowing and complete drying of the infested vines. Infestation is more severe during the post-monsoon period.

Management

Against root mealy bugs, Soil drenching is recommended with the EPF, *Lecanicillium lecanii* @ 20 g/L. This has to be repeated at intervals of 15 days. In case of severe infestation, soil drenching with chlorpyrifos @ 2.5 mL/L is recommended to reduce the infestation and after 30 days of insecticidal application, soil drenching with *Lecanicillium lecanii* @ 20 g/L has to be done and this has to be continued for prolonged control (Ummer and Kurien, 2021).

References

Devasahayam, S. 2000. Insect pests of black pepper. In: Ravindran, P.,N. (ed.) Black pepper, CRC Press, 336-362.

Devasahayam, S., & Koya, K. A. 1994. Field evaluation of insecticides for the control of mussel scale (Lepidosaphes piperis Gr.) on black pepper (Piper nigrum L.). Journal of Entomological Research 18 (3): 213-215.

Dhanush, M., and Patil, R. S. 2021. Field evaluation of insecticides and biopesticidesfor the control of marginal gall thrips, Liothrips karnyi (Bagnall) on Black pepper. Journal of Farm Sciences, 34(02), 220-222.

Prathapan, K. D. 2015. The case of pollu beetle in the Andaman Islands. Indian Journal of Entomology, 77(1), 71-75.

Ummer, N., and Kurien, S. 2021. Management of root mealybug in black pepper (Piper nigrum). Journal of Krishi Vigyan, 10(1), 157-163.

Verma, R., Gupta, P. K., & Kaur, M. (2023). Black pepper: diseases and pests.In: Pests and disease management of horticultural crops, New Delhi: Biotech Books, pp. 199-208.

Questions

1. Which of the following is the most serious pest of black pepper under shaded condition

   a) *Laspersia hemidoxa* b) *Longitarsus nigripennis*

   c) *Liothrips karnyi* d) *Myzus persicae*

2. The pest that bores into berries of black pepper causing 'Pollu' or hollow berries is:

   a) *Ferrisia virgata* b) *Longitarsus nigripennis*

   c) *Laspersia hemidoxa* d) *Liothrips karnyi*

3. *Top shoot borer* of black pepper is:

   a) *Cydia hemidoxa* b) *Dasynus piperis*

   c) *Cydia pomonella* d) *Dasychira mendosa*

4. Sucking pest of black pepper that forms a hard encrustation on the vines, berries and leaves of black pepper causing severe yield loss is

   a) *Pollu beetle* b) *Aspidiotus destructor*

   c) *Dasynus piperis* d) *Lepidosaphes piperis*

5. Population of ....scale insects seen on the upper leaf surface in black pepper

   a) *Lecanicillium* sp. b) *Coccus viridis*

   c) *Marsupicoccus marsupiale* d) *Aspidiotus* destructor

6. **Assertion (A):** The pollu beetle is a serious pest of black pepper causing economic loss.

   Reason (R): The grubs feed on berries causing yield loss

   a) Both A and R are true, and R is the correct explanation of A.

   b) Both A and R are true, but R is not the correct explanation of A.

   c) A is true, but R is false.

   d) A is false, but R is true.

7. **Assertion (A):** Shade lopping is recommended to manage Pepper polu beetle

   Reason (R): Shaded condition favours mass multiplication of polu beetle.

   a) Both A and R are true, and R is the correct explanation of A.

   b) Both A and R are true, but R is not the correct explanation of A.

   c) A is true, but R is false.

   d) A is false, but R is true.

8. **Assertion (A):** Scale insects are rarely seen in black pepper plantations.

   Reason (R): They are controlled effectively by natural enemies and oils.

   a) Both A and R are true, and R is the correct explanation of A.

   b) Both A and R are true, but R is not the correct explanation of A.

   c) A is false, but R is true.

   d) Both A and R are false.

Answer Key

1		2		3		4		5		6		7	
8													

12

Pests of Cardamom

Cardamom, often called the "Queen of Spices", is one of the most valuable and aromatic spices in the world. It belongs to the family Zingiberaceae and the genus Elettaria. Cardamom, which is indigenous to South India's Western Ghats, is grown for its tiny, fragrant, green pods that contain tiny seeds that are used in cosmetics, medicine, and cooking. Kerala, Karnataka, and Tamil Nadu are the main cardamom-growing states in India, which ranks among the world's top producers. The crop grows best in shady regions with evenly distributed rainfall, rich forest soils, and humid, tropical weather.

Sl. No.	Common name	Scientific name	Family and Order	Site of oviposition	Site of pupation
		Borers			
1	Shoot and capsule borer	*Conogethus punctiferalis/ Conogethus sahyadriensis*	Crambidae Lepidoptera	Tender plant parts	Shoot
2	Thrips	*Sciothrips cardamomi*	Thripidae, Thysanoptera	Plant tissues	In soil/plant debris
3	Root grub	*Basilepta fulvicorne*	Chrysomelidae Coleoptera	Soil	Soil
4	Redhairy caterpillars	*Euproctis lutifacia* *E. cardamom* *Eupterote spp.*	Erebidae Eupterotidae Lepidoptera	On the leaves of shade trees	Soil
		Sucking pests			
5	Whitefly	*Kanakarajiella (Dialeurodes) cardamomi*	Aleurodidae, Hemiptera		
6	Marginal gall thrips	*Liothrips karnyii*	Thripidae Thysanoptera		
7	Lacewing bug	*Stephanitis typicus*	Tingidae, Hemiptera		
8	Scales	*Aulacaspis elettaria*	Diaspididae, Hemiptera		
9	Mealybugs	*Xenococcus annandalei*	Pseudococcidae Hemiptera		
10	Red spider mites	*Tetranychus urticae*	Tetranychidae	Leaf tissues	

Shoot and capsule borer	:	*Conogethes punctiferalis* Guenee *Conogethes sahyadriensis*
Order	:	Lepidoptera
Family	:	Crambidae

Introduction

Shoot and capsule borer is a significant pest that infests a wide variety of wild and cultivated plants. Since larvae directly affect the reproductive plant parts, this pest becomes more significant in tropical and subtropical nations. Yellow peach moth, cardamom, or castor shoot and capsule borer are other names for the shoot and capsule borer (Thyagaraj, 2003).

Distribution: Tamil Nadu, Karnataka and Kerala. A serious pest of the nursery in cardamom

Host plants: Castor, turmeric, guava, mulberry, *etc.*

Biology: Adult moth lays eggs singly or in groups on delicate plant parts. Egg is oval, flat and pink in color. The egg period ranges from six to seven days. Larva is long and covered with tiny hairs that grow on warts. The larval head and pro- thoracic shield are brown in color. The larval period is about fifteen to eighteen days. The larva pupates in the larval tunnel made on the plant parts within the silken cocoon. The pupal period is seven to ten days. The adult is a medium- sized yellow moth with a number of minute black dots on its wings. They are about an inch long with a wingspan of about 1.5 inches. The life cycle lasts for three to thirty-five days (Doddabasappa *et al*., 2014).

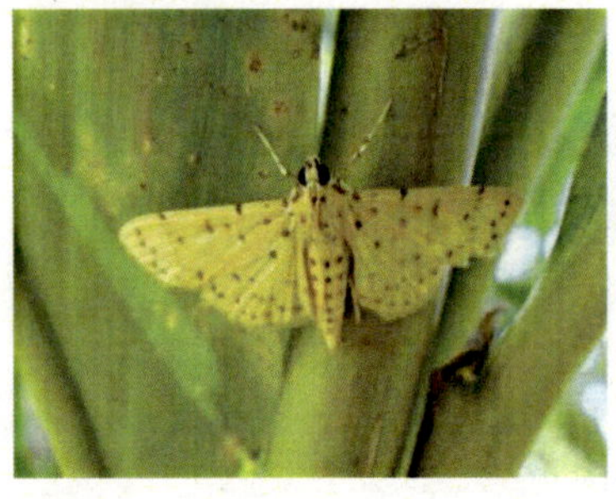

Adult

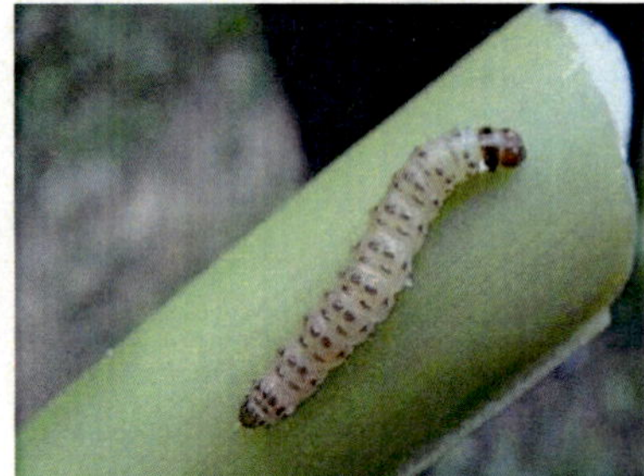

Larva

Nature of damage and symptoms

- Early stage of the larva bores the unopened leaf buds and feeds on the leaf tissue.
- Consume young seeds within immature capsules, leaving the capsules empty.

- At the early stage of the crop, caterpillars bore into the pseudostem, resulting in the death of the central spindle. This symptom is known as 'dead heart'.
- At the time of flowering, the caterpillars attack the panicles and spikes leading to flower shedding and drying of the affected portion.
- At later stage of the crop, they bore into young green pods, feed on tender seeds, and make them hollow.
- Oozing out of frass material at the point of tunnelling is an indication of the presence of larvae inside the plant parts.
- The incidence of this pest is noticed throughout the year but the pest attack is more severe during January- February, June, and September-October
- Pest abundance synchronizes with panicle production, fruit formation, and new tiller production.

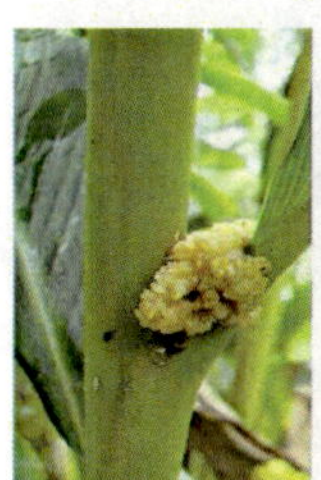
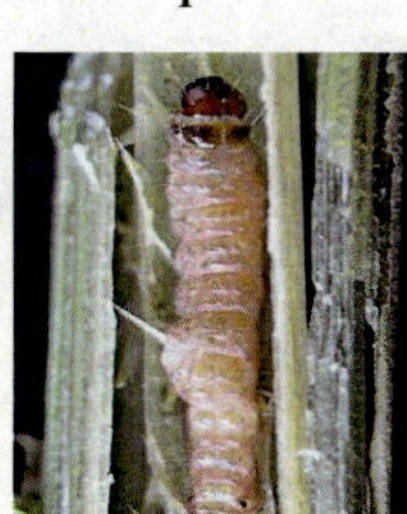
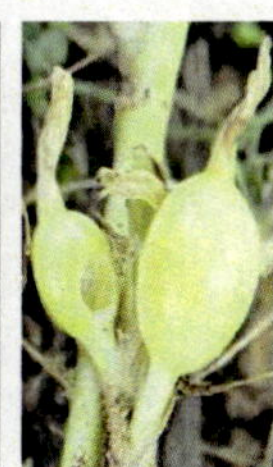
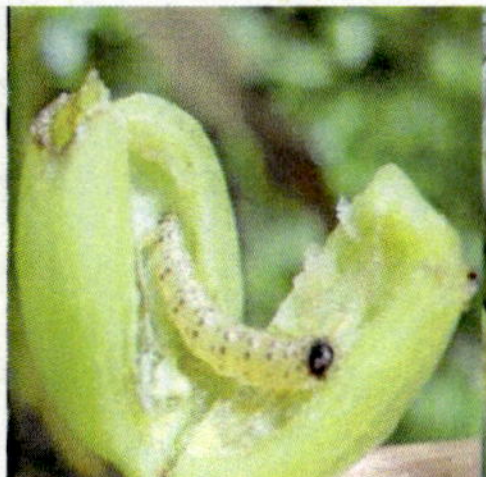
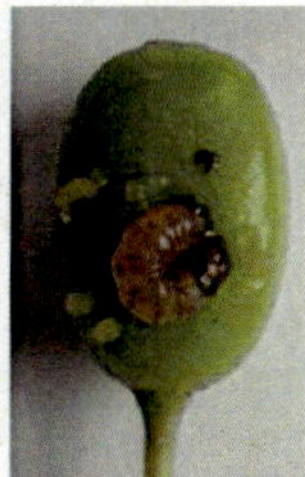

Symptoms on shoot and capsule

Integrated pest management

- Avoid excess use of fertilizers
- Remove alternate host plants (Castor, Ginger,Turmeric) from the field
- Discarding tillers showing 'dead heart' symptoms
- Trashing (removal of old and infested tillers) should be practiced twice a year
- At severe infestation-spray dimethoate 30 EC (1.5 mL/L)/ quinalphos 25 EC (2 mL/L)/ spinosad 45SC (3.5 mL/10 L)/ chlorantranilprole 18.5 SC (3mL/ 10 L)/ flubendiamide 39.35 SC (1 mL/10 L/ diafenthiuron (8 g/10 L)
- For effective management, the insecticides have to be targeted on early stages of the larvae, which are usually present within 15-20 days after adult emergence in the field.

Cardamom thrips : *Sciothrips cardamomi* Ramk.

Order : Thysanoptera

Family : Thripidae

Distribution: India and Papua New Guinea. Most destructive pest of cardamom in South India

Host range: Cardamom, tea, grapevine, castor, cotton *Prosopis juliflora*, ginger and turmeric.

Biology: The adult thrips have two pairs of fringed wings, are 1.25 to 1.5 mm in length, and are greyish brown in color. Females lay their eggs singly in incisions made on plant tissue. Eggs are kidney-shaped. After 12 days, the eggs hatch, and the larvae appear. The first two nymphal instars are active while the pre-pupae and pupae are inactive. They complete their life cycle in 21–32 days (Singh *et al.*, 1999).

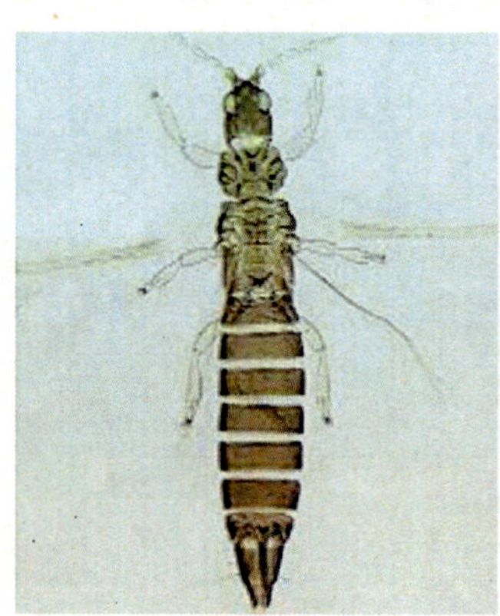

Adult – *S. cardamom*

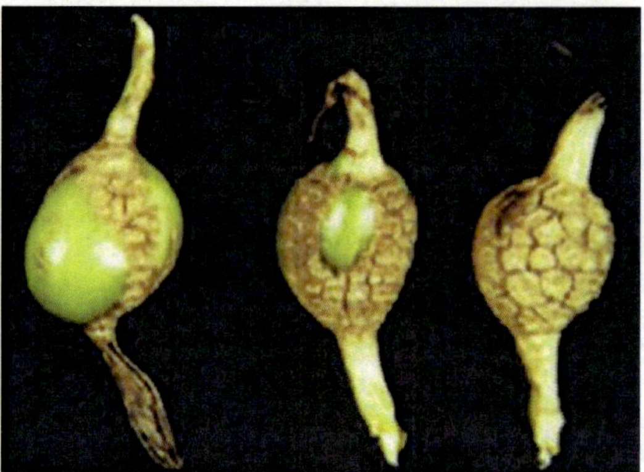

Thrips infestation on capsules

Nature of damage and symptoms

- Capsules: Warty/corky encrustations (scabs). Under sized, under weighed, malformed and shrivelled capsules. – "itch capsules"
- The seeds of the affected pods are underdeveloped and without the normal aroma.
- Both quantity and quality of the pods are affected

Integrated pest management

- Regulate shade (60-70% shade should be maintained)
- Severity of infestation - less in Malabar varieties
- Malabar varietis can be grown in hot spot areas

- Trashing should be done during the month of January-February and September-October
- Release predators like *Chrysoperla zasrowii* Zillemi
- Spray any one of the following insecticides - spinosad 45SC @ 3.3mL/L quinalphos 2 mL/L or dimethoate 1.5 mL/L or imidacloprid 0.5 mL/L or thiamethoxam 2 g/10 L
- 4 sprays during the dry months (January to May) (since population is high)
- Skip insecticidal application during heavy monsoon showers
- The insecticides may be applied 6 to 8 times at monthly intervals starting from January

Root grub : *Basilepta fulvicorne* Jacoby

Order : Coleoptera

Family : Chrysomelidae

Distribution: Kerala, Karnataka, Tamil Nadu

Host range: Jack, rose, Indian almond, mango, guava, ficus, cocoa, and dadaps

Biology: Adult beetles are greenish-blue or brownish-green. Females are bigger than males. Beetles can be seen during morning and evening hours. Eggs are laid on dry grasses, leaf sheaths, or on dry cardamom leaves. The minute creamy 'C' shaped white grubs hatch out from eggs, fall on the ground, reach the root zone, and start feeding the roots. Pupation occurs in the soil (Vijayan, 2018).

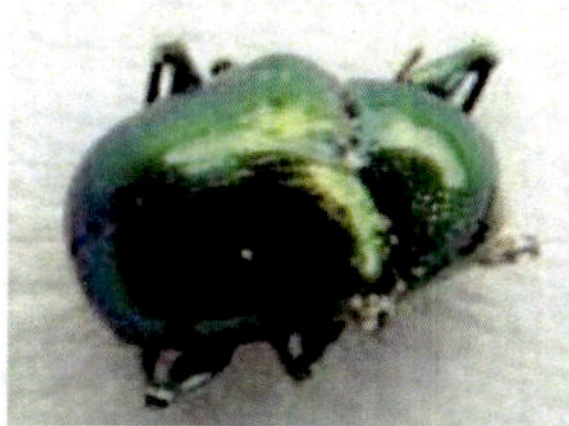
Adult beetle

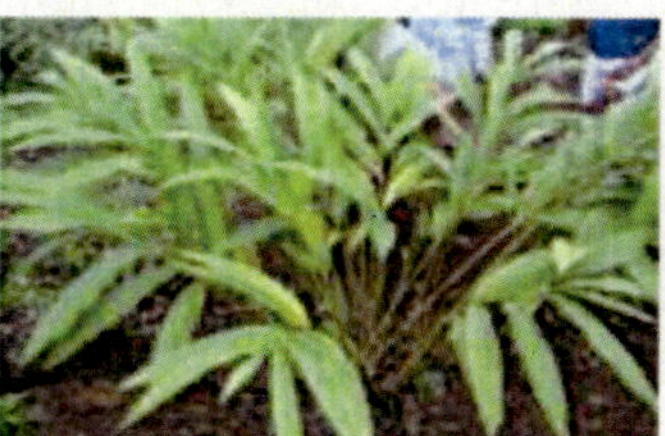
Root grub infested plant

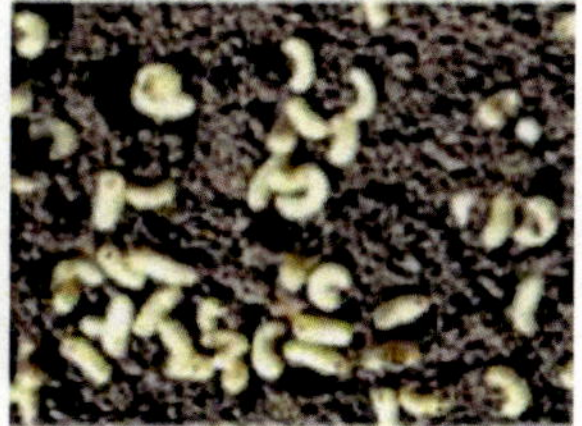
Grubs in soil

Nature of damage and symptoms

- The grubs feed throughout the length of the roots
- Reduction in the uptake of nutrients
- In the latter stages of an attack, the leaves also turn chlorotic due to damage to the roots
- Later drying up and death of the plant

Integrated pest management

- Ensure enough shade in the plantation
- Collection and destruction of adult beetle during the time of emergence (March-April and August-September)
- Avoid planting crops near alternate host trees (Mango tree, Jack, Ficus)
- Drench *Metarrhizium* (20 g/L) at the plant basin
- Apply EPN-infected cadavers @ 4 no's/plant
- Drench the soil with chlorpyriphos 0.04% (2 mL/ L) @ 5L/plant to kill grubs in the soil

Whitefly : *Kanakarajiella (Dialeurodes) cardamomi*

Family : Aleyrodidae

Order : Hemiptera

Serious pests in cardamom growing parts of Kerala.

Biology: Adults are tiny, white moth-like insects covered with waxy blooms. Nymphs range in color from pale green to greenish yellow. The life cycle is completed within two to three weeks.

Nature of damage and symptoms

- Nymphs and adults appear on the underside of the leaves and cause discoloration and yellowing by sucking the sap from the leaves
- Cause gradual yellowing and finally plant dry
- The infected plant eventually becomes stunted
- Sooty mould development occurs due to honeydew secretion

Integrated pest management

- Placing yellow sticky traps between rows of cardamom plants to monitor and trap adults
- Avoid excess application of nitrogen fertilizers
- Spray the lower surface of leaves with a mixture of neem oil (500 mL) and triton (500 mL) in 100 litres of water
- Spray *Verticillium / Lecanicilllium lecanii*
- *Aschersonia placenta* infect the pupal stage of the insects (Muraleedharan, 1985)
- Avoid repeated application of synthetic pyrethroids
- Spray dimethoate 30 EC (2 ml/l) or acephate (1.6 g/l). Repeat the spraying 2 or 3 times at 15 days interval

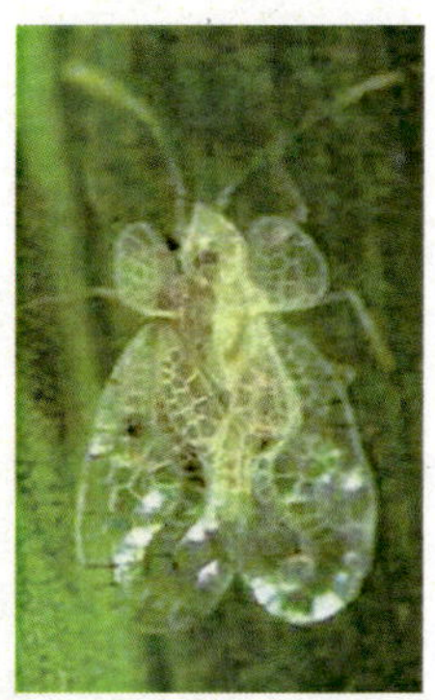

Lacewing bug : *Stephanitis typicus*
Order : Hemiptera
Family : Tingidae

Both adult and nymph suck sap from the leaves resulting in yellowing and discoloration of leaves. Adults are little, dull-colored insects with reticulate wings that are translucent and glossy. An average of 30 eggs are laid by females in leaf tissue. The egg and nymphal period are 12 days and 13 days respectively. As a result of feeding, white/yellow dots are formed on the upper surface, and on the severe infestation, drying up of leaves occurs. For managing the pests provide proper shading and spray dimethoate 30 EC (2 ml/l) or acephate (1.6 g/L).

Scale insect : *Aulacaspis elettaria* Joshi and Nafeesa
Order : Hemiptera
Family : Diaspididae

Initially, the infested part of the pseudostem shows yellowing and brown discoloration. Due to the pseudostem drying, the clump gets a sickly appearance. Browning, shrinkage, darkening, and drying of the entire panicle, including the flowers and capsules, were seen when the infestation got severe (Nafeesa and Murugan. 2024).

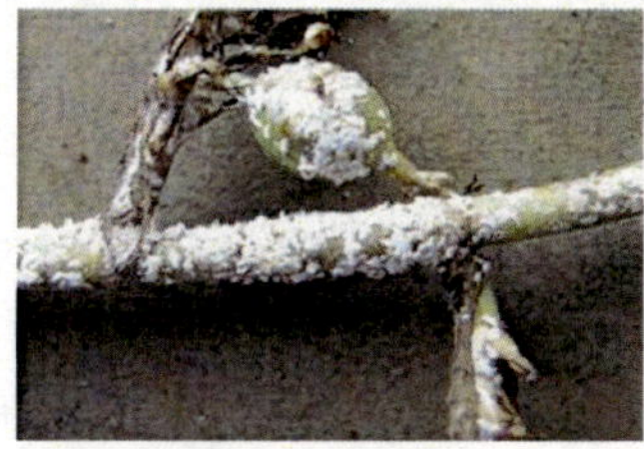

A. elettaria

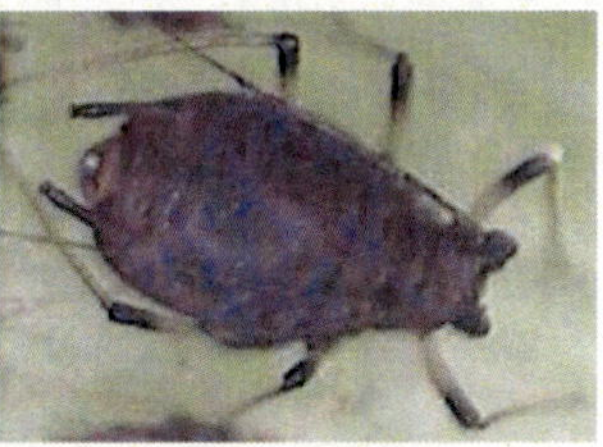

Pentalonia nigronervosa

Aphids : *Pentalonia nigronervosa* Coq.
Order : Hemiptera
Family : Aphididae

Distribution: India, Australia, Sri Lanka

Host range: *Colocasia* sp., *Alocasia* sp. and Banana

Both winged and wingless forms are present. Wingless aphids are dark brown and pyriform, and the winged ones have prominent black veins on their wings. Both adults and nymph suck sap from the plant. They can be seen concealed inside the leafsheaths of pseudostem. These are the vectors of Katte mosaic disease in cardamom.

Management

- Banana cultivation in and around the cardamom plantation should be avoided
- Monitoring and destruction of "kattae mosaic" affected plants
- Foliar spray with dimethoate 30EC @ 1.5 mL/L will reduce the pest population

Root Mealybugs : *Xenococcus annandalei* Silvestri.

Family : Pseudococcidae

Order : Hemiptera

Root mealybugs are mealybugs that infest the roots of crop plants. Damage is caused by nymphs and adults sucking sap from the root and rootlets. On the roots, nymphs and adults are seen congregating. These mealybugs inject poisonous saliva into the plant in addition to feeding. Plants that experience persistent desapping lose their vigour and eventually die from drooping, yellowing, and drying up. Deepthy *et al.* (2017) reported the root mealybug, *Xenococcus annandalei*, for the first time from the Idukki district.

Nature of damage and symptoms

Adults and nymphs congregate on the root zone and suck sap from the feeding roots of cardamom. Continuous desapping result in loss of vigour, yellowing, wilting and complete drying of plants.

Management

- Continuous monitoring is needed for effective management of root Mealybugs
- Monitoring and management of ants should also be done because ants are always seen in association with root mealybugs and also help them for dispersal to other areas
- Soil drenching of affected plants with chlorpyriphos 0.05% @ 5-7 litres per plant is recommended
- Drenching shall be repeated if the root mealybug persists
- Soil drenching with EPF, *Lecanicicillium lecanii* @ 20g/L (5-7 litres per plant) at regular intervals (application of EPF should be done at 25-30 days after chemical pesticide application) will reduce mealybug infestation

Root knot nematode : *Meloidogyne incognita* Kofoid & White.
Family : Heteroderidae
Order : Tylenchida

Nature of damage and symptoms

Root knot nematodes are found infesting cardamom roots, and the issue is more common in places with less shade. Symptoms of the root knot nematode infestation include knots or galls on the roots, yellowing of the leaves, and stunted plant growth as a result of the blockage in nutrient absorption. Infested plants frequently exhibit narrowing of the upper leaves, and the afflicted leaves become leathery.

Management

- Avoid planting of shade tree dadap and intercrops like banana and ginger should be avoided in cardamom plantation
- Neem cake application @ 250-1000g twice a year reduces the nematode population drastically
- Mulching of cardamom roots with Leaves of weed plants like wild sunflower, eupatorium, clerodendron *etc*. can be used as mulching materials in cardamom to reduce the nematode population in soil
- Soil application of *Trichoderma* spp. and *Paecilomyces lilacinus* reduced the nematode population to a greater extent

Hairy caterpillars

Cardamom is heavily defoliated as a result of the infestation of hairy caterpillars. Hairy caterpillars consume a lot of cardamom leaves, causing the pseudostem and midrib of leaves to become completely defoliated. The cardamom leaves are infested by a variety of hairy caterpillars, including *Euproctis lutifacia* Hamp., Walk., *Pericallia ricini* Fabr., *Eupterote canaraica* Moore, *E. cardamomi* Renga, *E. fabia* Cram., *E. testaceae* Walk., *E. undata*, *Linodera vittata* Walk (Deepthy *et al*., 2021)

Nature of damage and symptoms

Eggs are usually laid on the shade trees and the initial instars feed on the leaves of shade trees and later instars feed on the cardamom plants. Caterpillars are voracious feeders and cause severe defoliation.

Management

- Congregation of caterpillars can be seen on the bark of shade trees or
- cardamom leaves these should be destroyed

- In case of severe incidence spraying with quinalphos 25EC @ 2ml/l will reduce the incidence

Red Spider Mite : *Tetranychus urticae* Koch.

Family : Tetranychidae

Nature of damage and symptoms

Red coloured spider mites are seen infesting cardamom leaves. Both nymphs and adults cause damage by sucking plant sap especially from the lower leaf surface.

Management

- Adequate shade should be ensured in the plantation
- Predatory mites, *Amblyseius* sp. were found feeding on red spider mites of cardamom
- In case of severe infestation, apply spiromesifen 22.9SC @ 8mL/10L or wettable sulphur 80 WP @ 2.5 g/L is effective in reducing the mite population

References

Deepthy, K. B., Joshi, S., Manoj, V. S., Dhanya, M. K., Maya, T., Kuriakose, K. P., & Krishnaprasad, K. P. (2017). A new report of the myrmecophilous root mealy bug Xenococcus annandalei Silvestri (Rhizoecidae: Hemiptera)-a devastating pest. Entomon, 42(3), 185-192.

Deepthy, K., B., Sathyan, T., Dhanya, M., K., Murugan M., Sachin, G., P., and M. Murugan, Sachin G. Pai and O. M. Shana, O., M. 2021. Pest Complex in Cardamom and Their Management In: Asokkumar K., Murugan, M. and Dhanya, M., K. (eds.) Cardamo [Elettaria cardamomum (l.)Maton] Production, Breeding, Management, Phytochemistry and Health benefits Nova science publishers, Newyork 103:135

Doddabasappa, B., Chakravarthy, A.K. and Thyagaraj, N.E., 2014. Comparative biology of shoot and capsule borer, Conogethes punctiferalis (Guenee),(Crambidae: Lepidoptera) on castor and cardamom. Current Biotica, 8(3), pp.228-245.

Muraleedharan, N. (1985). A new disease of the cardamom whitefly. Trop.Pest Manage., 31, 234–235.

Nafeesa, M. and Murugan, M., 2024. Nature of Infestation and Management of Cardamom Scale Aulacaspis elettaria Joshi and Nafeesa on Cardamom. Indian Journal of Entomology, pp.1-5.

Singh, J., Sudharshan, M.R. and Selvan, M.T. (1999). Seasonal population of cardamom thrips (Sciothrips cardamomi (Ramk.) on three cultivar types of cardamom (Elettaria cardamomum Maton). Journal of Spices and Aromatic Crops 8: 19-22.

Thyagaraj, N.E. 2003. Integrated Management of some important cardamom pests of hill region of Karnataka, South India. Ph.D Thesis, Dr. B.R Ambedkar University, Uttara Pradesh, India. Pp. 213.

Vijayan, A.K., 2018. Small cardamom production technology and future prospects. International Journal of Agriculture Sciences, ISSN, pp.0975-3710.

Questions

1. Dead heart symptom in cardamom is caused by
   a) *Conogethes punctiferalis* b) *Pentalonia nigronervosa*
   c) *Basilepta fulvicorne*
2. Vector of Katte mosaic disease in cardamom
   a) *Dialeurodes cardamom* b) *Aulacaspis elettaria*
   c) *Pentalonia nigronervosa*
3. Trashing is usually practised in cardamom against
   a) *Sciothrips cardamom* b) *Dialeurodes cardamom*
   c) *Aulacaspis elettaria*
4. Scabs on the capsules of cardamom is an important symptom by
   a) *Conogethes punctiferalis* b) *Sciothrips cardamom*
   c) *Pentalonia nigronervosa*
5. Entomopathogenic fungi infecting the pupal stage of cardamom whitefly
   a) *Lecanicillium lecanii* b) *Aschersonia placenta*
   c) *Beauveria bassiana*

Answer Key

1		2		3		4		5					

13

Pests of Cinnamon

Cinnamon, commonly known is a highly valued spice crop obtained from the inner bark of the tree *Cinnamomum verum*, belonging to the family Lauraceae. It is native to Sri Lanka and Southern India, and widely cultivated in Kerala Tamil Nadu, and Karnataka. The spice is used globally in culinary, medicinal and aromatic industries. It thrives well in tropical humid climates with well-drained loamy soils and is generally propagated by seeds or cuttings. Though relatively hardy, cinnamon can be affected by a few key pests, especially when grown in monoculture or under poor management.

Sl. No.	Common name	Scientific name	Family and Order	Site of oviposition	Site of pupation
		Borers			
1	Cinnamon butterfly	*Chilasa clytia*	*Papilionidae Lepidoptera*	Leaves	Plant parts
2	Common blue bottle	*Graphium sarpendon*	Papilionidae Lepidoptera	Lower leaf surafce	Leaf, branches
3		*Ichneumenoptera cinnamomumi*	Sessidae Lepidoptera	Base of the stem	Beneath bark
4	Red borer	*Zeuzera coffeae*	Cossidae Lepidoptera	Plant	Inside stem
	Shot hole borer	*Xylosandrus compactus*	Curculionidae Coleoptera	Inside stem	Inside stem
	Leaf miner	*Conopomorpha civica*	Gracillaridae Lepidoptera	Leaf tissues	Leaf litter/ soil
	Root grub	*Anomala sp.*	Scarabidae Coleoptera		
		Sucking pests			
5	Psyllids	*Trioza cinnamomic*	Triozidae, Hemiptera	Leaves	Leaves/ shoot
6	Mites	*Eriophyes boisi*	*Eriophyidae*	Leaves	Leaves/ shoot

Cinnamon butterfly/
Common Mime : ***Chilasa clytia***

Order : Lepidoptera

Family : Papilionidae

Distribution: India and Sri Lanka

Host range: Cinnamon, Chinese cassia

Biology: There are two adult forms clytia and dissimilis. The clytia are blackish brown wings with a series of arrowhead shaped white spots on the outer margin, and the dissimilis are black winged with elongated white spots and a series of marginal arrowhead shaped spots. Adults lay spherical, waxy looking, and orange-yellow colored egg singly on the upper and lower surfaces of young leaves. The emerging larva resembles bird droppings (defensive mimicry) at the initial stages. The fully-grown larvae are pale yellow with dark stripes on the sides. There are five larval instars, and the larval period lasts for 11–17 days. The elongated, brownish-black pupa is joined to the host plant's stem by silky supports at the rear end. The pupal stage is 11–13 days long. The life cycle is completed in 24-36 days (Singh *et al.*, 1978).

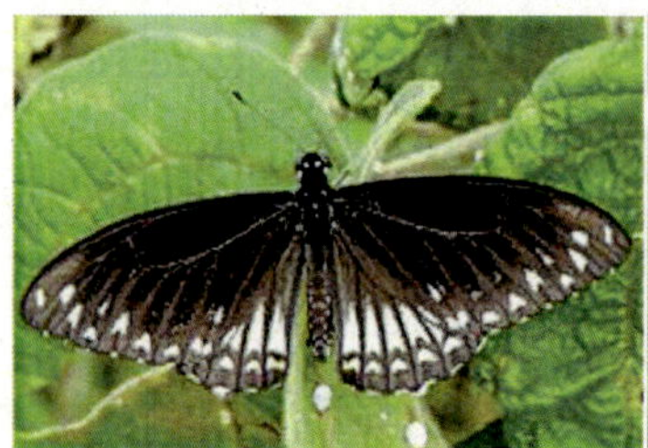

Chilasa clytia

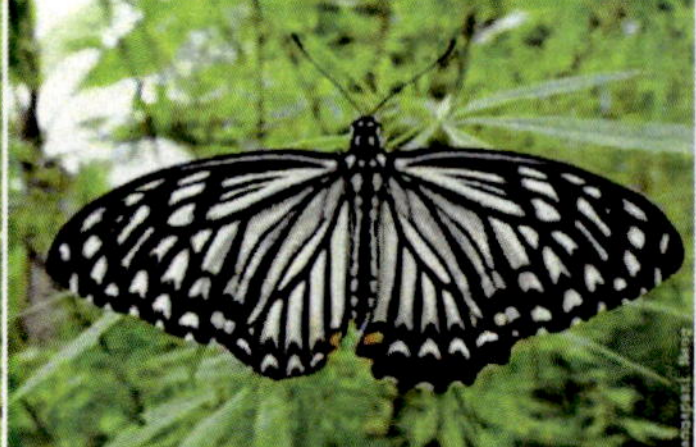

Chilasa dissimilis

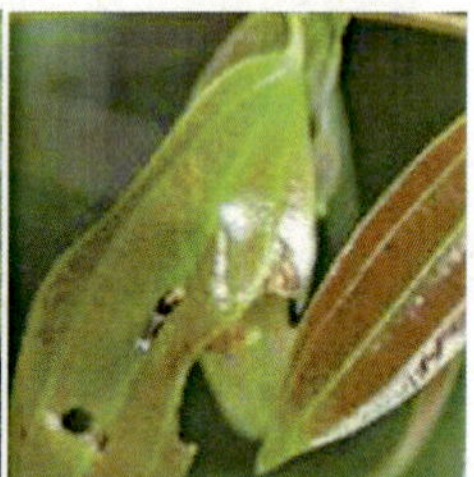

Symptom on the leaf

Nature of damage and symptoms

- The pest affects plants in plantations as well as young plants in nurseries
- Larva feed on tender and slightly mature leaves
- In severe cases of infestation, the entire plant is defoliated and only midribs of leaves with portions of veins are left

Management

- Hand picking the larvae and pupae from the field with the help of light trap
- Eggs are heavily parasitized by the egg parasitoid, *Telenomus remus* (Hymenoptera: Scelionidae)
- Spraying quinalphos (0.05%) 2 ml/L on tender and partly mature leaves

Common blue bottle : ***Graphium sarpendon***

Order : Lepidoptera

Family : Papilionidae

Distribution: India and Sri Lanka

Biology: The adult butterflies are large with blackish brown wings with elongated, pale greenish-blue patches in the middle of the fore and hind wings. Adults lay eggs on the lower surface of tender leaves. The egg period lasts for 5–6 days. The first instar caterpillar is smoky colored with spines on its body. There are five larval instars, which last 29–31 days. The larva pupates on the underside of the leaves, stalks, or small branches, and the pupal period lasts for 19–20 days. The life cycle is completed within 59–60 days (Rajapakse and Kulasekara, 1982).

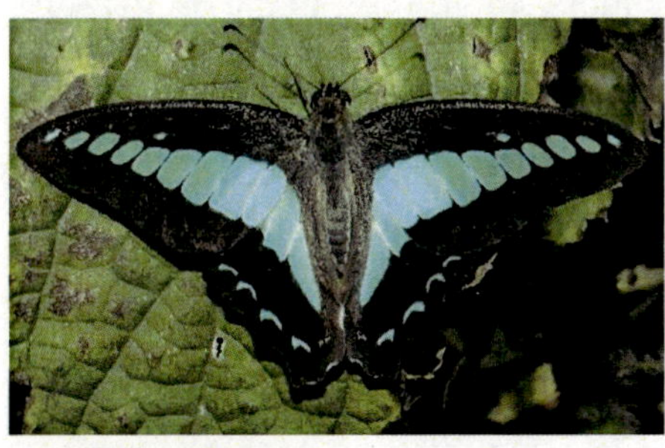

Adult – *G. serpedon*

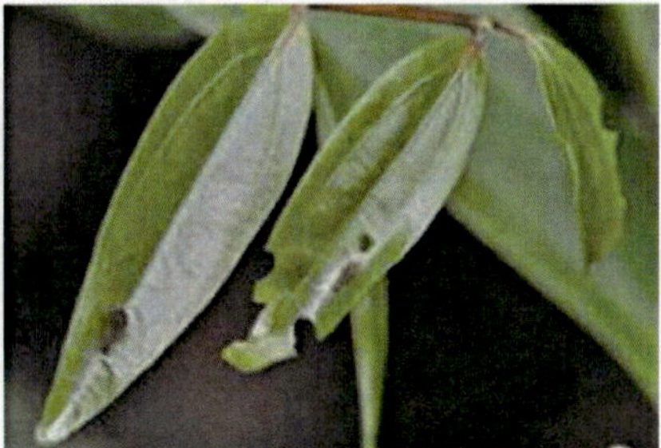

Infested leaf

Nature of damage and symptoms

- Larvae first feed on the undersurface of leaves, later they seem to favor the midrib on the upper surface of the cinnamon leaf

Management

- Remove and destruction of infested leaves
- Spraying quinalphos (0.05%) 2 ml/L on tender and partly mature leaves

Cinnamon Wood Borer : *Ichneumenoptera cinnamomumi*

Order : Lepidoptera

Family : Sesiidae

Distribution: Sri Lanka

Biology: Adult females deposit their eggs in crevices on the base of cinnamon bushes. Eggs are reddish to dark brown and 1 mm long. The egg period is about 1 week. There are five larval stages, with a larval period of about 40–55 days. Larvae have a light pink body with a dark brown head (pink stem borer).

Larval pupation takes place beneath the bark which lasts about 35–40 days Emerged adult moths survive for about 3–7 days (Dharshanee *et al.* 2008).

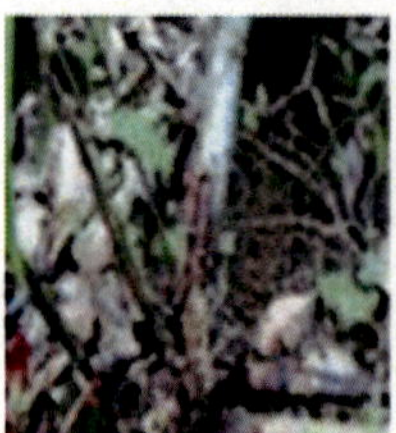
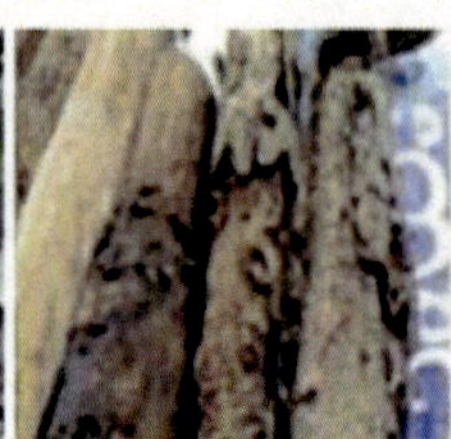
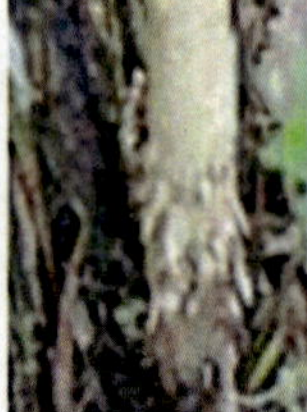
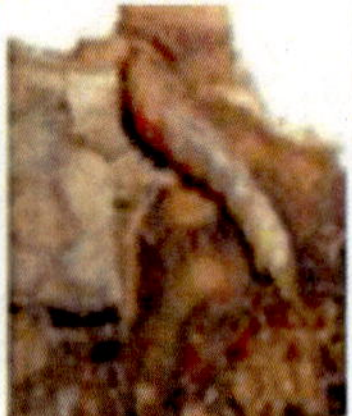
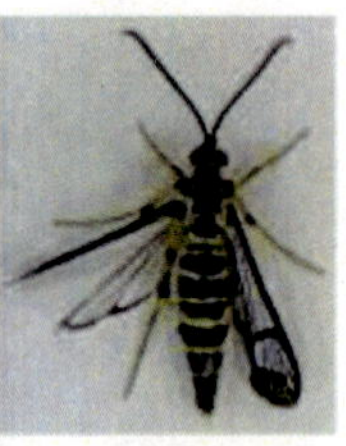

Nature of damage and symptoms

- The larvae feed and tunnel on the stem at ground level causing depletion of food reserves resulting in weakening and breakage of stems
- In severe cases cause die-back of shoots, and rotting of the pruned stems without producing new shoots
- Development of numerous adventitious roots, above the damaged point is the characteristic symptom (Jayasinghe *et al.*, 2020)

Management

- Heaping soil at the base of the cinnamon bush, earthing-up, minimizes laying of eggs on preferred sites
- Use of pheromone, [(E,Z)-3,13-octadecadien-1-ol and (E,Z)-3,13 octadecadienyl acetate] (Grassi *et al.*,2002; Jayasinghe *et al.*, 2006); that disrupts the mating pattern of the moth

Cinnamon red borer : *Zeuzera coffeae*

Order : Lepidoptera

Family : Cossidae

Biology: The adult moths are white in color, and males are comparatively smaller than females. The forewings and the outer margin of the hindwings are marked with small black dots. The abdomen is long and posteriorly. Female moths lay eggs in rows on host plants. the egg period is about 10 days. The emerging larvae are slender, soft, and red in color. Larvae bore into the stems or twigs and feed on the pith of plants, making tunnels. The larval period is completed within 4–5 months. The pupation occurs inside the boreholes, and the pupal period is about 3–4 weeks. The life cycle is completed within 5-6 months (Chang, 1984).

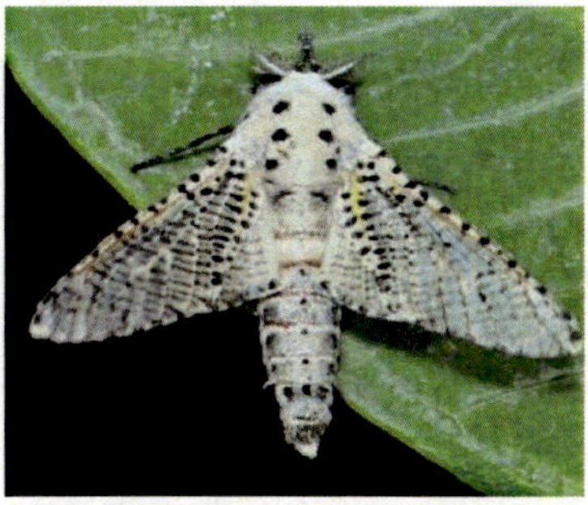
Adult moth

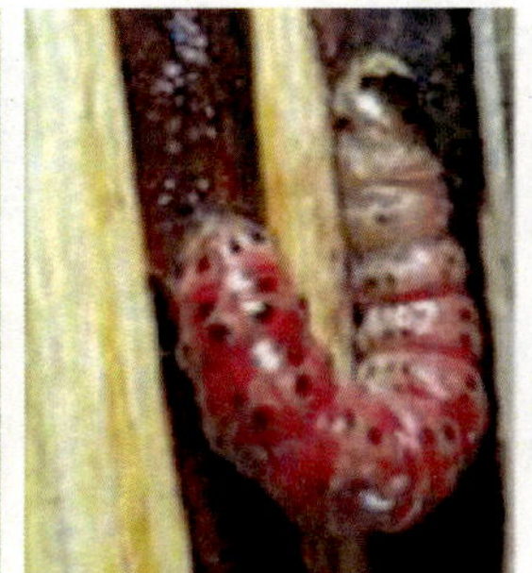
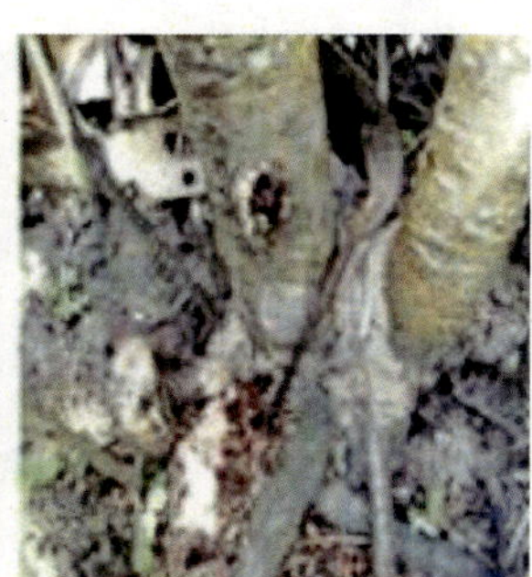
Larval feeding damage symptoms

Nature of damage and symptoms

- Caterpillars create tunnels inside the stem and root by boring into the bark and twigs
- Tunnelling of the stem leads to leaf withering and at a more severe stage, the stems or entire bushes eventually die off
- The dark brown excrement can be observed in the bore holes (Jayasinghe *et al.*, 2020)

Management

- Removing and burning of severely infested branches and twigs
- Cotton bud, soaked with an insecticide can be inserted into the tunnel

Cinnamon leaf gall makers

A. Upper Surface Leaf Galls

Psyllids	:	*Trioza cinnamomi*
Order	:	Hemiptera
Family	:	Triozidae

Nature of damage and symptoms

- Solitary galls are widely dispersed on the top surface of the leaf; however, they are not formed on the veins
- Galls are yellowish-green, firm, conical, and unilocular
- Each gall contains a single insect until it reaches maturity; later, they leave holes on the leaf's underside that cause the gall to become dry and brown (Mani, 1973)

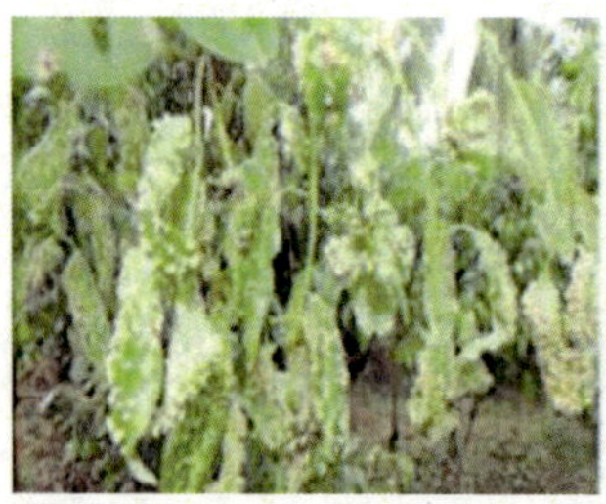 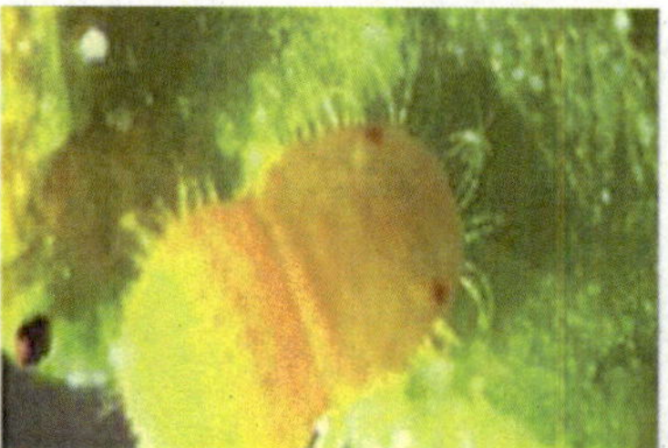 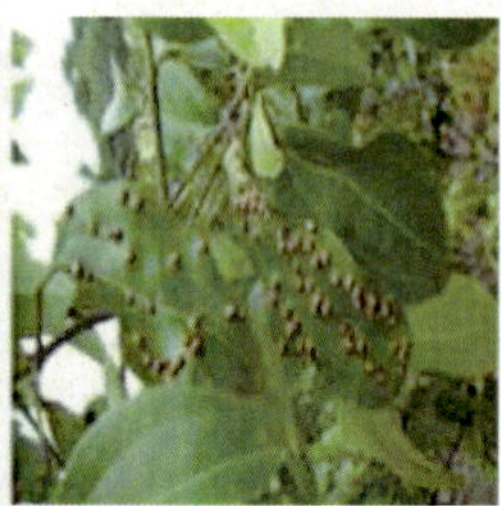

T. cinnamomi causing galls in cinnamon (Jayasinghe *et al.*, 2020)

B. Lower Leaf Galls

Mite : *Eriophyes boisi*

Order : Acarina

Family : Eriophyidae

Nature of damage and symptoms

- Large, irregular galls are formed on the lower leaf surface
- The mite-infested galls are ovoid or irregularly conical with a ridged surface, pinkish in color initially and becoming green on maturity
- Sometimes entire apical bud becomes a mite gall and does not develop into a leaf
- The lower surface is covered by a thin layer of cells which ruptures to permit the emergence of the adult (Mani, 1973)

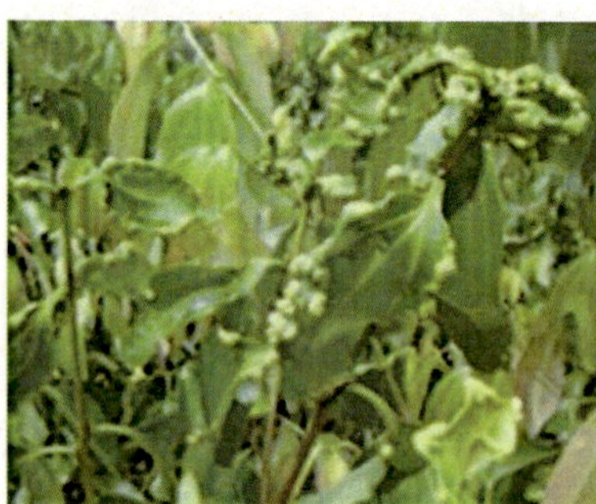 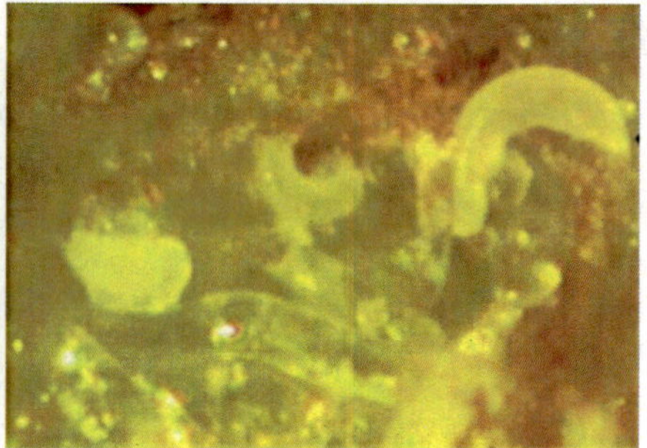

Damage symptoms caused by eriophyid mites (Jayasinghe *et al.*, 2020)

Management

- Pruning periodically to remove the gall-bearing shoots
- Insecticides/miticides must be applied to prevent further infestation when initial symptoms become apparent in a few newly emerged flushes

Cinnamon shot hole borer : *Xylosandrus compactus*
Order : Coleoptera
Family : Curculionidae (Scolytinae)

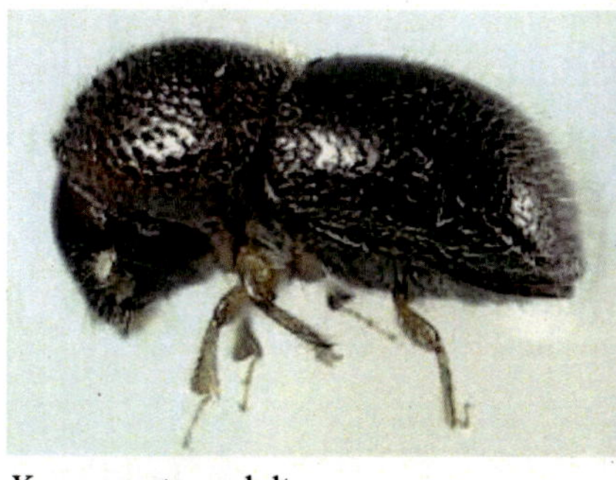

X. compactus- adult

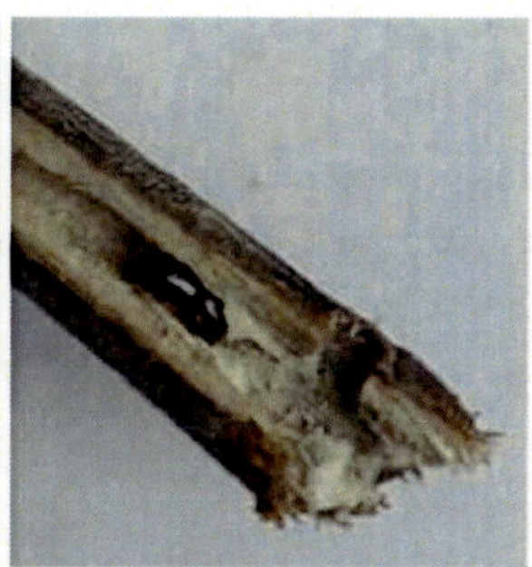

Damage symptom on the stem

Biology: The adult female beetles deposit their eggs inside the galleries made on mature stems. The eggs are off-white colored. The emerging larvae are legless C-shaped ones. The eggs, larva, and white pupa can be seen in the galleries (Jayasinghe *et al.*, 2020).

Nature of damage and symptoms

- Necrosis on the leaves and stems of infested seedlings extends from the entrance hole
- The twigs, branches, or entire plants begin to wilt five to seven days after the gallery formation
- At the site of infestation, the stem breaks down, causing cinnamon seedlings to collapse

Management

- Removal and destruction of infested plants is the most effective and recommended cultural practice
- Spray chlorpyriphos 20 EC

Leaf miner : *Conopomorpha civica*
Order : Lepidoptera
Family : Gracillaridae

The larvae are pale gray initially and later become pink. The adult moth is a minute silvery gray. The larva feeds on tissues between the upper and lower epidermis of tender leaves. Linear mines that end in 'blister' like patches. The infested leaves become crinkled, and the mined areas dry up, leading to the formation of large holes on the leaves.

Spraying quinalphos 0.05% during the emergence of new flushes is effective in preventing pest infestation

Cinnamon root grub : *Anomala sp.*

Order : Coleoptera

Family : Scarabaeidae

Soils that are heavy in organic matter have very high population of root grubs. Newly established young cinnamon plants are particularly susceptible to the pest. After a protracted dry spell, damage may be more severe when the rainy season begins because starved grubs begin to eat roots in large quantities after being dormant during the dry term (Jayasinghe *et al.*, 2020).

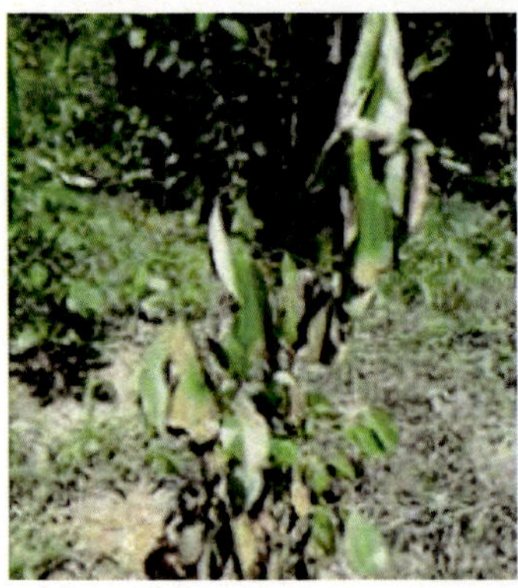
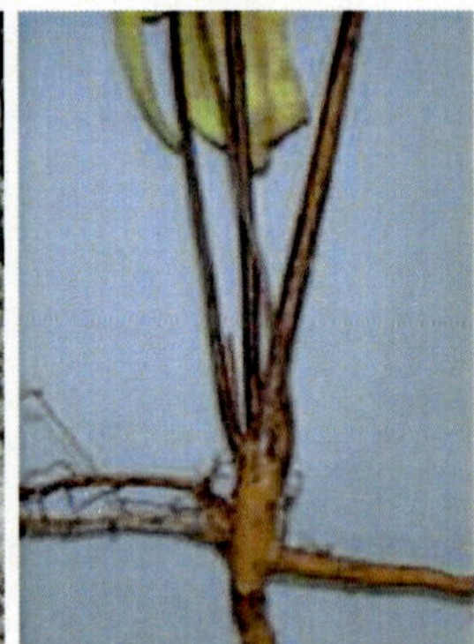
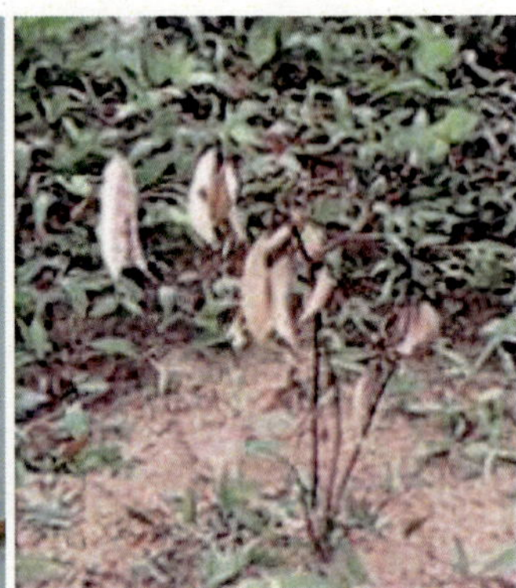

Symptoms of root grub infestation

References

Chang CP (1984) The morphology and life history of Zeuzera coffeae Nietner on grapevine in Taiwan. Plant Protect Bull Taiwan 26:145–153

Dharshanee HLC, Dharmadasa M, Nugaliyadda L, Wijesinghe KGG et al (2008) Development of a pheromone based management method for cinnamon wood boring moth (Ichneumoniptera cinnamomumi) (Lepidoptera: Sesiidae). Proc Natl Symp Fac Agric Univ Ruhuna Sri Lanka:31

Jayasinghe, G.G., Rajapakse, R.H.S., Kumara, K.W., Ratnasekera, D. and Adikaram, N.K.B., 2020. Pests and Diseases of Cinnamon (Cinnamomum zeylanicum Blume). Cinnamon: Botany, Agronomy, Chemistry and Industrial Applications, pp.201-232.

Mani, M. S. (1973). Galls on Some Unidentified Plants. In Plant Galls of India Palgrave Macmillan UK. 291-294.

Rajapakse, R.H.S. and Kulasekara, V.K. (1982) Some observations on the insect pests of cinnamon in Sri Lanka. Entomon, 7, 221–223.

Singh, V., Dubey, O.P., Nair, C.P.R. and Pillai, G.B. (1978) Biology and bionomics of insect pests of cinnamon. J. Plantation Crops, 6, 24–27.

Questions

1. Egg parasitoid of cinnamon butterfly
   a) *Trichogramma chilonis* b) *Anagrus* sp.
   c) *Telenomus remus*
2. Upper leaf galls in cinnamon leaves are caused by
   a) *Trioza cinnamomi* b) *Eriophyes boisi*
   c) *Conopomorpha civica*
3. Lower leaf galls in cinnamon leaves are caused by
   a) *Trioza cinnamomic* b) *Eriophyes boisi*
   c) *Conopomorpha civica*

Answer Key

1	a	2	a	3	b								

14

Pests of Ginger and Turmeric

Shoot borer : ***Conogethes punctiferalis***

Order : Lepidoptera

Family : Crambidae

Distribution: India, China, Bangladesh, Sri Lanka, Taiwan, Thailand

Host: Turmeric, ginger, cardamom, castor, guava, mango, cocoa *etc.*

Biology: Adult moths are yellowish medium-sized moths. Wings are pale yellowish with black spots on the wings. The female moth lays round yellowish eggs singly or in groups on the tender part of the plant. Larva is long, pale greenish with a pinkish tint dorsally, head and pro-thoracic shield brown in color, body covered with minute hair. Pupation takes place in a loose silken cocoon inside the larval tunnel (Chong *et al.*, 1991)

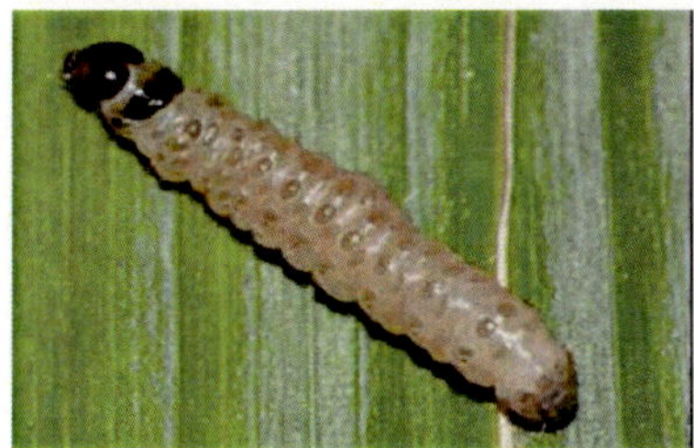
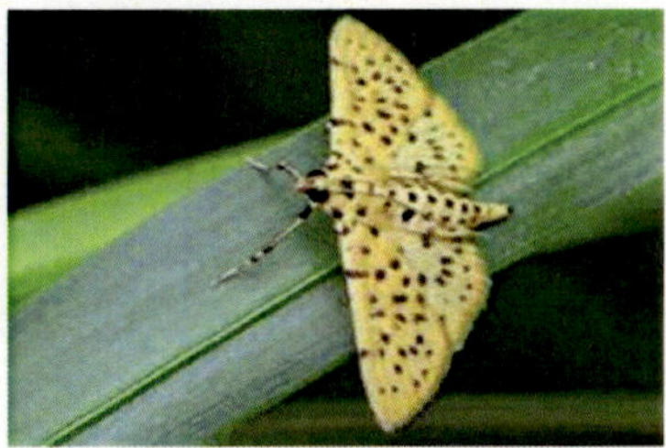

Larva and adult of *C. punctiferalis*

Nature of damage and symptoms

- Yellowing and drying of leaves of infested pseudostems
- Presence of a bore-hole on the pseudostem through which frass is extruded
- Withering and yellowing finally cause death of the central shoot (dead heart) (Devasahayam *et al.*, 2010 and Chong *et al.*, 1991)

Management

- Pruning and destruction of infected plant parts
- Application of neem oil 1%

- Spraying of dipel 0.3% (Devasahayam, 2000)
- A mermithid nematode was found parasitic to larvae of *Conogethes punctiferalis*
- Spraying dimethoate or quinalphos @ 2 ml/l

Rhizome scale : ***Aspidiotus hartii***

Order : Diaspididae

Family : Hemiptera

Distribution: India, West Africa, and West Indies

Host: Turmeric, ginger, elephant foot yam, and tannia

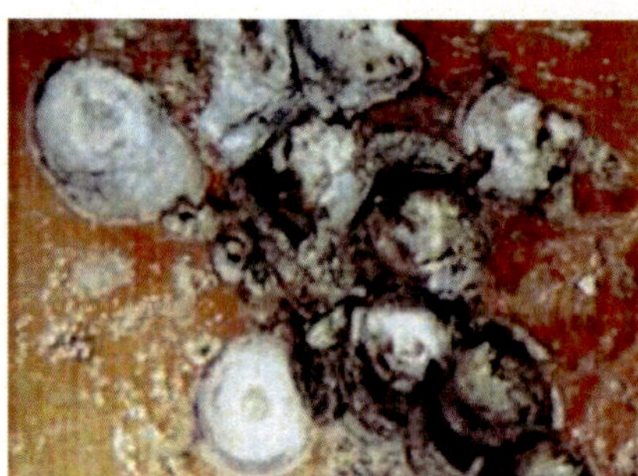

A. hartii

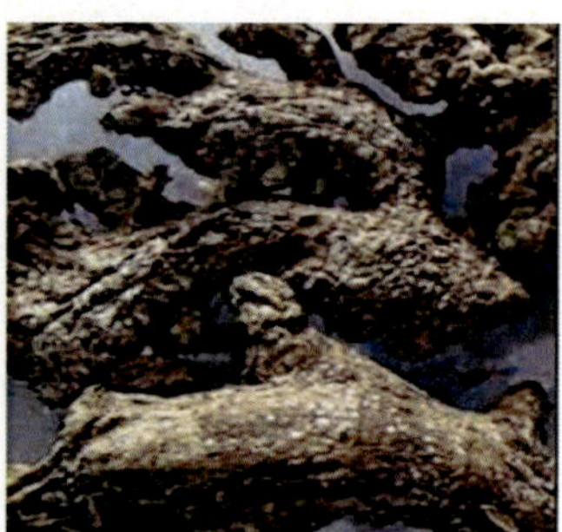

Damage symptoms on ginger

Biology: Scales are minute, circular, light brownish to grey with a thin pale membrane. Adult scales are yellow to deep yellowish in color. It reproduces either parthenogenetically or ovoviviparously. The female lays about 100 oval, yellowish eggs under the scale. The egg period lasts for one day and the nymphal period 30 days (Jacob, 1982, 1986).

Nature of damage and symptoms

- Field infestation: Plants look devitalized, pale, and withered before drying completely. At the time of harvest, minute yellowish crawlers can be seen moving in large numbers, which is the potential stage of dissemination
- Storage infestation: White-colored scales are scattered on rhizomes, and later they congregate near the growing buds. When the infestation is severe, the rhizome and buds shrivel, and ultimately, the entire rhizome dries

Management

- Discard and do not store severely infested rhizomes
- Collect and destroy damaged leaves

- Select healthy rhizomes free from scale infestation for seed materials
- Apply well rotten cow manure/poultry manure in two splits @ 10 tons/ha, first before planting and the second at the time of earthing up
- Rhizome scale are parasitized by *Physcus comperei* Hayat (Aphelinidae), *Adelencyrtus moderatus* Howard (Encyrtidae) (Jacob, 1986)
- Drench soil with dimethoate 30 EC @ 2ml/L of water
- Soak seed rhizomes, in insecticide solution of either dimethoate 30 EC, 1.5 ml/L for 15 min. for storing

Skipper butterfly : *Udaspes folus*

Order : Lepidoptera

Family : Hesperiidae

Distribution: Throughout India. Very common pest

Host: Turmeric, ginger, arrow root, cardamom, and wild lily

Biology: Adult butterfly is brownish-black with white spots on the forewings and one large patch on the hindwing. The female lays about 50 eggs on the underside of the leaves. The egg period is about 3-4 days. There are five larval instar stages. The full-grown larva is dark-green, and measures 36 mm in length. The larval period is about 12-21 days. Pupation occurs inside the leaf fold. The pupal period is 6-7 days. Insects are abundant from August to October. The duration from egg to adult was recorded as 28.6 days on ginger and 25.1 days on turmeric (Abraham *et al*., 1975).

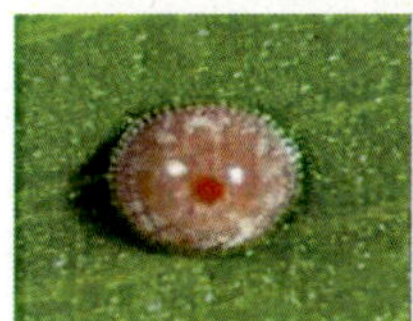
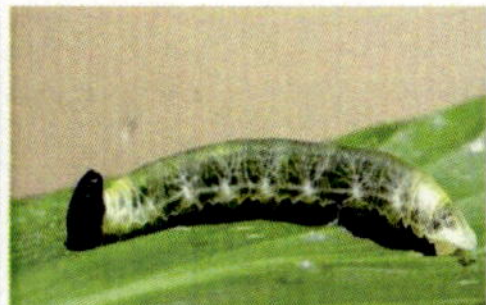
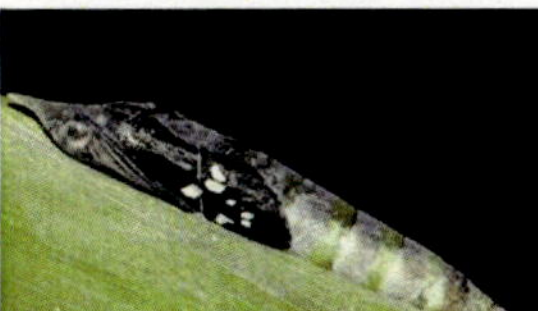
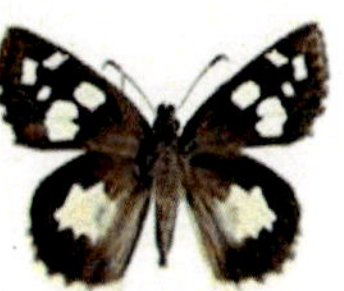

Egg, larva, pupa and adult of *U. folus*

Nature of damage and symptoms

- Larvae webs leaves with silken threads, fold the leaves into a tubular form and feed on them (Lefroy, 1906)
- Cause extensive defoliation

Management

- Hand pick and destroy the caterpillars
- Larval parasites recorded are *Ceromya* sp, *Apanteles* sp, *Sympiesis* sp and a mermithid nematode (Dubey *et al*. 1976)

- The pupal parasite recorded was the chalcid *Brachymena coxodentata* (Dubey *et al*., 1976)
- Apply malathion 50 EC 2 ml in L of water

Rhizome maggot

Formosina flavipes, Chalcidomyia atricornis (Chloropidae: Diptera), *Eumerus albifrons* (Syrphidae: Diptera), *Mimegralla coeruleifrons* (Micropezidae: Diptera), *Calobata sp.* (Micropezidae: Diptera), *Celyphus sp.* (Celyphidae: Diptera)

Distribution

- *Formosina flavipes, Chalcidomyia atricornis* - on turmeric and ginger in South India
- *Eumerus albifrons, Mimegralla coeruleifrons* - on ginger in Karantaka
- *Celyphus sp.* - on ginger in Kerala and Uttar Pradesh

Nature of damage and symptoms

- Maggots began eating on the collar area before moving into rhizomes and pseudostems and consuming the soft tissues ferociously (Premkumar *et al*., 1980)
- As a result of larval feeding, the leaves began to turn yellow, later the leaves and shoots dried up (Ghorpade *et al*., 1988)
- Additionally, the rhizomes were observed to be totally destroyed

Management

- Avoid using seed material from the infested fields
- Spray dimethoate 1.5 ml/L water per ha
- Soak seed rhizomes, in insecticide solution of either dimethoate 30 EC for 15 min. for storing

Flea beetle : *Lema praeusta*
Order : Coleoptera
Family : Chrysomelidae

Adult beetles lay eggs singly on leaves. Grub feed on leaves for 10-12 days. Pupation occurs in soil. adult emerge out from pupa, last for 15-25 days. Longevity for adults is 43-60 days. Both adult and grub feed on leaves.

Thrips : *Panchaetothrips indicus*
Order : Thysanoptera
Family : Thripidae

As a result of continuous feeding leaves become rolled up. Later, leaves turn pale and gradually dry up. For pest control, spray insecticides like quinalphos 0.025% or fenthion or phosalone 0.07%.

References

Abraham, V.A. and Pillai, G.B. (1974). Biology and bionomics of insect pests. Annual report for 1973, Central Plantation Crops Research Institute, Kasargod. pp.153.

Chong KK, Ooi PAC, Tuck HC (1991) Crop pests and their management in Malaysia. Tropical Press Sdn. Bhd, Kuala Lumpur, p 242

Devasahayam S (2000) Evaluation of biopesticides for the management of shoot borer (Conogethes punctiferalis Guen.) on ginger (Zingiber officinale Rosc). In: Proceedings of the centennial conference on spices and aromatic plants, Indian Society for Spices, Calicut, India, pp 276–277

Devasahayam S, Jacob TK, Abdulla Koya KM, Sasikumar B (2010) Screening of ginger (Zingiber officinale) germplasm for resistance to shoot borer (Conogethes punctiferalis). J Med Aromat Plant Sci 32(2):137–138

Dubey, O.P., Pillai, G.B. and Vijay Singh (1976). Biology and bionomics of insect pests of spices. Central Plantation Crops Research Institute, 1976, Annual Report for 1975. pp.154-155.

Ghorpade, S.A., Jadhav, S.S. and A j n, D.S. (1988). Biology of rhizome fly, Mimeqralla coeruleifrons Macquart (Micropezidae: Diptera) in India, a pest of turmeric and ginger crops. Tropical Pest Management. 2(1):48-51.

Jacob, S.A. 1980. Biology and binomics of ginger and turmeric scale Aspidiotus hartii Green. In: Nair, M.K, Preemkumar, T., Ravindran, P.N., and Sarma, Y.R., Proceedings, National Seminar on ginger and turmeric. Central plantation crop research institute, Kasargode, pp. 131-132.

Jacob, S.A. 1986. Important pests of ginger and turmeric and their control. Indian Cocoa Arecanut Spices J., 9, 61-62

Lefroy, H.M. (1906). Indian Insect Life. Agricultural Research Institute, Pusa. pp.432-631.

Premkumar, Sarma, Y.R. and Gautham, S.S.S. (1980). Association of dipteran maggots in rhizome rot of ginger. In: Proceedings of the National Seminar on Ginger and Turmeric, 8-9 April, 1980, Calicut, pp. 128-136

Questions

1. Dead heart symptom in ginger and turmeric is caused by
   a) *Conogethes punctiferalis* b) *Mimegralla coeruleifrons*
   c) *Udaspes folus*
2. Pupation of *Udaspes folus* occurs in
   a) Soil b) Leaf fold
   c) Bore holes

Pest of Ornamentals

15

Pests of Jasmine

In India, jasmine is one of the oldest traditional flowers cultivated. It is infested by a number of insect and mite pests. The lepidopteran pests like bud borer, gallery worm, and leaf web-worm, are of significant importance. Sucking pests like eriophyid mite, lace wing bug, and thrips also causes minor damage to the crop. Dipteran pest like blossom midge also infests the crop. This chapter outlines brief descriptions of insect pests along with their hosts, life cycle, nature of damage, seasonal incidence and overall integrated pest management.

Sl No.	Common name	Scientific name	Family and Order
1	Bud worm	*Hendecasis duplifascialis*	Pyralidae, Lepidoptera
2	Gallery worm	*Elasmopalpus jasminophagus*	Pyralidae, Lepidoptera
3	Web worm	*Nausinoe geometralis, N. neptis*	Pyralidae, Lepidoptera
4	Jasmine eriophyid mite	*Aceria jasmini*	Eriophyidae, Acarina
5	Jasmine Blossom Midge	*Contarinia maculipennis*	Diptera, Cecidomyiidae
6	Jasmine lace wing	*Corythauma ayyari,*	Tingidae, Hemiptera
7	Whitefly	*Dialeurodes kirkaldyi*	Aleyrodidae, Hemiptera
8	Thrips	*Thrips orientalis*	Thripidae, Thysanoptera

1. Bud worm: *Hendecasis duplifascialis*, Pyralidae, Lepidoptera

Budworm is an important pest of jasmine. Its damage ranged from 30 to 70 per cent, which had a significant impact on flower quality. The quality of opened flowers was affected by the silken tunnels and excretions created by budworm larvae inside the bud clusters (Gunasekaran, 1989 and Kamala and Kennedy, 2016).

The adult moths are small, pale white with wavy markings on wings and black patches on the wing margin. The moths lay eggs singly and glued on the unopened or immature buds, calyx and sometimes on the bud stalk, where the larvae eventually hatch and begin feeding.

Host range: Jasmine

Biology: Female moths lay eggs on the on the unopened or immature buds, calyx, and bud stalk. Freshly laid eggs are round and creamy white in colour which later turn yellow. They hatch in about 3-4 days. The neonate larva is creamy yellow in colour with a dark black head and prothoracic shield. There are five larval instars. Pupation mostly takes place inside the soil and sometimes on the leaves, at the junction of petioles and leaf blades.

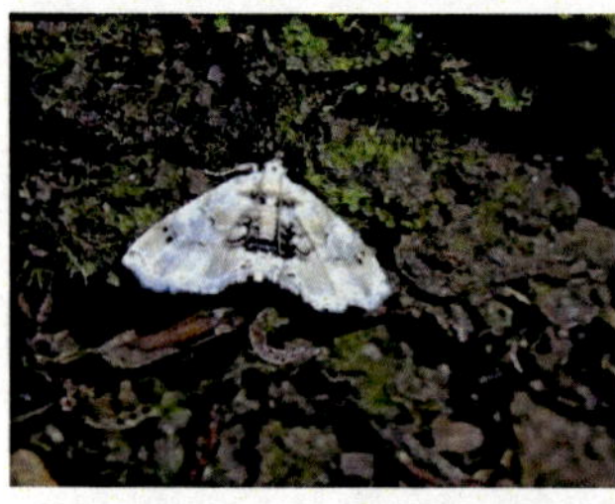
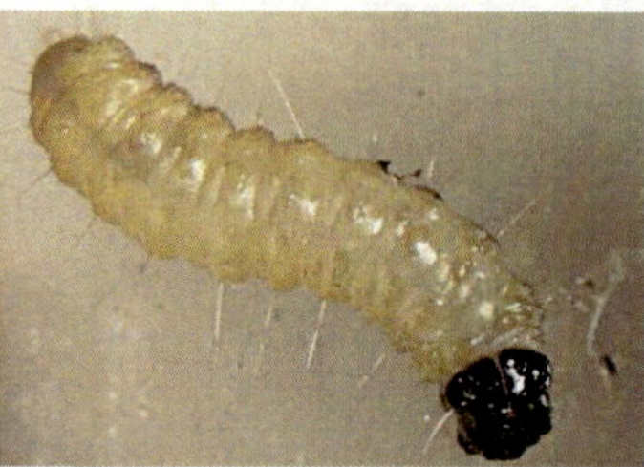

Adult and larva of *H. duplifascialis*

Nature of damage and symptoms

- Tiny caterpillar makes holes in the flower bud, feeds on the inner content of the bud (David, 1958)
- The larva emerges through circular holes made on the corolla tube and starts tunnelling into other buds of the same shoot (Reddy *et al.*, 1978)
- Infested flower turn violet in colour, and finally fall off
- In case of severe infestation, adjacent flower buds are webbed together by means of silken thread

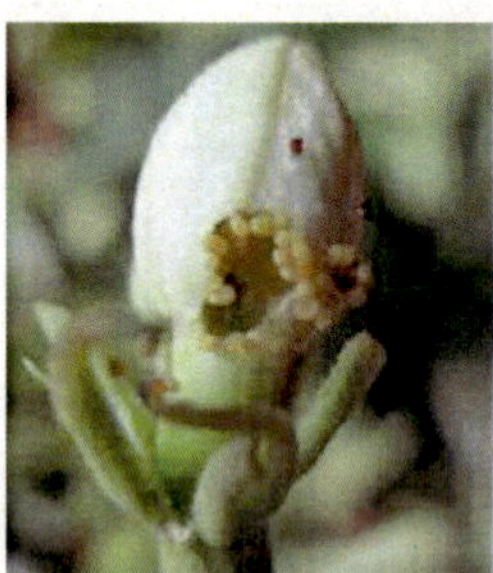
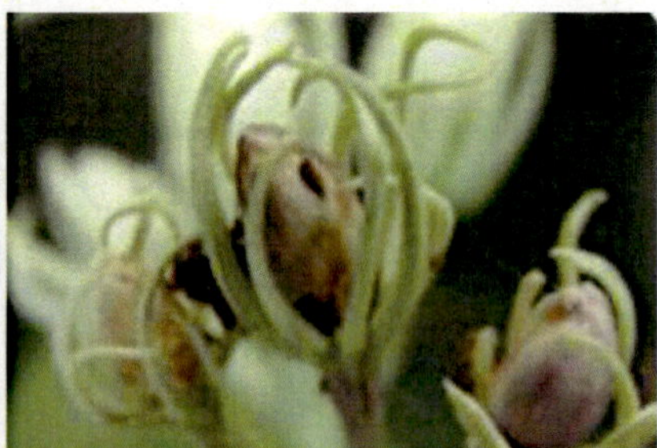

Damage symptoms of budworm

2. Gallery worm: *Elasmopalpus jasminophagus,* Pyralidae, Lepidoptera

The adult moth is small and dark grey, and the larva of the moth remains inside the silken web formed on the bud and starts feeding them. Jasmine gallery worm infestations varied from 5.96 to 21.64 per cent (Sudhir, 2002).

Host range: Jasmine

Biology: The eggs of gallery worm are creamy white in colour. The initial instars are pale green with latero- dorsal brown streaks and turned to complete brown in their later stages. They fed on the buds and remained inside the silken tunnels outside the buds. There are five larval instar stages. Pupation occurs within the galleries formed.

Nature of damage and symptoms

- Caterpillar web together the terminal leaves, shoots, and flower heads and feed on them
- Initial instars prefer feeding on green buds whereas the late larval instars feed on matured white buds (Shobitha, 2001)
- Faecal matter can be seen attached to the silken web

3. Web worm: *Nausinoe geometralis, N. neptis*, Pyralidae, Lepidoptera

Adult is a medium sized moth, having light brownish wings with white spots. The caterpillar is green with dark warts and starts feeding within the webs formed on the surface of the leaves.

Biology: The female moth lays about 15-30 greenish-yellow eggs on the leaf lamina. The egg period ranges from 3-4 days. The caterpillar is green with dark warts. The larval period is about 12-15 days. Pupation occurs within the leaf web. The pupal period is 6-7 days. The life cycle is completed in 22-24 days.

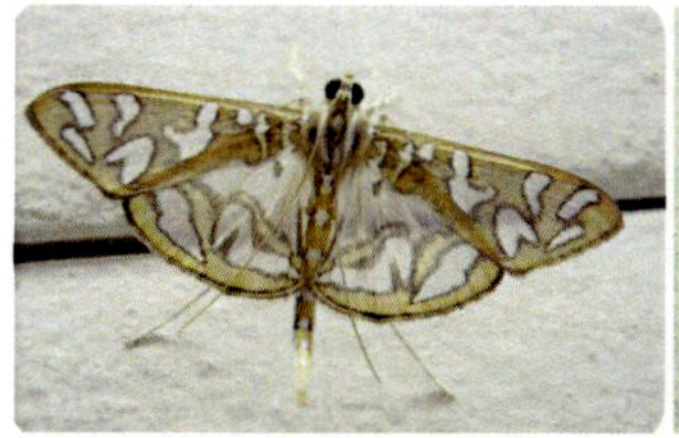
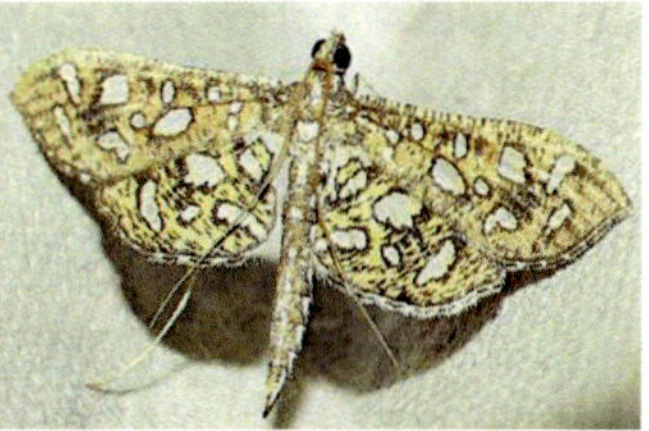

Nature of damage and symptoms

- The maximum infestation of jasmine leaf webworm occurs during November (12.70%) (Gunasekaran, 1989)
- Caterpillar attack leaves mostly in the lower bushy and shaded portions
- The leaves are webbed in an open and loose manner
- The silk threads can be seen as a cobweb on the surface of the leaves
- Larvae skeletonize the leaves by eating away the parenchyma
- Plants with severe infestations had burnt-up symptoms and reduced vigour, which in turn decreased flower yield (Sandhu and Shukla, 1984)

4. Jasmine eriophyid mite: *Aceria jasmini*, Eriophyidae, Acarina

Host range: Jasmine, *Jatropha intergrima*

Biology: The female is cylindrical and vermiform with two pairs of legs and measures about 150-160 µm long and 44 µm thick.

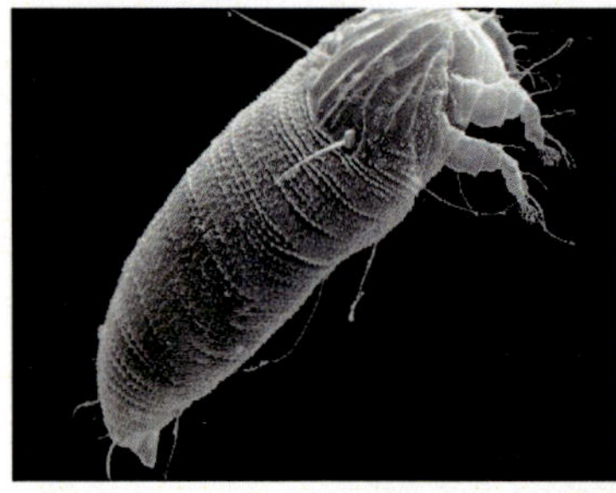

Aceria jasmini

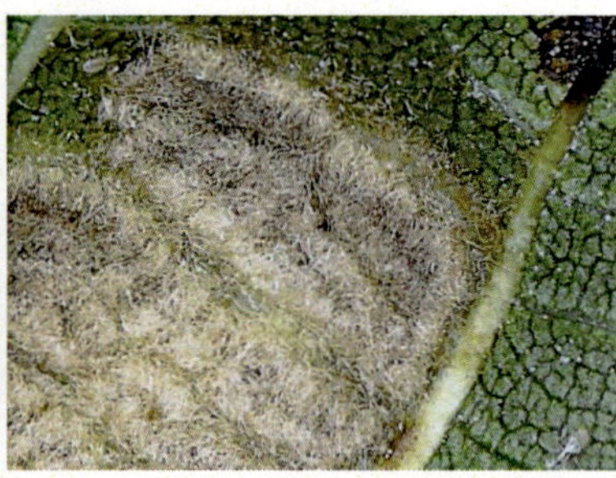

Symptom on leaf - erineum

Nature of damage and symptoms

- Forms felt-like webs that resemble white, hairy growths on the surface of leaves, tender stalks, and flower buds (David, 1958)
- The surface of leaves, tender stems, and flower buds develop felt-like hairy outgrowth (Erineum) as a result of feeding

5. Jasmine Blossom Midge: *Contarinia maculipennis* Felt. Diptera, Cecidomyiidae

Biology: The adult midges are delicate with bright orange coloured abdomen, and the maggot of blossom midge was white, which later turned yellowish.

Nature of damage and symptoms

- Maximum incidence of blossom midge was reported during October (29%) (Gunasekaran, 1989)
- Maggots enter the buds through the base of the corolla and feed within them, resulting in shrivelled and swelled up base of the buds
- Feeding results in the formation of pinkish to purple discoloured buds and flowers which gradually dry up

Management

- Collection and destruction of infested plant parts
- Use light trap to attract and kill the adult moths
- Spray NSKE 5% or malathion 0.05% Proper pruning and hygienic maintenance of bushes
- Spraying of cypermethrin 0.05% or deltamethrin 0.0015%

6. Jasmine lace wing: *Corythauma ayyari*, Tingidae, Hemiptera

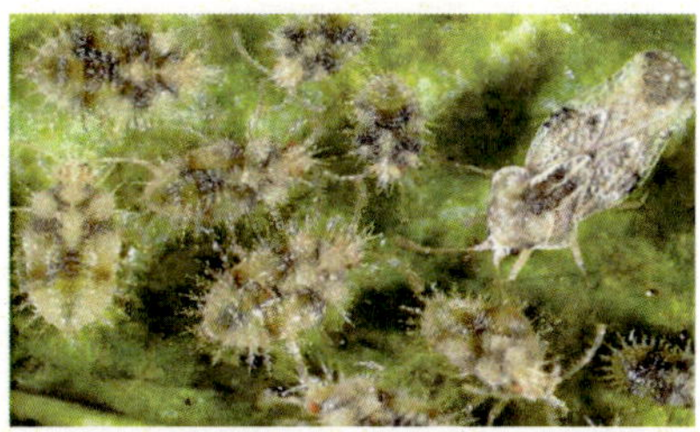

Corythauma ayyari – Nymphs & adults

The brown-coloured adults of tingids lay their eggs on the underside of leaves or midribs that were partially pushed into the plant tissue. The insect began by feeding on the underside of the leaves before moving on to the younger stems. Premature defoliation and the development of discoloured leaves from black excretions were the main symptoms (Nair and Nair, 1974 and Haouas *et al*., 2015).

7. Whitefly: *Dialeurodes kirkaldyi*, Aleyrodidae, Hemiptera

The adults and nymphs of whiteflies can be seen on the ventral side of leaves, along with hundreds on the veins and midrib. Continuous sap sucking results in the yellowing of the leaves. Sooty mold formation can also be observed on the underside of leaves due to honeydew excretion (Govindarajan *et al*., 1974 and Rabeena *et al*., 2020).

8. Thrips: *Thrips orientalis* Bagnall, Thripidae, Thysanoptera

T. orientalis is black-colored and infests both buds and flowers. Feeding causes elongated brownish streaks on buds and flowers. The second fortnight of April is reported to have the highest thrips population (Neelima, 2005).

References

Biotica Res. Today 2(6):414-415.

David, S. K. 1958. Insects and mites affecting jasmine in Madras state. Madras Agric. J. 45:146-150.

Govindarajan, R., David, B. V., Srinivasan, P. M., and Subramaniam, T. R. 1974. Aleurotrachelus sp. A new whitefly pest of Jasminum auriculatum and its control. S. Indian Hortic. 22(1): 24-25.

Gunasekaran, V. 1989. Studies on the bio-ecology of jasmine pest complex. M. Sc (Ag) thesis, Tamil Nadu Agricultural University, Coimbatore, 160p.

Haouas, D., Guilbert, E., and Halima-Kamel, B. M. 2015. First report of Corythauma ayyari (Drake) (Hemiptera: Tingidae) on arabian and spanish jasmine in Tunisia. EPPO Bull. 45(1): 144-147.

Kamala, I. M. and Kennedy, J. S. 2016. Evaluation of microbial agents against jasmine budworm, Hendecasis duplifascialis Hampson in jasmine (Jasminum sambac L.). Curr. Biot. 10(3): 230-240.

Nair, C. P. R. and Nair, M. R. G. K. 1974. Studies on the biology of the lacewing, Corythauma ayyari Drake a pest of jasmine. Aggric. Res. J. Kerala 12: 172-173.

Neelima, Y. 2005. Bioecology and management of jasmine pests. Ph.D thesis, Acharya NG Ranga Agricultural University, Rajendranagar, Hyderabad, 260p

Rabeena, I., Bose, A. S. C., and Sathyan, T. 2020. Pests of jasmine and their management.

Reddy, A. S., Krishnamurthy, B. H. R., and Wilson, Y. 1978. Chemical control of jasmine pests.

Sandhu, G. S. and Shukla, G. K. 1984. Chemical control of jasminum leaf webworm. Pestology 8(1): 17-19.

Shobitha, C. A. 2001. Studies on the bud borer complex of jasmine. M. Sc.(Ag) thesis, University of Agricultural Science, Bengaluru, 127p.

South Indian Hort. 26: 25-27.

Sudhir, B. 2002. Survey and management of insect and mite pests of Jasminum spp. M.Sc. thesis, University of Agricultural Science, Dharwad, 139p.

Questions

1. Webbing of flower buds with silken threads and feeding inside them is the characteristic symptom of
   a) *Hendecasis duplifascialis*
   b) *Elasmopalpus jasminophagus*
   c) *Nausinoe geometralis*
2. Pupation of bud worm occurs mostly in
   a) Leaf web b) Buds
   c) Soil
3. Pupation of the jasmine web worm occurs in
   a) Leaf web b) Soil
   c) Flower bud
4. Feeding of which pests results in the formation of felt-like hairy outgrowth (Erineum) on the surface of leaves, tender stem, and flower buds of jasmine
   a) Bud worm b) Eriophyid mite
   c) Jasmine lacewing bug
5. *Elasmopalpus jasminophagus* is the scientific name of
   a) Jamine bud worm b) Jasmine web worm
   c) Jasmine gallery worm

Answer Key

1	a	2	c	3	a	4	b	5	c				

16

Pests of Rose

Rose, one of the most popular cut flowers of the world known as the queen of flowers owing to its fragrance and aesthetic value. The rose has represented love, affection, innocence, and other noble traits for thousands of years. Roses are used for bouquets, flower arrangements, garlands, and worship. Apart from these, it is widely used in ayurvedic preparations, perfumes, soaps, cosmetics and also as flavouring agents in soft drinks and beverages.

Sl No.	Common name	Scientific name	Family and Order
1	Rose thrips	Rhipiphorothrips cruentatus	Thripidae, Thysanoptera
2	Red Scale	Lindingaspis rossi	Coccidae, Hemiptera
3	Aphids	Macrosiphum rosaeformis	Aphididae, Hemiptera
4	Red spider mite	Tetranychus cinnabarinus	Tetranychidae, Acarina
5	Leafcutter bee	*Megachile anthracina*	Megachilidae, Hymenoptera
6	Blackfly	*Aleurocanthus spiniferus, A. rosae*	Aleyrodidae, Hemiptera
7	Hairy caterpillar	Euproctis fraterna	Lymantriidae, Lepidoptera
8	Flower chaffer beetle	Oxycetonia versicolor	Cetoniidae, Coleoptera

1. Rose thrips: *Rhipiphorothrips cruentatus,* Thripidae, Thysanoptera

Adults are blackish brown in colour while nymphs are reddish in colour. Both adult and nymph lacerates leaves from the under surface and also on flower and flower buds.

Host range: Rose, grapes, *Lagestoemia indica, Punica granatum.*

Biology: Adult thrips lay about 45-55 eggs. Eggs are inserted into the plant tissues. The nymphal period is about 2-3 weeks, and the adult period is about five days.

Nature of damage and symptoms

- The undersurface of leaves and flower buds are lacerated by nymphs and adults
- Continous feeding results in the formation of white streaks on the leaf surface (Ananthakrishnan, 1973)
- The leaves get deformed, display brown patches, eventually wither, and fall off
- Infested flowers do not open, they fade and fall off

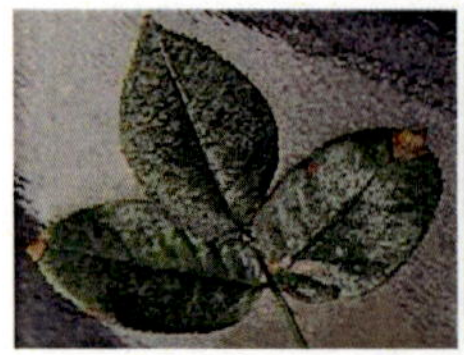
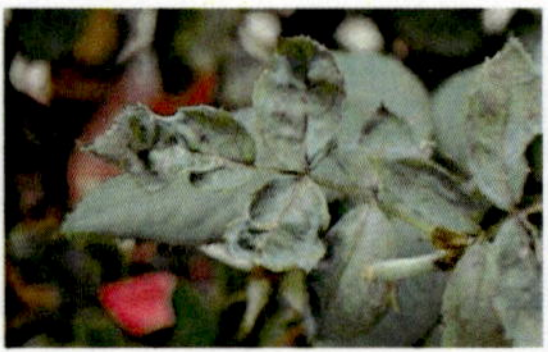
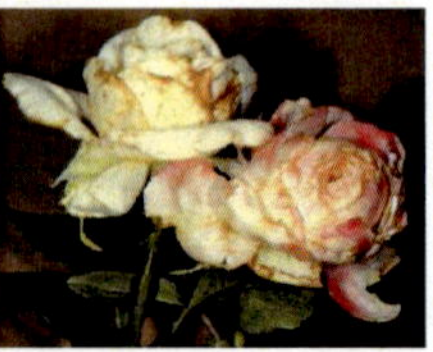
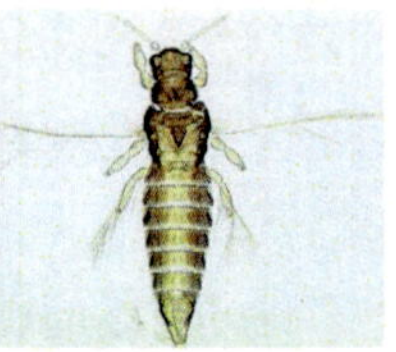

Damage symptoms on leaf and flower *R. cruentatus*

Management

- Remove and destroy the damaged leaves, twigs, and flower buds along with the pest
- Use blue sticky traps at 15/ha to monitor the pests
- Spray neem oil 3%
- Spray methyl demeton 1ml/ L or Spinosad 45 SC 3.3 ml/L or acetamiprid 20 SP 1-2g/L

2. Red Scale: *Lindingaspis rossi*, Coccidae, Hemiptera

Host range: Rose, raspberries, lemon grass, black berry

Biology: Males with extended wings migrate to fertilize the female scale, while females are wingless, bigger, and settle in suitable feeding locations.

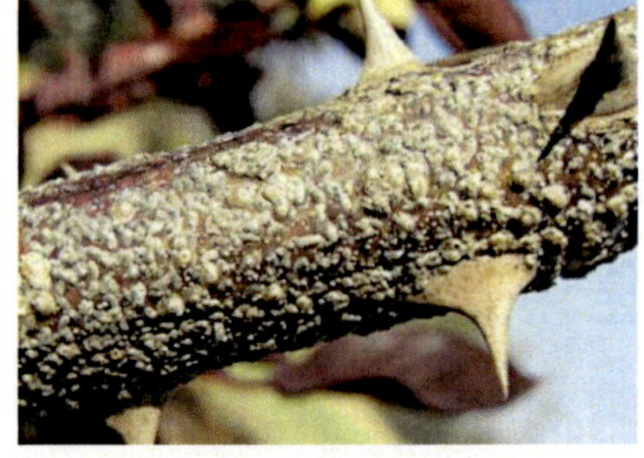

Red scale infestation on stem

Nature of damage and symptoms

- The stem gets entirely covered with reddish-brown, waxy scales, particularly on the lower part of the older stem and younger branches (Nair, 1975)
- The affected stems have tiny dots that resemble pox spots in scurvy-like areas
- The affected plant portions dry out and deteriorate
- In case of severe infestation, the entire plant dies

Management

- Cut and burn affected branches
- Rub off scales with cotton soaked in kerosene or diesel
- Spray malathion 2 ml/L at time of pruning
- Spray fish oil resin soap 25g/L

3. Aphids: *Macrosiphum rosaeformis,* Aphididae, Hemiptera

Host range: Rose

Biology: Aphids are small, soft-bodied, pear-shaped, and range in colour from pale green to dark blackish green. Large red eyes, black cornicles, a yellowish-green tip at the abdomen, and an elongated body are characteristics of the apterous type. For apterous forms, nymphal development takes 11–14 days, but for alate forms, it takes 14–19 days

Nature of damage and symptoms

- Nymphs and adults are found in clusters on the tender shoots, flowers and buds and suck sap
- Withering of tender shoots
- Buds fall off prematurely and the flowers show fading

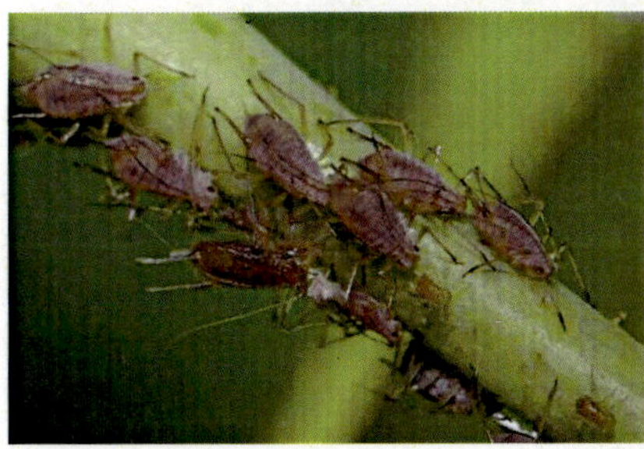
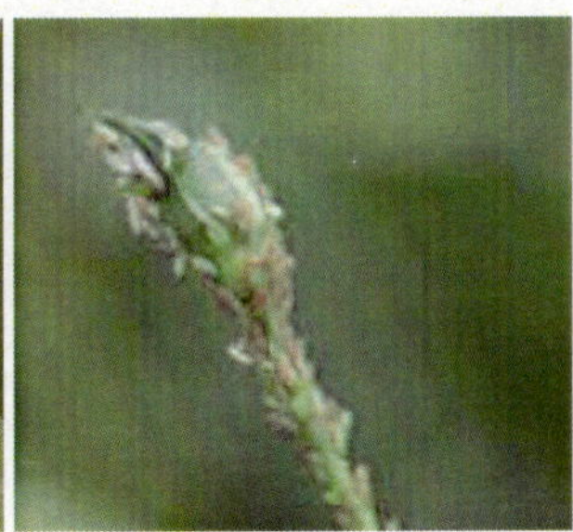

Aphid clonies on rose stem and flower bud

Management

- Spray dimethoate 30EC @ 1.5 mL/L after pruning of affected branches

4. Red spider mite: *Tetranychus cinnabarinus*, Tetranychidae, Acarina

Biology: Adults and nymphs are both red in colour. About 200 spherical, white eggs are laid on the ventral surface of the leaves. Larval and pupal phases are 3-5 and 8-12 days, respectively, whereas the egg period is 4-7 days. There are 15 generations annually, and the life cycle is completed within 15 to 20 days.

Nature of damage and symptoms

- Feed on the undersurface of leaves and are covered with silken webs
- Yellow spots appear on the upper surface and leaves turn reddish due to feeding
- Affected leaves finally wither
- Growth and flower production are adversely affected

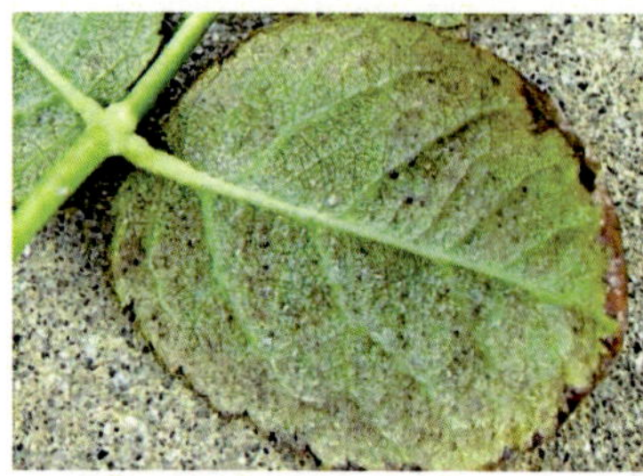
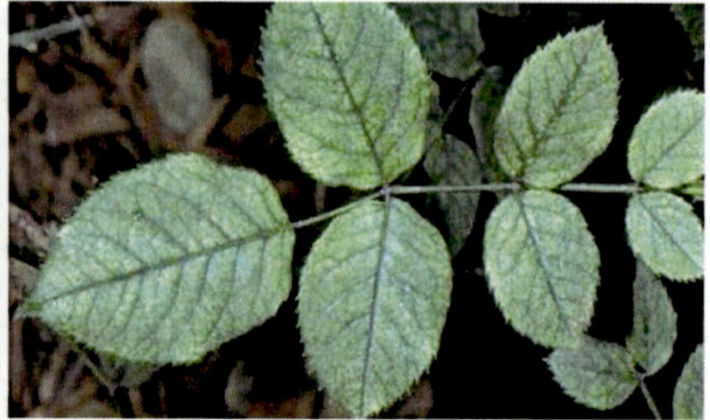

Mite infestation on leaves

Management

- Remove and destroy the damaged leaves along with mites
- Spray dicofol 2 ml or wettable sulphur 2g/L

5. Leafcutter bee: *Megachile anthracina*, Megachilidae, Hymenoptera

Host range: Red gram, rose

Biology: Adults are hairy, medium-sized dark insects. The base of the insect's abdomen is tinged with a red-brown colour. They build cells in crevices and cavities in hedges, dead wood *etc.*

Nature of damage and symptoms

- Leafcutter bees cause characteristic damage to rose leaves **(Ayyar, 1940)**
- Cut neat circular or oval patches from the leaf margin
- Cut bits of leaves are used for nest cell construction

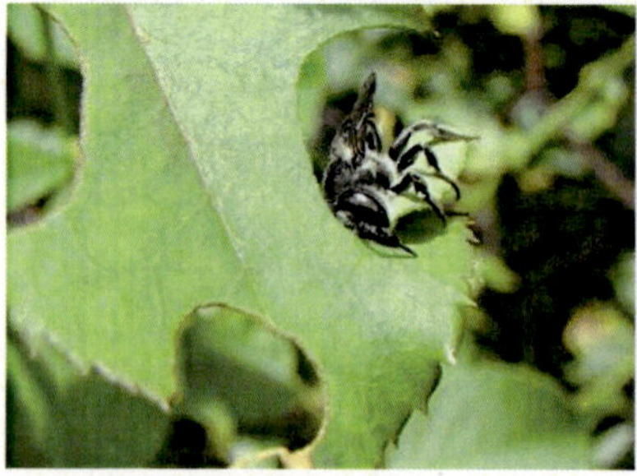
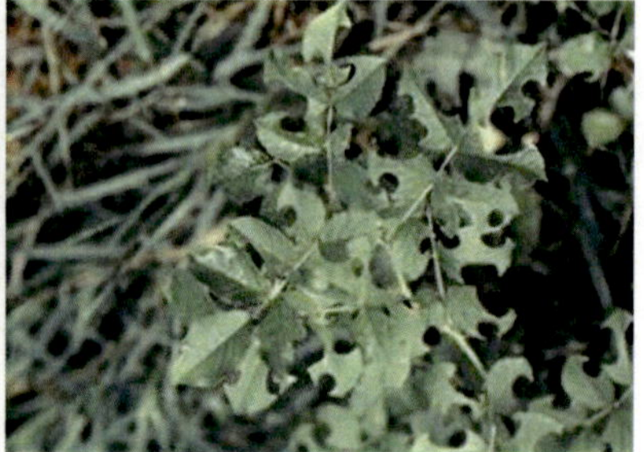

Damage symptoms on leaves

Management

- Insecticides are ineffective in preventing leafcutter bees
- Cover susceptible plants with cheesecloth or loose netting to prevent leaf injury

- Breeding sites should be eliminated
- Application of sawdust on the tunnel or thick-stemmed plants with a hollow opening

6. Blackfly: *Aleurocanthus spiniferus, A. rosae*, Aleyrodidae, Hemiptera

Adult flies lay eggs on the undersurface of leaves. The nymphs are brownish yellow and the pupa is black with cotton fringes around. Nymphs and adults suck the sap of the leaves, causing crinkling. Black oval puparia can be seen on the undersurface of leaves (Nair, 1975).

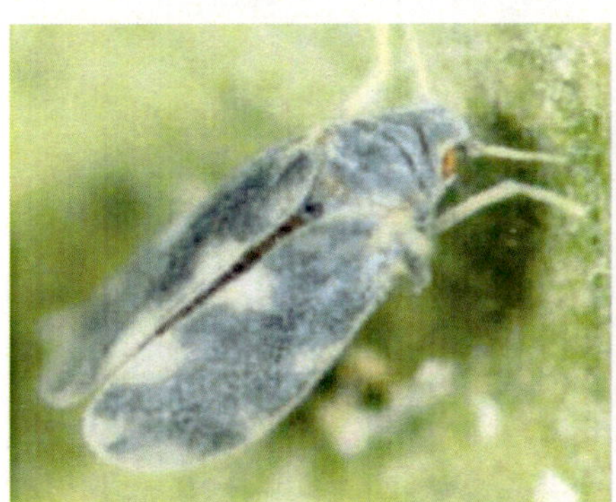
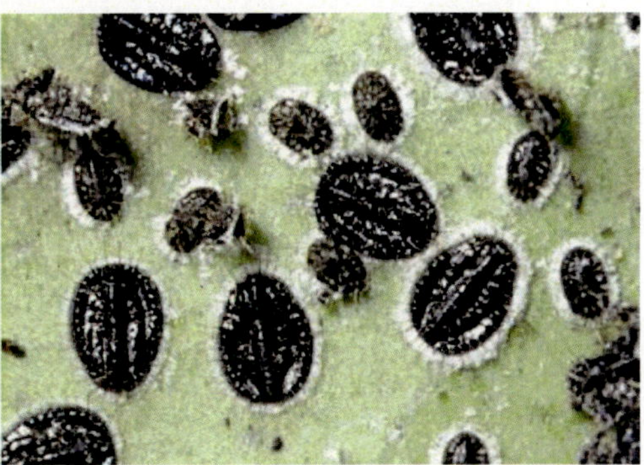

Adult and nymphs of *A. spiniferus*

7. Hairy caterpillar: *Euproctis fraternal*, Lymantriidae, Lepidoptera

Host range: Polyphagous, castor, mango, red gram, linseed, ground nut, grapevine, phalsa, pomegranate, and pear

Larva is reddish brown with red head surrounded by white hairs arising on warts and a long preanal tuft. Adult moths are yellowish with pale transverse lines on the forewings. Larval feeding results in defoliation.

8. Flower chaffer beetle: *Oxycetonia versicolor*, Cetoniidae, Coleoptera

Adult beetles are red-coloured with black markings. Feeding results in buds and flowers with irregular feeding marks. Causes girdling of twigs (Ayyar, 1940).

References

Ananthakrishnan, T.N. 1973. Thrips. Biology and control. Mac Millan Co. of India Ltd. 120p.

Ayyar Ramakrishna, T.V. 1940. Handbook of economic entomolgy for South India.

Nair, M.R.G.K. 1975. Insects and mites of crops in India. ICAR, New Delhi. 4p.

Questions

1. Leaves with yellow patches and black spots of excreta on rose are caused by
   a) *Rhipiphorothrips cruentatus* b) *Tetranychus cinnabarinus*
   c) *Lindingaspis rossi*
2. Circular or semi-circular cuttings on rose leaves are characteristic symptoms of
   a) Leafcutter bee b) Flower chaffer beetle
   c) Hairy caterpillar
3. Buds and flowers with irregular feeding marks is due to
   a) Leafcutter bee b) Flower chaffer beetle
   c) Hairy caterpillar
4. Silken webs on the undersurface of the rose leaf are caused by
   a) *Rhipiphorothrips cruentatus* b) *Tetranychus cinnabarinus*
   c) *Lindingaspis rossi*

Answer Key

1	a	2	a	3	b	4	b

17

Pests of Anthurium

Anthurium is a famous decorative cut flower and pot plant in the Araceae (order Spathiflorae) genus because of its extended vase life and beautiful, long-lasting inflorescences. After orchids, anthurium sales are the second-highest in the world.

Anthurium Thrips	:	*Chaetanaphothrips orchidii* Moulton
Order	:	Thysanoptera
Family	:	Thripidae

Biology: *Chaetanaphothrips orchidii* are small, pale yellow thrips commonly found in unopened anthurium buds and flowers. These pests are also commonly found in orchids. Females reproduce parthogenetically and on an average 80-100 eggs are laid by each female (Hata and Hara, 1998). Eggs are inserted inside the flower bud or leaf sheath. Nymphs are light yellowish in colour and are similar to the adults. Pupation takes place beneath the host plant in the soil or growing media. The entire life cycle lasts approximately 28 to 32 days but can extend up to 3 months, depending on the temperature. Increased temperatures and humidity, along with new growth of host plants, seem to promote thrips feeding and reproduction, resulting in heavier infestations and greater damage during the summer months

Nature of damage

Thrips typically favour feeding on young, succulent, immature flowers, and foliage. As soon as the bud appears from the leaf axil, both adult and juvenile thrips start feeding inside the unopened anthurium spathe.

Symptoms

Damage to anthurium appears as white streaks or scarring on the front and back of the spathe, deformed spathes, and with age, bronzing of injured tissue. Generally, white streaks and scarring on spathes caused by anthurium thrips are wider than those caused by banana rust thrips which is a closely related species. In severe cases, anthurium spathes fail to open, foliage may be deformed with bronzing and streaking, and reduced plant growth may occur.

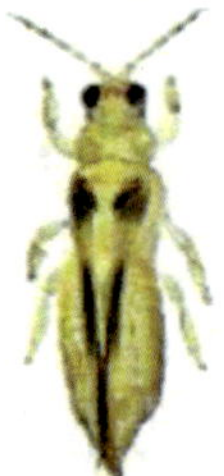
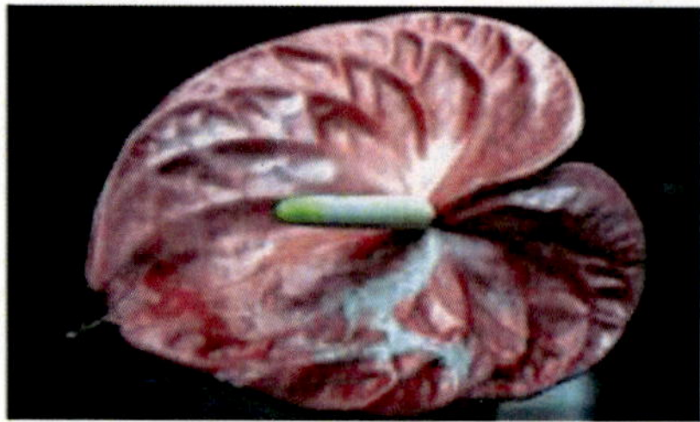
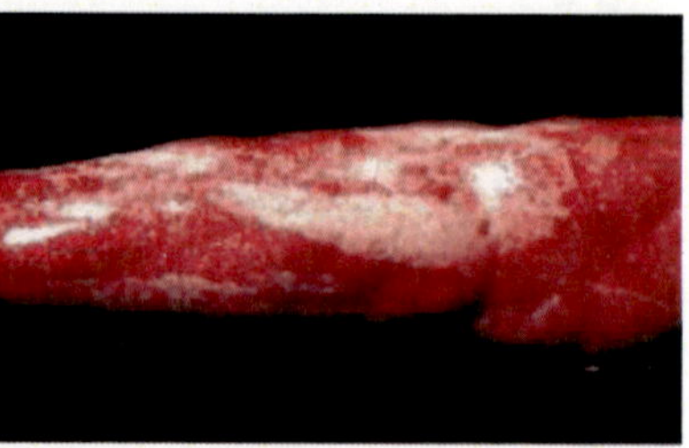

Chaetanaphothrips orchidii Symptoms on flower and flower bud

Management

- Thrips infested plant parts should be clipped off and destroyed
- In netted areas, insecticide granules are very effective in decreasing injury to flowers by *C. orchidii*
- Foliar sprays cyfluthrin 2.0 EC and chlorpyriphos 1ml/lit are effective in reducing the number of injured flowers.
- Spraying of dimethoate 30 EC @ 1 ml/l also controls thrips.
- Field release of predatory mite *Amblyseius cucumeris* 500,000/ha is effective in reducing thrips infestation

Red spidermites : *Tetranychus cinnabarinus* Boisduval

Subclass : Acari

Family : Tetranychidae

Nymphs and adults are red in colour. Eggs are laid on the ventral surface of the leaves and are whitish, spherical in shape

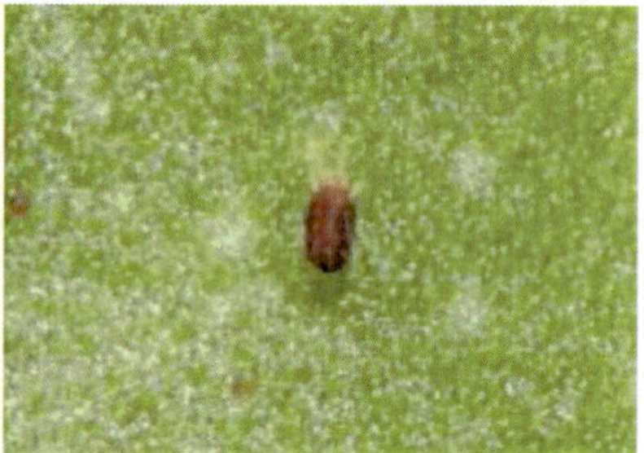

Tetranychus cinnabarinus adult

Nature of damage and Symptoms

- Colonies of nymphs and adults are seen on undersurface of leaves and inside spathes
- Feeding cause motling and wilting of affected parts
- Leaves shrivel and turn brown
- A fine web spun on the undersurface of leaves

Management

- Spraying the affected plants with dicofol 18.5 EC @ 3 ml/l of water.
- Field release of predatory mite - *Phytoseiulus persimilis* 6/ m2

Aphids : *Myzus circumflexus*

Order : Acari

Family : Aphididae

Myzus circumflexus is a polyphagous aphid species reported to infest Anthurium, particularly under humid, protected conditions like greenhouses and shade houses, where the environment supports aphid multiplication.

Nature of damage and Symptoms

- Nymphs and adults suck the plant sap
- Yellowing, curling and distortion of leaves and poor growth
- Honeydew excretion causes black sooty mould fungus

Management

- A formulation containing pyrethrum extract gave effective control
- Field release of parasitic wasp *Aphidius colemani* 5/m2 per week
- In case of severe infestation, spraying with imidacloprid 17.8 SL @ 3ml/10l or thiamethoxam @ 2g/10l is effective

References

Hata, T. Y., & Hara, A. H. (1992). Anthurium thrips, Chaetanaphothrips orchidii (Moulton): biology and insecticidal control on Hawaiian anthuriums. International Journal of Pest Management, 38(3), 230-233.

Hara, H. A., Jacobsen, C. and DuPonte N.R.2002. Anthurium thrips damage to ornamentals in Hawaii Cooperative Extension Services

18

Pests of Orchids

Orchids belong to the family Orchidaceae, one of the largest and most diverse families of flowering plants, with over 28,000 species and more than 100,000 hybrids worldwide. They are renowned for their exotic beauty, structural diversity, and ornamental value. Orchids, a diverse and prized group of ornamental plants, are sensitive to a variety of insect and mite pests. These pests affect orchids grown both under protected conditions (greenhouses, polyhouses) and in open environments.

Sl No.	Common name	Scientific name	Family and Order
1	Brown Soft Scale	*Coccus hesperidium*	Coccidae, Hemiptera
2	Elongate Soft Scale	*Coccus longulus*	Coccidae, Hemiptera
3	Boisduval Scale	*Diaspis boisduvali*	Diaspididae, Hemiptera
4	Long-tailed mealybug	*Pseudococcus longispinus*	Pseudococcidae, Hemiptera
5	Citrus mealybug	*Planococcus citri*	Pseudococcidae, Hemiptera
6	Solanum mealybug	*Phenacoccus solenopsis*	Pseudococcidae, Hemiptera
7	Western flower thrips	*Frankliniella occidentalis*	Thripidae, Thysanoptera
8	Chilli thrips	*Scirtothrips dorsalis*	Thripidae, Thysanoptera
9	Orchid thrips	*Dichromothrips spp*	Thripidae, Thysanoptera
10	Green peach aphid	*Myzus persicae*	Aphididae, Hemiptera
11	Cotton aphid	*Aphis gossypii*	Aphididae, Hemiptera
12	Banana aphid	*Pentalonia nigronervosa*	Aphididae, Hemiptera
13	Gray garden slug	*Deroceras reticulatum*	Stylommatophora
14	Giant African snail	*Achatina fulica*	Stylommatophora
15	Common garden snail	*Cornu aspersum*	Stylommatophora
16	Two-spotted spider mite	*Tetranychus urticae*	Tetranychidae
17	Carmine spider mite	*Tetranychus cinnabarinus*	Tetranychidae

Scales

Brown Soft Scale : *Coccus hesperidium*

Elongate Soft Scale : *Coccus longulus*

Family : Coccidae

Boisduval Scale : *Diaspis boisduvali*

Family : Diaspididae

Order : Hemiptera

Distribution: Kerala, Tamil Nadu, Karnataka, West Bengal, Assam, Sikkim, Maharashtra

Biology: Eggs are laid under the female's shell and may remain after death. Crawlers are mobile and settle to feed, secreting protective coverings. Females remain stationary; males, where present, are short-lived and winged. Multiple overlapping generations per year occur under warm, humid conditions. Crawlers are the most susceptible to control treatments (Smith *et al.*, 2018).

Brown Soft Scale – *Coccus hesperidium* Linn

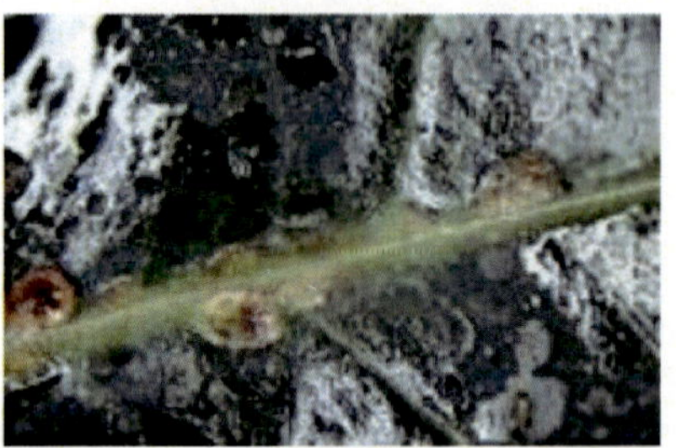

Adult females: Oval, convex, with a smooth shell, yellow to dark brown, 3–4 mm.

Males: Winged, rare.

Crawlers: Yellowish-pink, flat, mobile.

Elongate Soft Scale – *Coccus longulus* Douglas

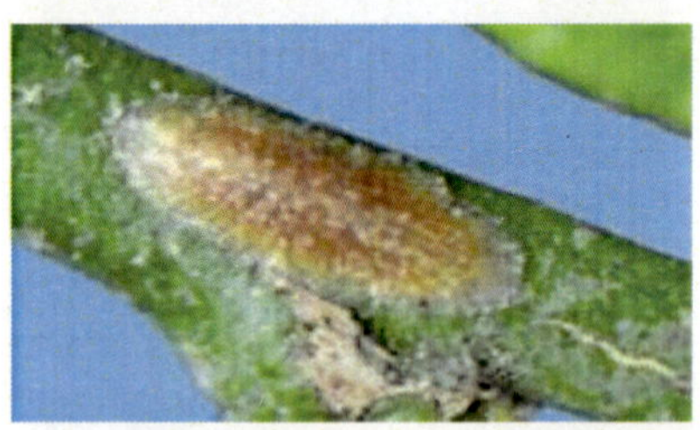

Adult females: Elongated oval, soft-bodied, tan to brown, up to 5 mm.

Surface: Smooth and slightly glossy.

Crawlers: Similar to *C. hesperidium*.

Boisduval Scale – *Diaspis boisduvali*

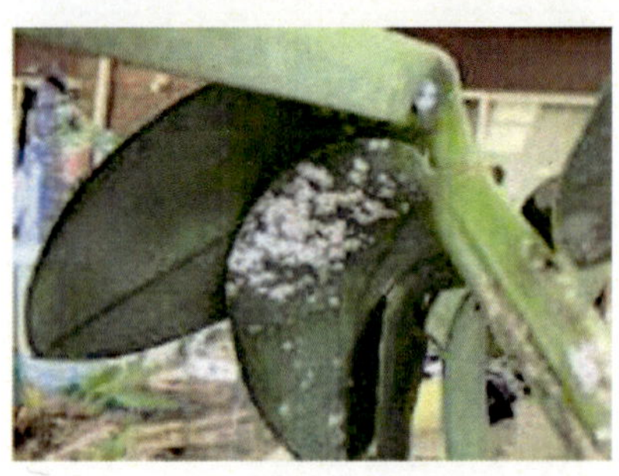

Adult females: Rounded, pale yellow to white with hard armored cover.

Males: Cottony aggregations, often confused with mealybugs.

Crawlers: Tiny, yellow to pink, briefly mobile

Nature of damage and symptoms

Shell-like bodies appear on leaves, stems, flowers, and roots. Feeding leads to yellowing, wilting, poor vigor, and flower drop. Soft scales excrete honeydew, which promotes sooty mould. Boisduval scale does not excrete honeydew but forms dense colonies at plant bases. Severe infestations can cause decline or death, especially in young or stressed plants (Jones & Lee, 2010).

Management

- Regular monitoring of pests, especially in leaf axils, undersides, and pseudobulbs
- Isolate newly acquired or infected plants to prevent spread
- Manually remove adults with alcohol swabs or soft brushes
- Prune and destroy heavily infested plant parts.
- Apply horticultural oils, neem oil, or insecticidal soap with full coverage
- Imidacloprid 17.8 SL @ 3ml/10l / dimethoate 30 EC @ 1.5 ml/l

Mealybugs

Long-tailed mealybug	:	*Pseudococcus longispinus*
Citrus mealybug	:	*Planococcus citri*
Solanum mealybug	:	*Phenacoccus solenopsis*
Family	:	Pseudococcidae
Order	:	Hemiptera

Distribution: Kerala, Tamil Nadu, Karnataka, West Bengal, Assam, Sikkim, Maharashtra

Biology: Mealybugs are small, soft-bodied, oval insects covered with a white, waxy, mealy secretion that gives them a cottony appearance. Adults are pale pink to gray underneath and measure about 1–4 mm depending on species. Nymphs resemble smaller versions of adults and are similarly wax-coated. Females lay hundreds of eggs in cottony sacs hidden in leaf axils or crevices. The life cycle includes egg, nymph, and adult stages, with no pupal stage. Depending on temperature and species, they mature and begin reproducing in 24–73 days. Males, if present, are winged and short-lived. Mealybugs feed on phloem sap, reducing plant vigor and secreting honeydew, which fosters black sooty mold (Patel & Kumar, 2015). Their waxy covering repels water and makes them resistant to many contact insecticides. Infestations typically develop under warm, humid conditions and spread easily via tools, containers, or infested plant material.

Nature of damage and Symptoms

Suck sap from the phloem, causing reduced vigor, stunted growth, leaf yellowing, flower and bud drop. Excrete honeydew, attracting black sooty mold and interfering with photosynthesis. Infest leaf axils, undersides, pseudobulbs, buds, and flower stems. Heavy infestations distort new growth and may lead to plant decline.

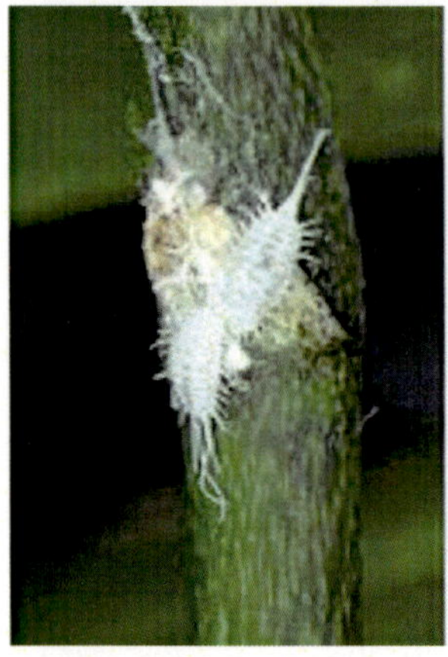
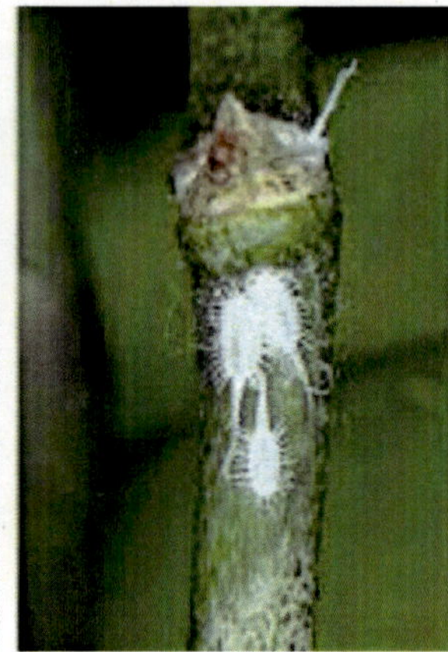

P. longispinus on shoots

Management

- Isolate infested plants promptly.
- Apply insecticidal soap or horticultural oil after disrupting mealy layer (Martin & Brown, 2012).
- Use systemic insecticides (e.g., imidacloprid) for phloem-level control.
- Perform 3–4 treatments at 3–7 day intervals.
- Maintain good sanitation and monitoring to prevent reinfestation.

Thrips

Western flower thrips	:	*Frankliniella occidentalis*
Chilli thrips	:	*Scirtothrips dorsalis*
Orchid thrips	:	*Dichromothrips spp*
Family	:	Thripidae
Order	:	Thysanoptera

Distribution: Kerala, Tamil Nadu, Karnataka, Maharashtra, West Bengal, Sikkim, Assam

Biology: Thrips are slender, minute insects (1–2 mm), with fringed wings and rapid, agile movement. They feed by rasping plant tissues and sucking up cell contents, leading to silvering or scarring. Adults are usually yellowish, brown, or black depending on species, while nymphs are wingless and paler. Thrips complete their life cycle in as little as two weeks under warm conditions, and pupate in soil or debris.

Nature of damage and symptoms

- Both nymphs and adults suck sap from leaves and floral parts
- Silvery or bleached streaks and scratch patterns on leaves
- Distorted and decimated flowers, often failing to open properly (Walker *et al.*, 2017)
- Black specks of frass and shiny excretory trails on foliage
- Bud blasting or aborted flower development
- Feeding sites often lead to necrotic patches and leaf curl
- Capable of transmitting viruses between orchid plants Aesthetic and commercial value of flowers severely reduced

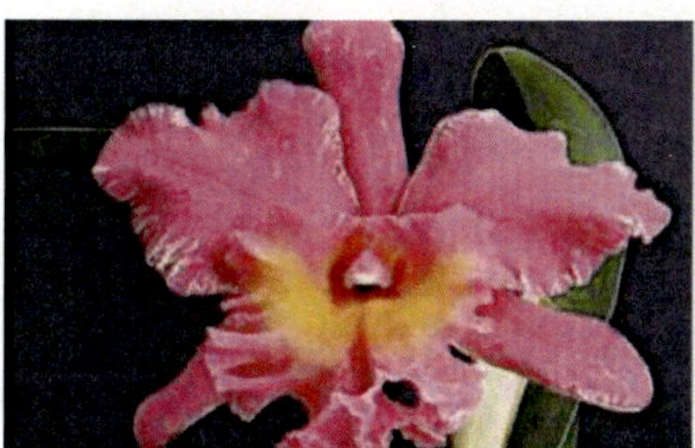
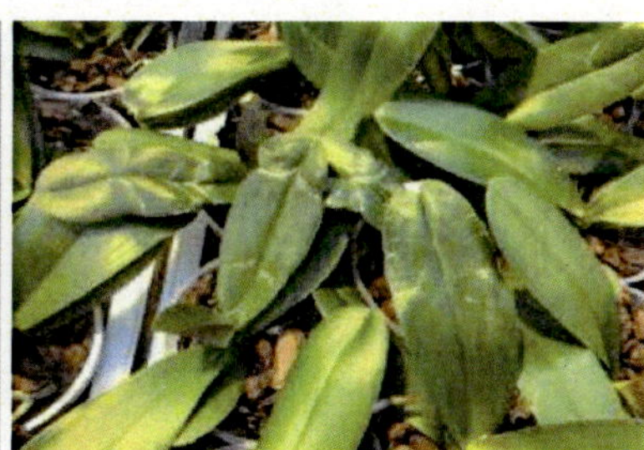

Frankliniella occidentalis -Orchid flower Symptoms on leaves

Management

- Collection and destruction of heavily infested plant parts
- Biological control: Release predatory mites (*Amblyseius cucumeris*) weekly for 2–3 rounds; they consume thrips and spider mites effectively
- Use insecticidal soaps and apply thoroughly and repeatedly
- Use blue sticky traps to monitor and reduce adult populations
- Thrips are resistant to most systemic insecticides; rely on contact sprays (Nguyen *et al.*, 2019)
- Treat soil with compatible insecticide to target pupating stages
- Pongamia oil 2% spraying or neem oil emulsion 2% is effective during the initial stage of infestation
- Spraying of acephate 0.1% or chlorpyriphos 0.02% when crawling of ants are noticed

Aphids

Green peach aphid : *Myzus persicae*

Cotton aphid : *Aphis gossypii*

Banana aphid : *Pentalonia nigronervosa*

Family : Aphididae

Order : Hemiptera

Distribution: Kerala, Tamil Nadu, Karnataka, Maharashtra, West Bengal, Assam, Sikkim

Biology: Aphids are small, soft-bodied insects (1–3 mm long), often green, black, brown, or yellow, and found in dense colonies on new growth, buds, and the undersides of leaves. They are sap-sucking pests that reproduce rapidly by parthenogenesis; a single female can produce 60–100 live nymphs daily for 20–30 days. Nymphs mature into reproductive adults in 7–10 days. In favorable greenhouse conditions, colonies grow rapidly year-round. Overcrowding triggers the development of winged forms, which migrate and start new infestations. In autumn, sexual reproduction leads to overwintering eggs. Aphids also shed white exuviae during molts, which often accumulate on plant surfaces (O'Connor, 2008).

Nature of damage and symptoms

- Curled or distorted leaves and stunted growth
- Sticky honeydew on leaves and stems
- Black sooty mold growing on honeydew
- Wilting, yellowing, and early leaf drop
- Deformed buds and mottled flowers if aphids feed on them (Lopez & Garcia, 2009).
- White cast skins on leaf surfaces

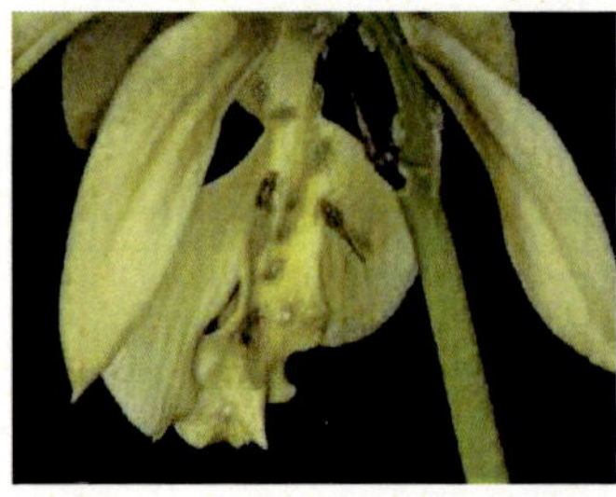
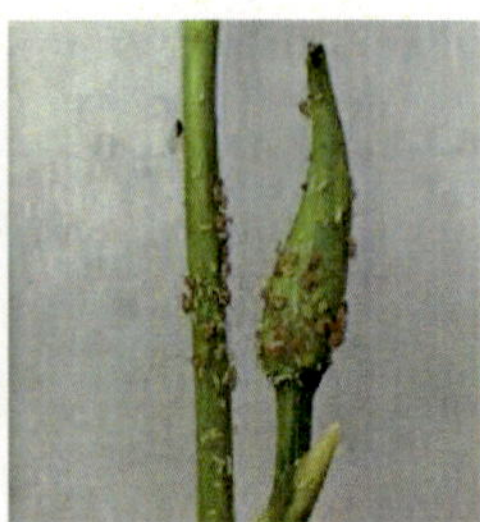

Symptoms on leaves, shoots and flower buds infestations

Management

- Isolate infested plants immediately
- Maintain good cultural hygiene and inspect new plants
- Use sugar-based ant baits to eliminate ant colonies

- Ensure greenhouse airflow control to limit aphid spread
- Biocontrols like lady beetles or lacewings can help in outdoor setting
- If the infestation is severe use imidacloprid 17.8 SL@ 3mL/10L or thiamethoxam25WG @ 2g/10L

Snails and slugs

Gray garden slug : *Deroceras reticulatum*

Giant African snail : *Achatina fulica*

Common garden snail : *Cornu aspersum*

Order : Stylommatophora

Distribution: Kerala, Tamil Nadu, Karnataka, Maharashtra, West Bengal, Sikkim, Assam

Biology: Slugs and snails are soft-bodied molluscs covered in mucus, requiring constant moisture to survive. They are hermaphrodites, meaning each individual can mate and lay eggs. In temperate regions, they overwinter in soil and debris, while in tropical and southern climates, they remain active year-round. Maturity is reached in about 3 to 6 months, after which they lay oval, translucent eggs in clusters of 3 to 40 in soil cracks or beneath debris. They are nocturnal, feeding at night or during cool, moist conditions, and avoiding dry, dusty environments. Movement is aided by a slimy trail, which also serves as a telltale sign of their presence. Because of their external mucus and non-insect physiology, slugs and snails are unaffected by insecticides and require separate management (Evans & Patel, 2006).

Nature of damage and symptoms

- Chew large, irregular holes with smooth edges in leaves, flowers, and buds
- Young and adult stages feed on leaves especially during night
- Scrap leaves, leaving only veins, cut holes on leaves and flowers, cut tender shoots
- Leave slimy mucous trails on foliage, pots, and benches (Roberts & Singh, 2014)
- Damage is more severe in wet or humid conditions
- May completely consume seedlings or severely deform flowers
- Often hide under pots, mulch, or leaf litter during the day

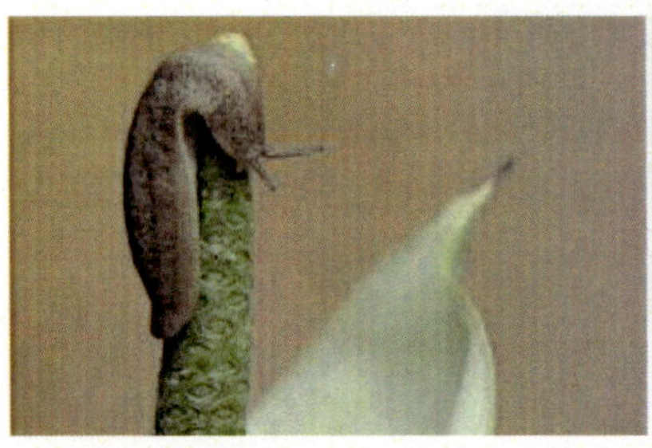

Deroceras reticulatum

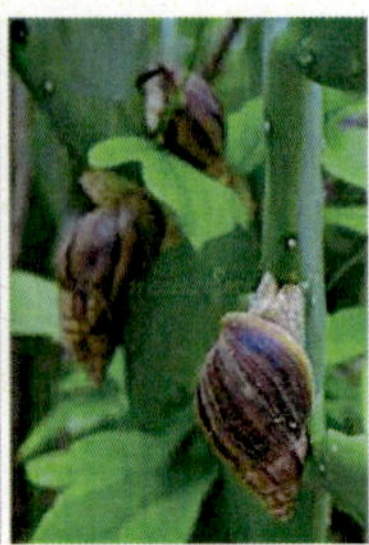

Achatina fulica

Management

- Use iron phosphate baits (e.g., Sluggo) as primary control
- Handpicking of grown up stages and killing them by dropping in 5% salt solution
- Trap the adults using wet jute bags
- Apply copper tape or sheeting around greenhouse bench legs
- Diatomaceous earth or ash barriers can help but fail when wet
- Use manual removal during night inspections
- Ensure greenhouse floors are sealed and dry
- Employ natural predators like ducks or chickens in open settings
- Spreading of 3% metaldehyde pellets in the field or 5% metaldehyde dust on plants

Spider mites

Two-spotted spider mite : *Tetranychus urticae*

Carmine spider mite : *Tetranychus cinnabarinus*

Family : Tetranychidae

Distribution: Kerala, Tamil Nadu, Karnataka, Maharashtra, West Bengal, Sikkim, Assam

Biology: Spider mites are extremely small arachnids, nearly invisible to the naked eye, measuring about 0.3–0.5 mm. They thrive in warm, dry environments and feed by puncturing individual leaf cells to extract contents (Chen & Davis, 2013), leaving behind pale speckling. Their life cycle is highly temperature-dependent, ranging from 40 days at 13°C (55°F) to just 5 days at 24°C (75°F). Females can lay up to 200 eggs, often on the undersides of leaves, and populations explode rapidly under favorable indoor or greenhouse conditions. Spider mites are most problematic on thin-leafed orchids and bright, sunlit parts of plants, especially during active growth or bloom periods.

They disperse through air currents or by hitchhiking on clothing. Webbing, pale stippling, and black specks of frass are the main visible signs of infestation.

Symptoms and nature of damage

- Undersides of leaves may have silken webbings
- Fine silky webbing on leaves, buds, and stems
- Leaves may be streaked or spotted due to lack of chlorophyll
- The upper surface becomes sunken and turns brown
- Pale speckled dots (stippling) caused by cell feeding
- Black frass spots scattered across infested areas
- Leaf yellowing, drying, and eventual leaf drop in severe cases
- Spider mites prefer thin-leaved orchids, but flowers of all orchids are susceptible (Alvarez *et al.*, 2011).

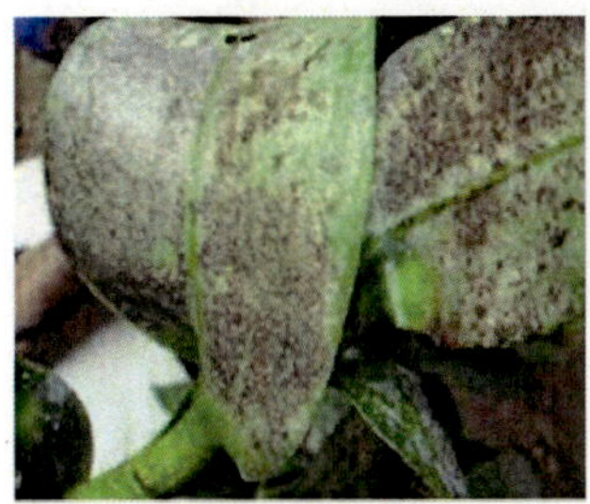

Symptoms on leaves

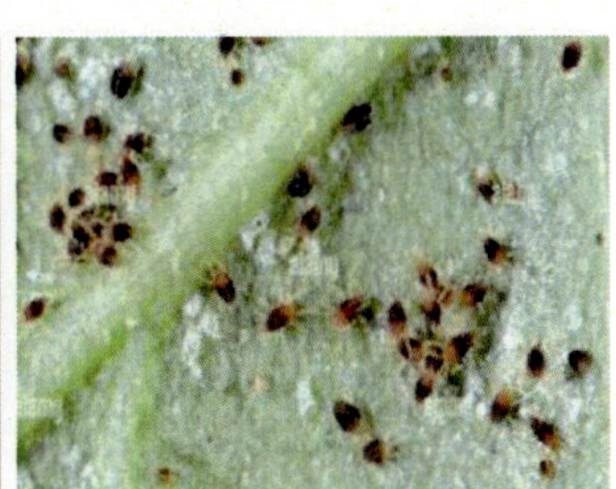

Population of spider mites – lower leaf surface

Management

- Mist or wash plants regularly to dislodge mites
- Use shaded net houses to reduce temperature spikes
- Release predatory mites such as *Phytoseiulus persimilis* and *Amblyseius cucumeris* for effective control
- Neem oil (0.5–1%) Suffocates mites and acts as an anti-feedant
- Abamectin 1.8 EC@0.5 ml/l or spiromesifen @ 1ml/l or propargite @ 2ml/l spray reduce mite infestation

References

Alvarez, M. J., Fernandez, R., & Lopez, D. 2011. Spider mite outbreaks in greenhouse orchids: temperature and humidity dynamics. Journal of Horticultural Pests, 22(3): 145–152.

Chen, S., & Davis, T. 2013. Feeding mechanics of spider mites on orchid foliage. International Journal of Plant Protection, 29(1): 25–31.

Evans, L., & Patel, R. 2006. Biology and management of slugs and snails in ornamental horticulture. Mollusk Management Journal, 5(2): 82–91.

Jones, P., & Lee, M. 2010. Scale insect infestations in young orchid seedlings. Orchid Science Journal, 14(4): 200–208.

Lopez, J., & Garcia, H. 2009. Aphid salivary toxins and damage in orchids. Plant Pathology Research, 17(2): 99–105.

Martin, G., & Brown, E. 2012. Resistance of mealybug wax coverings to contact insecticides. Entomology Today, 8(1): 12–18.

Nguyen, V., Tran, P., & Holmes, A. 2019. Thrips control in orchids: efficacy of contact agents vs systemic insecticides. Journal of Integrated Pest Management, 9(2): 85–93.

O'Connor, S. 2008. Parthenogenetic reproduction in aphids on orchids. Aphidology Research, 10(3): 50–57.

Patel, N., & Kumar, S. 2015. Honeydew and sooty mold development on orchids due to mealybug infestation. Mycology and Plant Health, 12(5): 210–218.

Roberts, A., & Singh, P. 2014. Molluscan feeding damage on ornamental orchids. Garden Pest Review, 6(3): 140–147.

Questions

1. Which orchid plant part is most commonly infested by aphids during active growth?

   a) Mature pseudobulbs b) Root tips

   c) New shoots and flower buds d) Leaf margins

2. What damage symptom is typically seen on orchid flowers due to thrips feeding?

   a) Petals turning translucent

   b) Blisters and necrotic rings

   c) Petal distortion and failed opening

   d) Purple discoloration on sepals

3. Spider mites are more likely to infest which type of orchids?

   a) Epiphytic orchids with thick leaves

   b) Orchids with bulbous stems

   c) Orchids with thin leaves and sun exposure

   d) Orchids grown in full shade

4. Which of the following pests is most likely to infest the base of orchid pseudobulbs and axils?

   a) Boisduval scale b) Western flower thrips

   c) Green peach aphid d) Carmine spider mite

5. What visual clue indicates early mealybug infestation on orchids?

   a) Brown crusts along midrib

   b) Cottony white masses near leaf axils

   c) Trdansparent tunnels in leaves

   d) Yellow leaf margins with red veins

6. Which pest's honeydew secretion on orchids can lead to black sooty mold development?

   a) Spider mites b) Aphids

   c) Thrips d) Boisduval scale

7. What is a likely consequence of orchid root infestation by soft scale insects?
   a) Pseudobulb cracking
   b) Leaf necrosis
   c) Sudden wilting and root rot symptoms
   d) Malformed flower spikes
8. How do slugs typically damage orchids?
   a) By laying eggs inside roots
   b) By chewing irregular holes in leaves and flowers
   c) By sucking phloem from buds
   d) By injecting toxins into tissue
9. Why is alcohol not recommended for controlling mealybugs on orchids?
   a) It promotes fungal infections
   b) It attracts more mealybugs
   c) It strips the protective epidermis of orchid tissues
   d) It reacts with potting medium and releases fumes
10. Which pest can be effectively controlled on orchids by releasing *Amblyseius cucumeris* mites indoors?
    a) Aphids
    b) Snails
    c) Thrips
    d) Mealybugs
11. What common pest signs might you find under orchid pots or trays?
    a) Scale colonies
    b) White cast skins
    c) Slug trails and fecal pellets
    d) Silk webbing
12. Which orchid pest can cause bud blasting, where buds drop before opening?
    a) Spider mites
    b) Aphids
    c) Thrips
    d) Snails

13. Which management practice is best to prevent aphid spread in orchid greenhouses?
    a) Use of sodium chloride drench
    b) High-nitrogen fertilization
    c) Isolating infested plants and using airflow control
    d) Deep irrigation during noon
14. Which orchid pest is known to migrate between plants when colonies become overcrowded, including forming winged morphs?
    a) Scale insects
    b) Aphids
    c) Mealybugs
    d) Spider mites
15. Why are systemic insecticides ineffective against spider mites on orchids?
    a) They develop resistance quickly
    b) They feed externally without ingesting phloem
    c) They are protected by hard exoskeletons
    d) They reproduce only in leaf crevices

Answer Key

1	c	2	c	3	c	4	a	5	b	6	b	7	c
8	b	9	c	10	c	11	c	12	c	13	c	14	b
15	b												

19

Pests of Gladiolus

Gladiolus is a genus comprising around 260 species of perennial flowering plants in the iris family (*Iridaceae*). Commonly known as "sword lilies," the name derives from their long, blade-like leaves—*gladius* being the Latin word for "sword." These plants grow from underground storage organs called corms and feature tall, unbranched stems that bear vibrant, trumpet-shaped flowers arranged in a single-sided spike. Their striking appearance makes them highly valued both in gardens and as cut flowers.

Most gladiolus species are native to sub-Saharan Africa, particularly South Africa, though some are also found in Europe and Asia. The flowers come in a wide variety of colors, forms, and often display intricate patterns or ruffled edges. Each flower is bisexual and sits between green bracts, with its tepals forming a characteristic funnel-shaped corolla. Known for their bold inflorescences and extended vase life, gladiolus flowers are a popular choice in floral design and landscaping worldwide

Sl. No.	Common name	Scientific name	Family and order	Siteof oviposition	Site of pupation
1.	Melon aphid	*Aphis gossypii*	Aphididae, Hemiptera		
2.	Potato aphid	*Macrosiphum euphorbiae*	Aphididae, Hemiptera		
3.	Gladiolus thrips	*Taeniothrips simplex, Taeniothrips traegardhi*	Thripidae, Hemiptera	Tissues of leave and flowers	
4.	Tarnished plant bug	*Lygus lineolaris*	Miridae, Hemiptera	Tender stems	

Melon aphid : *Aphis gossypii* Glover

Family : Aphididae

Order : Hemiptera

Biology: ***Aphis gossypii***, part of the Aphididae family, exhibits a wide range of colors that change with the season and host plant conditions. Females, which can be winged or wingless, are better described than males. The wingless females are live-bearing, about 1.5–1.8 mm long, with pear-shaped bodies varying from pale yellow to dark green or black. Yellow forms are smaller and appear in warm weather, while larger green forms occur in cooler temperatures or low populations. Color can also shift depending on the host plant. Their antennae have five or six pale segments with dark tips, and the head is smooth between the antennae. The eyes are dark brown, legs pale with darker joints, and the cauda varies from pale to dark with several setae. Cornicles are dark, cylindrical, and longer than the cauda. Winged females are more slender, 1.2–1.8 mm long with a 4.5–6.0 mm wingspan. Their antennae are longer, with the sixth segment longest and the third segment carrying 3–15 secondary rhinaria (Edde, 2022). *Aphis gossypii* usually reproduces without eggs except in colder regions, where eggs overwinter and hatch in about 4 days. Nymphs pass through five instars, molting four times before becoming adults. Adults can be winged or wingless; wingless females reproduce without mating, giving live birth. They live about 15 days reproductively, then 5 days post-reproductively. Under good conditions, females produce around 3 nymphs daily, with crowding and nutrition triggering winged forms for dispersal.

Nature of damage and symptoms

The damage can cause flower deformities and slow down plant growth, particularly in young plants. Aphids feed by sucking sap, resulting in stunted growth and weakened vigor. Infestations mainly target tender shoots and leaf undersides, causing leaves to curl, crinkle, and become distorted.

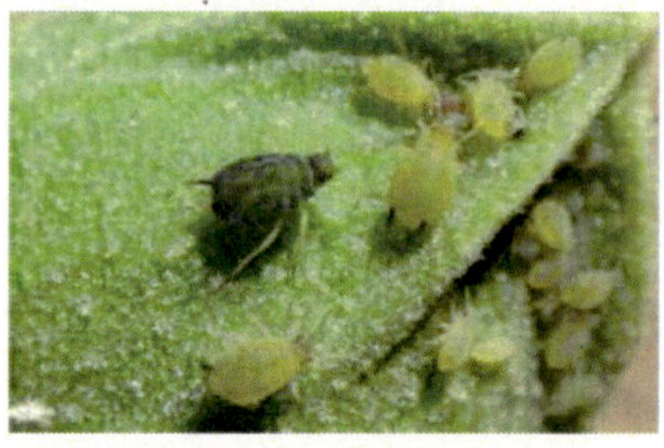

A. gossypii nymphs and adults

Potato aphid :
Macrosiphum euphorbiae Thomas

Family : Aphididae

Order : Hemiptera

Biology and lifecycle: The potato aphid is a medium to large-sized insect, typically green in color, though some forms may appear pink or magenta with reddish eyes. Originating from North America, this polyphagous species feeds on nearly 200 plant species across 20 different families, including several from the Solanum genus. The aphid often reproduces without a sexual phase but can occasionally have a complex life cycle involving different host plants. Its main hosts are rose species, although eggs may also be laid on various herbaceous plants (Saguez *et al.*, 2013). Throughout the growing season, reproduction is mostly asexual, with wingless females giving birth to live young without mating. Each female can produce between 50 and 67 offspring, and the time it takes for a nymph to reach reproductive maturity varies from 6 to 12 days, influenced by temperature. Multiple generations occur simultaneously each year, and in warm conditions, nymphs can mature in as little as 2 to 3 weeks. When food supplies dwindle or populations become overcrowded, some nymphs develop wings and fly off to colonize new plants.

Nature of damage and symptoms

Both the nymph and adult stages of *Macrosiphum euphorbiae* feed by sucking sap from plants, which reduces nutrient availability and disrupts the balance of growth hormones. This feeding causes slowed development, stunted plants, and misshapen leaves and stems. Common symptoms include yellowing or discoloration of leaves, overall decline in plant health and yield, and in severe infestations, young plants may die if attacked early in the growing season. Additionally, aphids produce honeydew, a sticky substance that encourages the growth of black sooty mold on plant surfaces.

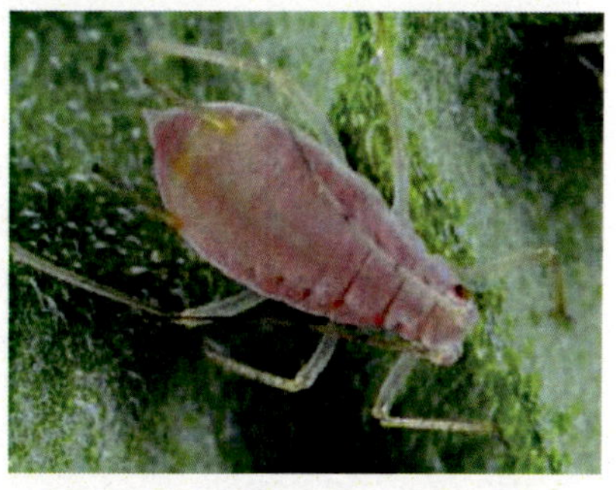

Adult of *Macrosiphum euphorbiae*

Gladiolus thrips : *Taeniothrips simplex* Morison.
Taeniothrips traegardhi Trybe.

Family : Thripidae

Order : Thysanoptera

Biology and lifecycle: *Taeniothrips simplex:* Adult thrips are tiny insects, approximately 1/16 inch in length, with dark brown bodies, lighter-colored leg tips, and a gray stripe across their wings. Males tend to be slightly smaller and paler than females. The larvae are light yellow with red eyes and are smaller than the adults. They undergo two pupal stages, both of which are dark orange in color and also have red eyes. Female thrips have a lifespan of 35–40 days, during which they lay between 100 and 200 tiny, white, kidney-shaped eggs within plant tissues such as leaves, flowers, or corms. The larvae are pale yellow with red eyes and feed on plant tissue, typically residing in buds or leaf sheaths before dropping to the ground to pupate. The pupal stage consists of two phases, both dark orange with red eyes, and while mostly inactive, they can move if disturbed. Adults initially appear milky-white but quickly darken to brown, featuring lighter leg tips and a gray band on their

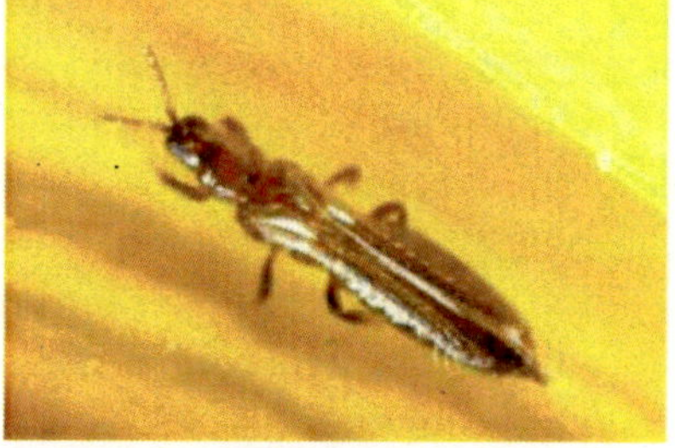

Taeniothrips simplex

wings, with females being slightly larger than males. Females outnumber males, and parthenogenetic reproduction is common. In warm conditions, the development cycle from egg to adult takes 2–4 weeks, allowing for nine or more generations in a single growing season.

Taeniothrips traegardhi: Adult thrips are small and slender, with males resembling females but having slight differences in their antennae. Females lay eggs inside plant tissues such as flowers or leaves, with incubation lasting 3 to 16 days depending on temperature. The larvae go through two feeding stages, mainly within flowers, before entering non-feeding pupal stages in concealed areas like flower parts or soil debris. The pupal phase can last from several days to over a week, influenced by environmental factors. Once adults emerge, they begin feeding, mating, and laying eggs. While most thrips reproduce sexually, some species can reproduce without fertilization. Females lay eggs soon after maturing, enabling multiple generations each year, especially in warm environments.

Nature of damage

Both larvae and adults feed by lacerating the plant tissues and extracting cell contents from leaves and flower spikes, resulting in direct damage and impaired plant growth. Initial symptoms include silvery marks on leaves that eventually turn brown and distorted. Flower buds can become misshapen or fail to open, and damaged spikes may produce poor blooms.

Tarnished plant bug : *Lygus lineolaris*

Family : Miridae

Order : Hemiptera

Biology and lifecycle: Adults measure around 6.5 mm and display varying colors, featuring a distinctive light "V" mark on their backs. The nymphs are wingless, yellow-green, and develop dark spots and wingpads as they grow. Adults survive the winter in protected areas and become active in early spring, feeding on buds before moving to crops. Females deposit single, flask-shaped eggs within plant tissue, which hatch in 7–10 days. Nymphs pass through five stages, reaching maturity in 2–3 weeks in warm conditions. The complete life cycle ranges from 18 to 30 days, with one to three generations annually depending on the climate. Egg-laying occurs throughout the growing season, with adults living 17–39 days and producing more eggs at higher temperatures.

Nature of damage and symptoms

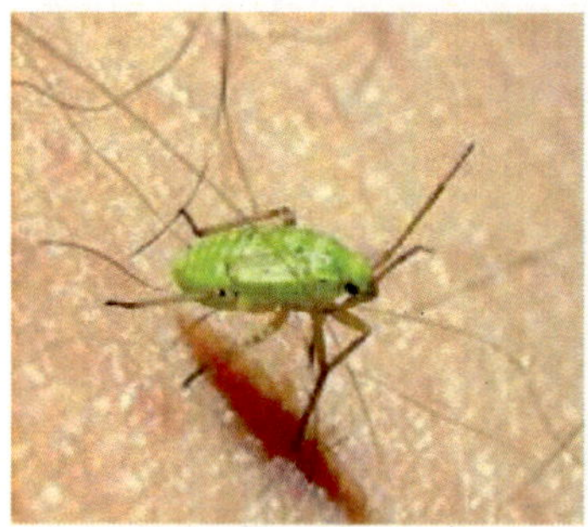
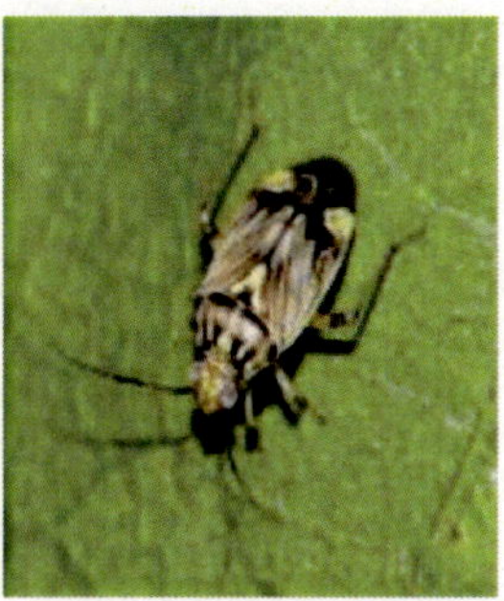

Nymph and adult of Lygus lineolaris

Both nymphs and adults of *Lygus lineolaris* harm plants by piercing and extracting sap from terminal shoots, buds, and young leaves, releasing toxic saliva that interferes with normal growth. In gladiolus, this leads to damage of the terminal shoot, early flower drop, mottled or injured leaves, stunted and distorted growth, and a general decline in plant health, resulting in poor flowering and malformed buds.

References

Edde, P.A., 2022. Arthropod pests of cotton (Gossypium hirsutum L.). Field Crop Arthropod Pests of Economic Importance, pp.208-274.

Saguez, J., Giordanengo, P. and Vincent, C., 2013. Aphids as major potato pests. Insect Pests of Potato: Global Perspectives on Biology and Management; Giordanengo, P., Vincent, C., Alyokhin, A., Eds, pp.31-63.

Questions

1. Which of the following is the most common and serious pest of gladiolus?
   a) Thrips
   b) Aphids
   c) Red spider mites
   d) Cutworms
2. Gladiolus thrips *(Thrips simplex)* primarily damage which part of the plant?
   a) Roots
   b) Corms
   c) Leaves and flowers
   d) Stems
3. Which pest of gladiolus causes silvery streaks, flower deformation, and reduced aesthetic value?
   a) Whiteflies
   b) Thrips
   c) Aphids
   d) Leaf miners
4. Aphid infestation in gladiolus results in:
   a) Tunneling in corms
   b) Leaf curling and virus transmission
   c) Stunted root growth
   d) Formation of galls
5. The most effective method for managing gladiolus thrips in storage is:
   a) Neem extract spray
   b) Gamma irradiation
   c) Treating corms with insecticides before storage
   d) Fumigation with ethylene
6. Which of the following natural enemies is effective against aphids in gladiolus?
   a) *Trichogramma chilonis*
   b) *Chrysoperla carnea*
   c) *Telenomus remus*
   d) *Habrobracon hebetor*

Assertion-Reasoning Questions

7. **Assertion (A):** Thrips are considered the most destructive pest of gladiolus.

   Reason (R): They suck sap from floral parts and cause flower deformation.

   a) Both A and R are true, and R is the correct explanation of A.

   b) Both A and R are true, but R is not the correct explanation of A.

   c) A is true, but R is false.

   d) A is false, but R is true.

8. **Assertion (A):** Aphids infest gladiolus mainly during the early flowering stage.

   Reason (R): Aphids prefer young, succulent plant tissues for feeding.

   a) Both A and R are true, and R is the correct explanation of A.

   b) Both A and R are true, but R is not the correct explanation of A.

   c) A is true, but R is false.

   d) A is false, but R is true.

9. **Assertion (A):** Cutworms damage gladiolus by boring into corms.

   Reason (R): They are primarily foliage feeders and do not affect underground parts.

   a) Both A and R are true, and R is the correct explanation of A.

   b) Both A and R are true, but R is not the correct explanation of A.

   c) A is true, but R is false.

   d) A is false, but R is true.

Answer Key

1	a	2	c	3	b	4	b	5	c	6	b	7	a
8	a	9	c										

20

Pest of Chrysanthemum

Chrysanthemum (*Chrysanthemum spp.*), popularly known as "mum" or "guldaudi", is a major commercial ornamental plant grown for cut flowers, loose flowers, and garden display. Belonging to the family Asteraceae, it is valued for its vibrant colors, diverse flower shapes, and long vase life. Chrysanthemum is attacked by several insect and mite pests, affecting both foliage and floral quality, leading to reduced aesthetic and commercial value.

Sl. No	Common name	Scientific name	Family and order	Site of Oviposition	Site of Pupation
1	Chrysanthemum Lace Bug	*Corythuca marmorata, Cadmilos retiaris*	Tingidae, hemiptera	Upper surface of leaves	-
2	Chrysanthemum Mealy Bug	*Phenacoccus gossypii, Nipaecoccus filamentosus, Phenacoccus madeirensis*	Pseudoc-occidae, Hemiptera	plant tissue	Plant
3	Thrips	*Thrips tabaci, Thripiphorothrips sp. Microce-phalothrips abdominalis, Frankiniella sp*	Thripidae, Thysanoptera	Singly in plant tissue	-
4	Whitefly	*Bemisia tabaci Aleurodicus dispersus*	Aleyrodidae, Hmeiptera Aleyrodidae	Leaves	-
5	Variagated Cutworm	*Peridroma saucia*	Noctuidae, Lepidoptera	Leaves	Soil
6	Chrysanthemum bud borer	*Helicoverpa armigera*	Noctuidae, Lepidoptera	Leaves	Soil
7	Leaf caterpillar	*Spodoptera litura*	Noctuidae, Lepidoptera	Leaves	Soil
8	Bihar hairy caterpillar	*Spilosoma obliqua*	Arctiidae, Lepidoptera	Underside of leaves	Soil

Chrysanthemum Lace Bug : *Cadmilos retiaris*, *Corythucha marmorata*

Family : Tingidae

Order : Hemiptera

Distribution: Widely distributed in India wherever chrysanthemum and sunflower are grown.

Biology: The eggs are laid singly on the upper surface of leaves, obliquely inserted into the tissue, with opercula appearing as whitish or brown dots. The incubation period for the eggs lasts about 5 to 7 weeks. Following hatching, the nymphs undergo hemimetabolous development (no true pupal stage). The nymphal period spans 2 to 3 weeks, during which the nymphs moult five times before reaching adulthood. Adult insects are approximately 4 mm long, with blackish bodies and lace-like transparent wings (Rizkawati *et al.*, 2023).

Nature of Damage

Both nymphs and adults suck plant sap. Piercing-sucking feeding on leaf tissue causes pale speckling (chlorotic stippling), premature leaf yellowing or drop.

Symptoms

Infestation leads to several noticeable symptoms, including curling of leaves and a yellowish-brown discoloration and pale metallic spotting. Black tar like excretion under leaves. Affected leaves may eventually dry up and fall off the plant. In addition to foliage damage, the flowers become discolored and distorted, significantly reducing their aesthetic appeal and overall market value.

Management

- Removal and destruction of infested plant parts
- Wash off nymphs/adults with strong water spray
- Spray of 0.05% Dimethoate or 0.03% Malathion

Chrysanthemum Mealy Bug : *Phenacoccus gossypii*, *Nipaecoccus filamentosus*, *Pseudococcus citriculus*, *Phenacoccus madeirensis*

Family : Pseudococcidae

Order : Hemiptera

Distribution: Found throughout India; more common in the south.

Biology: The eggs are laid in a protective waxy mass on the plant, with an incubation period of 10 to 20 days. After hatching, the amber-colored nymphs, covered in a waxy coating, undergo development over a nymphal period of 6 to 8 weeks. Male nymphs pupate inside a cotton-like cocoon, with the pupal stage lasting 2 to 3 weeks. Adult females are wingless, while males are winged and non-feeding. The complete life cycle for females takes about 8 to 11 weeks, and multiple overlapping generations occur throughout the season.

Nature of Damage

Nymphs and adult females suck sap from the tender parts of the plant, which impairs overall growth and reduces flower quality. Their honeydew excretion promotes the development of sooty mould, further affecting the plant's appearance and health.

Symptoms

Infestation leads to weak plant growth due to continuous sap sucking by the pests. The honeydew they excrete encourages the development of sooty mold, which further hampers photosynthesis. As a result, both flower yield and quality are significantly reduced (Chong *et al.*, 2003).

Management

Removal and destruction of infested plant parts

Spray 0.03% Malathion or Azadirachtin

Release of predatory insects like Ladybird beetles, lacewing larvae

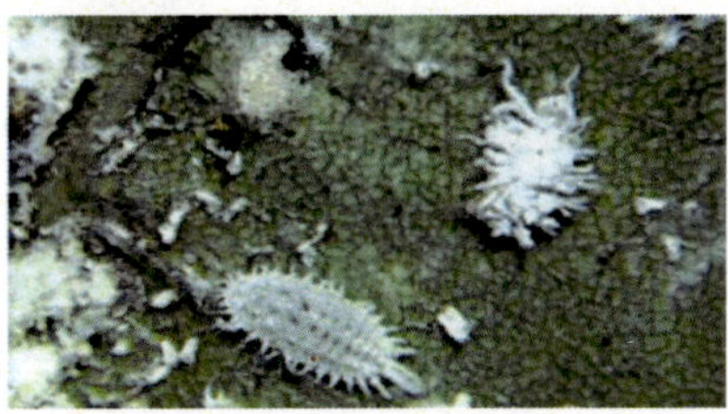

Phenacoccus gossypii

Thrips : *Thrips tabaci*, *Thripiphorothrips* spp.

Family : Thripidae

Order : Thysanoptera

Biology: The egg is bean-shaped and laid singly within the plant tissues. Upon hatching, minute sap-sucking nymphs emerge and begin feeding on the plant. The insect undergoes incomplete metamorphosis, with a non-typical pupal stage. Adults are approximately 1 mm long, with brown bodies and narrow, fringed wings. The entire life cycle—from egg to nymph, pupa, and adult—occurs on the plant.

Nature of Damage

Nymphs and adults suck sap from tender plant parts.

Symptoms

Infestation results in noticeable symptoms such as leaf curling and the development of pale, discolored flowers. These effects, combined with continuous sap loss, lead to stunted plant growth and a significant reduction in overall yield.

Management

Apply 0.03% Azadirachtin or 0.01% Dichlorvos

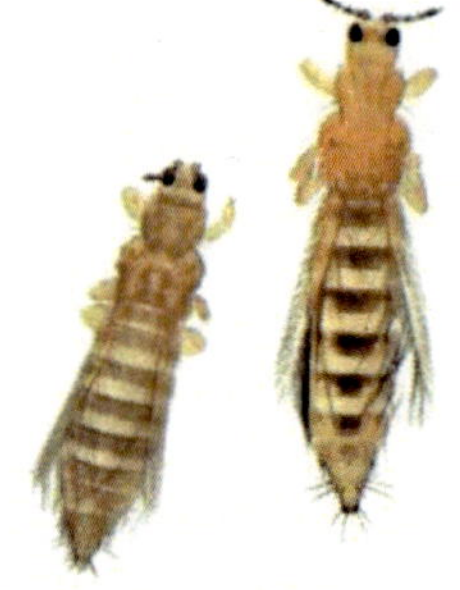

Thrips tabaci

Variagated Cutworm : *Peridroma saucia*

Family : Noctuidae

Order : Lepidoptera

Biology: The life cycle begins when moths lay their eggs on plant leaves. Upon hatching, the larvae emerge with three pairs of thoracic legs and several abdominal prolegs, actively feeding on the foliage. After completing larval development, they pupate in the soil, forming brown, obtect pupae, with the pupal stage lasting 6 to 12 days. The adult stage is a moth, which continues the cycle by laying eggs on the leaves. The species completes multiple generations within a growing season.

Nature of Damage

Larvae consume foliage heavily and can sever seedlings at the soil line at night. Caterpillars skeletonize leaves.

Symptoms

Seedlings cut at the base. Coiled larvae use to coil and hide in soil during daylight. Infestation is characterized by the appearance of holes in the leaves, which progressively leads to severe defoliation. In advanced stages, the damage results in skeletonized plants, where only the veins and midribs remain intact, severely impacting plant health and productivity.

Management

Clean tillage to remove residues and overwintering sites; weed control; trenches/barriers to prevent larval migration

Manual collection and destruction of pests.

Release of lacewing fly

Spray Malathion 0.03% or Azadirachtin 0.03%

Pyrethroids or granular soil insecticides targeting early-stage larvae; Bacillus thuringiensis (Bt) for small larvae.

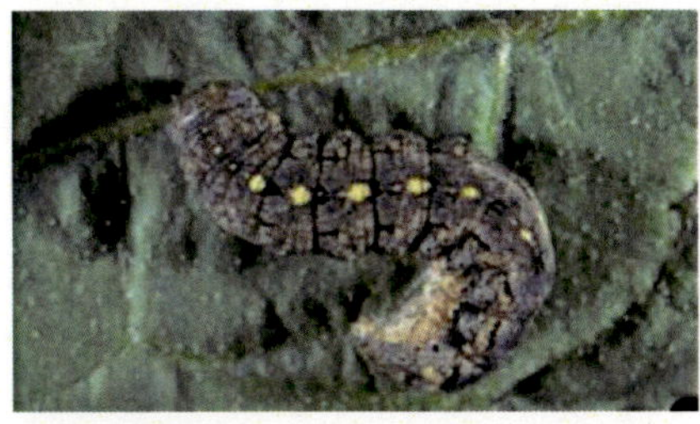
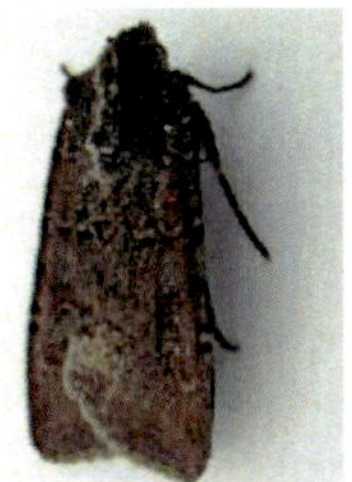

Adult and larvae of *Peridroma saucia*

Whitefly : *Bemisia tabaci, Aleurodicus dispersus*

Family : Aleyrodidae

Order : Hemiptera

Biology: Eggs are laid on the leaves of the host plant, from which short, wax-coated nymphs emerge. These nymphs develop into adults after a pupal period of 2 to 5 days. The adult insect is small and moth-like, with clear wings and two distinctive black spots. The entire life cycle takes about 21 to 31 days, with multiple generations occurring throughout the year.

Nature of Damage

Both nymphs and adults suck sap from plant tissues.

Symptoms

Infestation leads to yellowing of the leaves and weak overall plant growth. Affected plants often exhibit deformed flowers, further reducing their ornamental or economic value. Additionally, the pests excrete honeydew, which promotes the growth of sooty mould on plant surfaces, compounding the damage (Sridhar *et al.*, 2022).

Management

Removal of infected plant parts

Spray 0.03% Malathion or 0.03% Azadirachtin

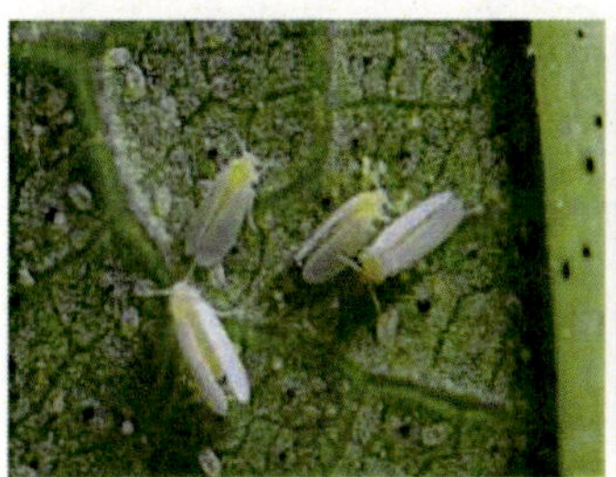
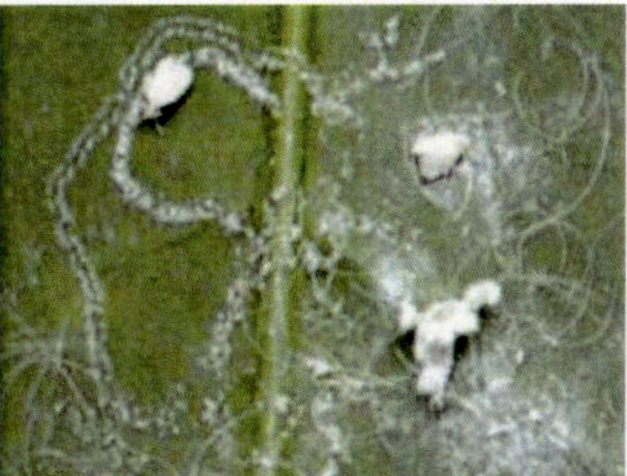

Bemisia tabaci and *Aleurodicus dispersus*

Chrysanthemum bud borer : *Helicoverpa armigera*
Family : Noctuidae
Order : Lepidoptera

Nature of damage

The larvae primarily feed on tender terminal shoots, young leaves, and developing flower buds and heads. Their feeding creates distinct round holes in the buds and flower heads (Sreedhar *et al.*, 2020).

Leaf caterpillar : *Spodoptera litura*
Family : Noctuidae
Order : Lepidoptera

Nature of damage

Newly hatched larvae feed in groups, scraping the underside of leaves. As they mature, they disperse and feed heavily on foliage, mainly during the night. Their feeding results in irregularly shaped holes on the leaves.

Bihar hairy caterpillar : *Spilosoma obliqua*
Family : Arctiidae
Order : Lepidoptera

Nature of damage

Initial stage of larvae feed gregariously on the under surface of leaves and causes defoliation. In severe cases only stems are left behind.

References

Chong, J. H., Oetting, R. D., & Van Iersel, M. W. (2003). Temperature effects on the development, survival, and reproduction of the Madeira mealybug, Phenacoccus madeirensis Green (Hemiptera: Pseudococcidae), on chrysanthemum. Annals of the Entomological Society of America, 96(4), 539-543.

Hara, A. H., & Matayoshi, S. (1990). Parasitoids and predators of insect pests on chrysanthemums in Hawaii.

Rizkawati, V., Sakai, K., Tsuchiya, T., & Tsukada, M. (2023). Different egg size in the chrysanthemum lace bug corythucha marmorata (Hemiptera: Tingidae) in response to novel host plant cultivars. Applied Entomology and Zoology, 58(1), 93-103.

Sreedhar, M., Vasudha, A., & Khudus, S. (2020). Insect-pests complex studies on chrysanthemum in Pantnagar region. Journal of Entomology and Zoology Studies, 8(2), 1644-1646.

Sridhar, V., Naik, S. O., Swathi, P., & Mani, M. (2022). Pests and Their Management in Ornamental Plants: (Rose, Jasmine, Chrysanthemum, Crossandra, Marigold, Tuberose, Carnation, China aster, Gerbera, Gladiolus, Hibiscus, etc.). Trends in Horticultural Entomology, 1189-1237.

Questions

1. Which of the following insects belongs to the family Tingidae?
   a) *Helicoverpa armigera* b) *Corythucha marmorata*
   c) *Spodoptera litura* d) *Bemisia tabaci*

2. Oviposition site of *Spilosoma obliqua* is:
   a) On flower buds b) Inside plant tissues
   c) On upper side of leaves d) On underside of leaves

3. Which pest produces black tar-like excretion under the leaves of chrysanthemum?
   a) Mealy bug b) Thrips
   c) Lace bug d) Whitefly

4. Which of these pests undergoes complete metamorphosis?
   a) Lace bug b) Thrips
   c) Mealybug d) *Peridroma saucia*

5. Whitefly adults are described as:
   a) Wingless and brown
   b) Moth-like with clear wings and black spots
   c) Small, beetle-like
   d) Large with colorful wings

6. Name the pest that shows coiled larvae hiding in soil during the day:
   a) *Helicoverpa armigera* b) *Spilosoma obliqua*
   c) *Peridroma saucia* d) *Bemisia tabaci*

7. Thrips are characterized by:
   a) Long antennae and clubbed wings
   b) Narrow fringed wings and small size
   c) Scale-like wings and spines
   d) Robust body and piercing mouthparts

8. **Assertion (A):** *Spilosoma obliqua* causes severe defoliation in chrysanthemum plants.

   Reason (R): The larvae feed gregariously on the leaves and later disperse.

a) A and R are true, and R is the correct explanation of A.

b) A and R are true, but R is not the correct explanation of A.

c) A is true, R is false.

d) A is false, R is true.

9. **Assertion (A):** Thrips damage results in pale, discoloured flowers in chrysanthemum.

   Reason (R): Thrips feed on roots and stems of the chrysanthemum plant.

   a) A and R are true, and R is the correct explanation of A.

   b) A and R are true, but R is not the correct explanation of A.

   c) A is true, R is false.

   d) A is false, R is true.

10. **Assertion (A):** *Spodoptera litura* larvae feed mostly during the day.

    Reason (R): The larvae are photophobic and hide during the night.

    a) A and R are true, and R is the correct explanation of A.

    b) A and R are true, but R is not the correct explanation of A.

    c) A is false, R is true.

    d) A and R are false.

Answer Key

1	b	2	d	3	c	4	d	5	b	6	c	7	b
8	a	9	c	10	d								

21

Pests of Carnation

Carnation (*Dianthus caryophyllus* L.) belonging to the family Caryophyllaceae is very remarkable as a cut flower crop all over the world. It is well known for its attractive flowers with fragrance and varying colors. In India, the area under its cultivation is 2190 ha with a production of 8940 tones. But its production is affected by a number of insect pests and spider mite.

Sl no	Common name	Sc. name	Family and Order	Site of oviposition	Site of pupation
			Borers		
1	Spider mites	*Tetranychus urticae*	Acari, Tetranychidae	Underside of leaves	-
2	Bud borer	*Helicoverpa armigera*	Noctuidae, Lepidoptera	Near flower buds & pods	Soil, leaf, pod and crop debris.
3	Thrips	*Thrips tabaci* *Thrips florum* *Thrips hawaiiensis* *Frankliniella schultzei*	Thripidae, Thysanoptera	Flower buds	Soil
4	Aphids	*Myzus persicae*	Aphididae, Hemiptera	Under leaf surface	-

Spider Mites : *Tetranychus urticae* Koch

Family : Acari

Order : Tetranychidae

It is the two spotted spider mite or red spider mite which is considered as one of the most serious pests of carnation. High temperatures and low relative humidity favor the multiplication of these mites. These mites are found to be persisting throughout the year under polyhouse conditions.

Host range

Citrus, grapes, apples, pears, tomatoes, okra, potatoes, eggplant, beans, cucumbers, peppers, roses, jasmine, tea, coffee etc.

Biology: Adults of these mites are about 1/60 inch long, red or orange, sometimes reddish yellow to greenish yellow in colour. They are found to lay transparent to pale yellowish eggs. The different life stages of these mites consist of egg, larval, two nymphal and adult stage. The life cycle is completed in 1 to 2 weeks. There can be several overlapping generations in a year. The adult lives up to 3 to 4 weeks.

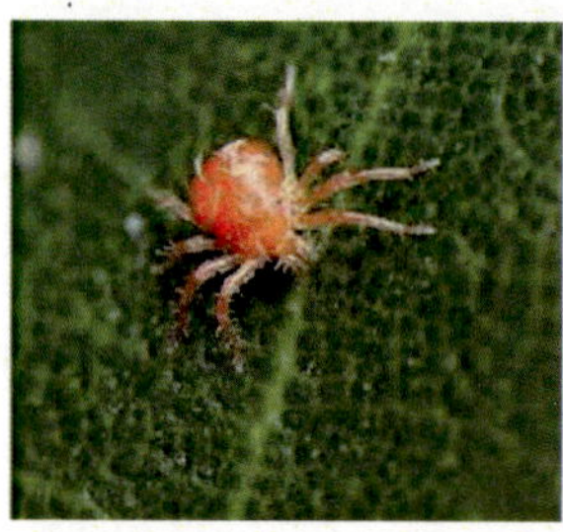 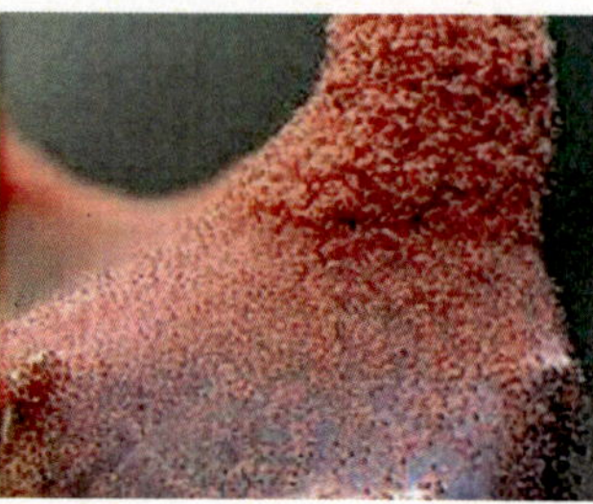

Nature of damage and symptoms

- The nymphs and adults suck sap from underside of the leaves which lead to yellowing or greying of leaves, necrotic spots are also found in initial stages.
- Infestation is found under leaf surface initially and they gradually cover the whole leaves as the infestation progresses.
- Mites also infest on flowers.
- When the infestation is high, severe webbing is found on the leaves as well as on flowers and flower buds and also observed on iron poles or other structures inserted in the field to support carnation shoots.
- This can affect the photosynthetic ability of plants leading to deterioration of the quality as well as aesthetic value of the flowers.

Management

- Make proper ventilation and irrigation in the crop.
- Regular observation in the field against the incidence of mites.
- Use of varieties having straight and flat leaves, which are proved to be resistant.
- Destroy the affected plants and weeds around the crop.
- Vigorous water jet spray directed towards the plant can remove mites.
- The use predatory mites like *Neoseiulus longispinosus* and *Phytoseiulus persimilis*.
- Use of chemicals such as propargite 57 EC @ 1.0 mL/L or abamectin 1.9 EC @ 0.5 mL/L followed by fenazaquin 10 EC @ 1.0 mL/L.
- Spraying dicofol 18.5 EC @ 2 ml/L or wettable sulphur @ 3 g/L.

Bud borer : *Helicoverpa armigera* (Hubner)
Family : Noctuidae
Order : Lepidoptera

Most devastating insect pest, with a widespread distribution and a polyphagous pest which cause immense crop loss. It also exhibits significant migratory behavior. It covers large distances in search of suitable host plants.

Host range

Cotton, tomato, chickpea, soybean, peas, maize, groundnut, sunflower, lentils, mung bean, crucifers, okra, popper, rice, apple, papaya, citrus.

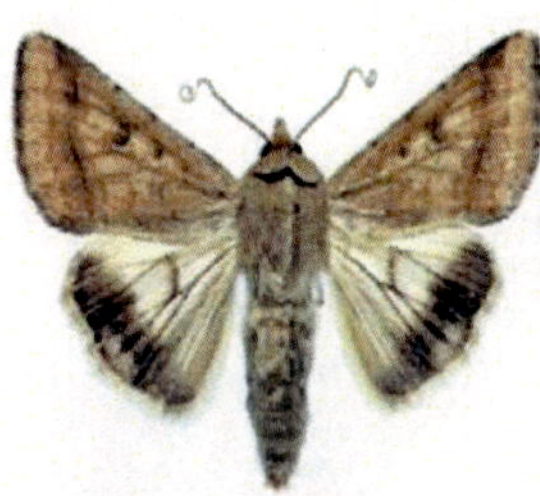

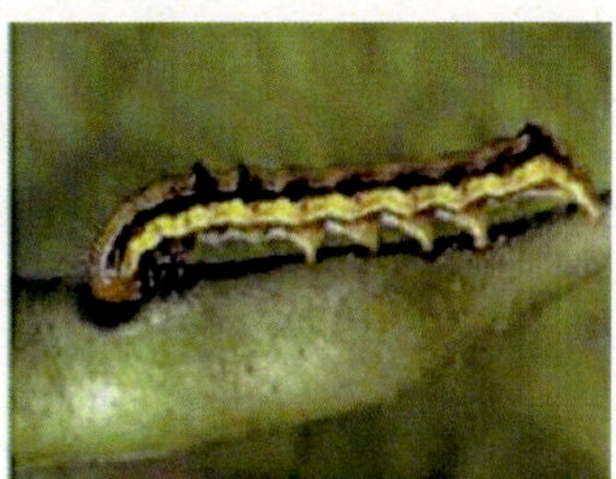

Biology: Adult moths appear brown to orange-brown in colour and the males are greyish-green in colour. Dots are present in series on the margins of forewings and black marking in comma shape in the middle of underside of each forewing. Eggs are laid singly and it can lay as many as 400-500 eggs/female in its life cycle. Initially eggs are yellowish-white and before hatching it turn brown. Larvae have six developmental stages. It has dark brown grey lines on the body with lateral white lines and also has dark band. Pupa is brown in colour, occurs in soil, leaf, pod and crop debris. Under favorable conditions, the pest can complete its life cycle in 4-6 weeks.

Nature of damage and symptoms

- Larvae bore into the bud and feed on the internal contents of bud and makes them hollow.
- It affects flowers and buds most and the presence of round holes in buds or flower heads is the characteristic damage symptom of this pest.

Management

- Expose the overwintering pupae by raking of soil before.
- Collection and destruction of larvae from the plants.
- Use of biocontrol agents such as egg parasitoid *Trichogramma* spp. and HaNPV @ 250 LE/ha followed any neem formulations spray at 1.0 – 2.0 mL/L.

- Entomopathogenic fungi such as *Beauveria* spp., *Metarhizium* spp., and *Nomuraea* spp., can also be used for its management.
- Applying Novaluron @ 3mL/L, Indoxacarb 14.5 SL @ 1mL/L.

Thrips: *Thrips tabaci, Thrips florum, Thrips hawaiiensis, Frankliniella schultzei*

They are minute, slender insects with fringed wings. Approximately 7,700 species have been described. They weak fliers instead they exploit an unusual mechanism, clap and fling, to create lift using an unsteady circulation pattern with transient vortices near the wings.

Biology: The entire life cycle takes 14-18 days. Eggs are laid in the flower buds. Pupation in soil.

Nature of damage and symptoms

- Nymphs suck sap from the leaves, making them yellow, and occasional black streaks with slight crinkling.
- Streaks are also developed on flowers rendering them unsuitable for the market.
- Overall plant growth is also affected.
- It also acts as vector of a number of plant viruses.

Management

- Monitor the activity of thrips using traps such as yellow or blue sticky traps.
- Spraying of acetamiprid 20 SP @ 0.4 g/L or oxydemeton methyl 25 EC @ 2.0 mL/L at fortnightly interval.

Aphids : *Myzus persicae* (Sulzer)
Family : Aphididae
Order : Hemiptera

This aphid causes substantial damage to the crop. It is known as the green peach aphid, or the peach-potato aphid. It can also act as a vector for the transport of plant viruses such as cucumber mosaic virus (CMV), potato virus Y (PVY) and tobacco etch virus (TEV). This aphid is found worldwide but is likely of Asian origin.

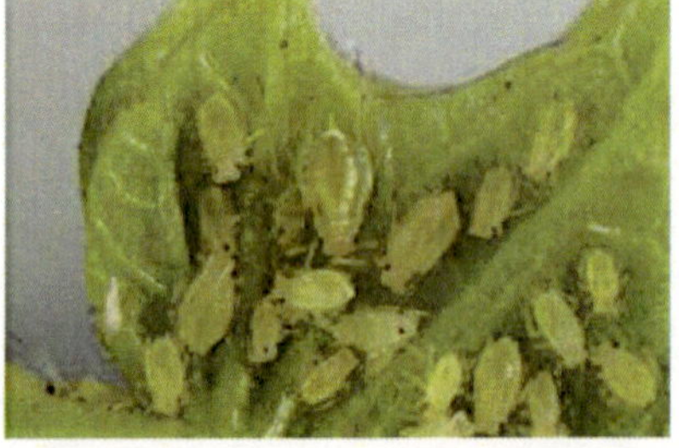

Host range

Peach, potato, cabbage, radish, mustard, tomato, pepper, etc.

Biology: They exhibit alternation in life cycles. Average length of life is approximately 23 days. The worst damage on plants is in the early summertime for the aphid breeding peak.

Nature of damage and symptoms

- Aphids suck sap from the leaves of developing plants resulting in a decrease in plant vigour.
- Secretion of honeydew on the leaves and flower buds causes sooty mould and blackening of leaves may also occur due to which the cut flowers become unmarketable.
- They also transmit carnation ring spot and carnation mosaic viruses.

Management

- Proper sanitation of the feld is to be maintained.
- Timely weeding helps reducing the pests.
- Use of yellow sticky traps.
- Release and conserve the natural enemies such as coccinellids, syrphids, Chrysoperla, etc.
- Spray with Thiomethoxam 1mL/L or Acetamiprid 1mL/L or Imidacloprid 17.8 SL 0.1 g/L.

References

Adhikari, D., and Pun, U. (2018). Major Insects and Diseases of Carnation Cut Flowers and their Management in Nepal. Nepalese Horticulture, 13(1): 44-51.

Gharge, C.P., S. G.angadi, N. Basavaraj and A. Patil (2012).Performance of standard carnation (Dianthus caryophyllus L.) varieties under naturally ventilated poly house. Karnataka. J. Agric. Sci. 24(4): 487-489.

Raina, V., Nain, M. S, Sharma, R., Khajuria, S., Kumbhare, N. V., and Bakshi, M. (2017). Floriculture in Jammu and Kashmir: Performance, problems and prospects. J. Pharm. Phyt. 1: 287-293.

Raj, V. P., Abu Manzar, A. M., Ahmad, M. J., Nazki, I. T., Bhat, Z. A., Imran Khan, I. K., and Mudasir Magray, M. M. (2019). Seasonal incidence of major insect pests and mite on carnation under protected conditions in Kashmir. 1197:1202.

Questions

1. Which of the following is an important pest of carnation?
    a) Fruit fly b) Spider mite
    c) Plume moth
2. Which of the following is a sucking pest of carnation?
    a) *Helicoverpa armigera* b) Tetranychus urticae
    c) Spodoptera litura
3. *Helicoverpa armigera* belongs to which family?
    a) Noctuidae b) Pyralidae
    c) Sphingidae
4. Which is the damaging stage of bud borer?
    a) Nymph b) Grub
    c) Caterpillar
5. Where do thrips pupate?
    a) Soil b) Leaves
    c) Stem

Answer key

1	2	3	4	5
b	b	a	c	a

22

Pests of Lily

Lily (*Lilium spp.*) is a high-value bulbous ornamental plant prized for its large, attractive, and often fragrant flowers. Belonging to the family Liliaceae, lilies are widely grown for cut flowers, landscape decoration, and potted plant markets. Despite its beauty, lily cultivation is often challenged by several insect and mite pests that reduce aesthetic quality, market value, and bulb health.

Sl No.	Common name	Scientific name	Family and Order
1	Lily caterpillar	*Polytela gloriosae*	Noctuidae, Lepidoptera
2	Lily beetle	*Lilioceris lilii* (Scopoli)	Chrysomelidae, Coleoptera
3	Crescent-marked lily aphid	*Neomyzus circumflexus*	Aphididae, Hemiptera
4	Purple-spotted lily aphid	*Macrosiphum lilii*	Aphididae, Hemiptera

Lily caterpillar : *Polytela gloriosae* F.

Family : Noctuidae

Order : Lepidoptera

Biology: Eggs are laid in clusters or singly on the undersides of lily leaves. They are yellowish to pale white, round, and smooth. Incubation lasts for about 3–6 days, depending on temperature and humidity. There are typically 5–6 larval instars. Newly hatched larvae are small and yellowish, later turning bright orange-red with black bands and spots. Caterpillars feed gregariously at first, skeletonizing leaves, then disperse to bore into stems or bulbs in later stages. The larval stage lasts for about 12–20 days. Pupation occurs in the soil, where larvae form a silken cocoon often mixed with soil particles. The pupal stage lasts 7–14 days. Pupae are reddish-brown and cylindrical. The adult is a medium-sized, metallic blue-black moth with bright yellow bands on the forewings and orange markings on the thorax. Adults are nocturnal and feed on nectar. Adult lifespan is around 4–6 days, during which female mate and lay eggs (Sathe, 2015).

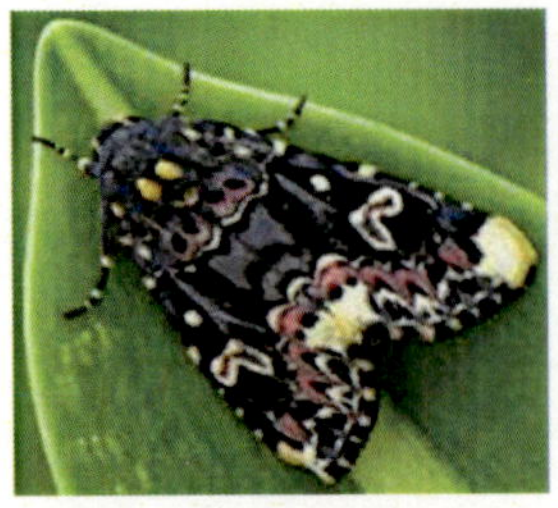
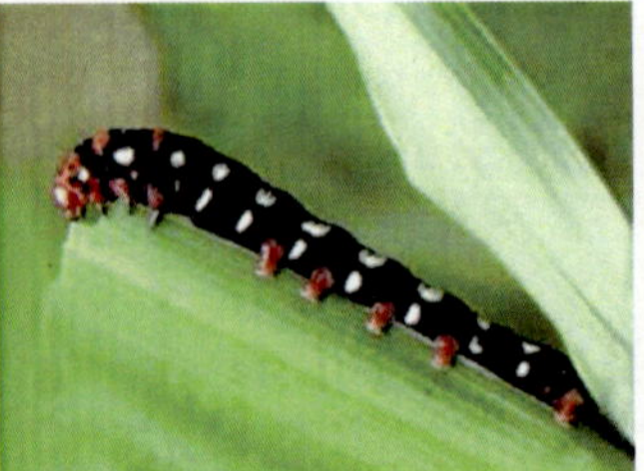
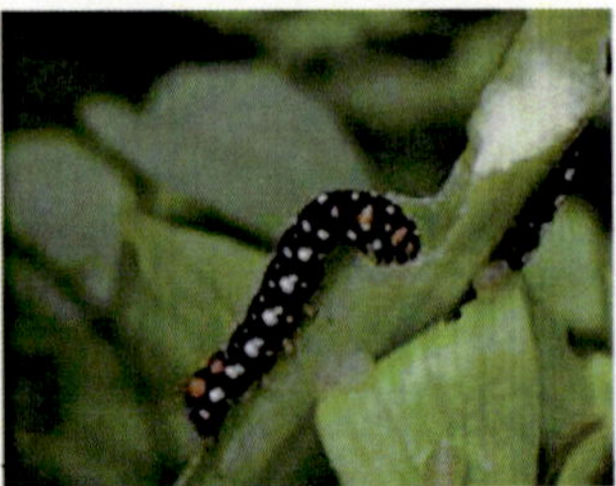

Polytela gloriosae Caterpillar feeding on leaves

Nature and symptoms of damage:

Early instars feed on chlorophyll of the leaves and later instars feed voraciously leaving only the hard stem of the plant resulting in complete defoliation.

Management

- Hand picking and destruction of the caterpillars
- Summer ploughing to expose pupae to hot sun and natural enemies and predatory birds
- During the initial stages, application of NSKE 5%

Lily beetle : *Lilioceris lilii* (Scopoli)

Family : Chrysomelidae

Order : Coleoptera

Biology

Eggs are reddish-orange and laid on the underside of leaves, hatching within 5–10 days. Larvae are slug-like, yellow-orange to brown, and cover themselves with their own faeces as a defense (LeSage, 1984). Pupation occurs in the soil. Adults are 6–8 mm, shiny red with black legs, antennae, and undersides. They overwinter in plant debris or soil and emerge in early spring adults emerge in about 2–3 weeks. Typically, 1–2 generations occur per year, though up to three generations have been observed under ideal conditions (Fox & Collins, 2006).

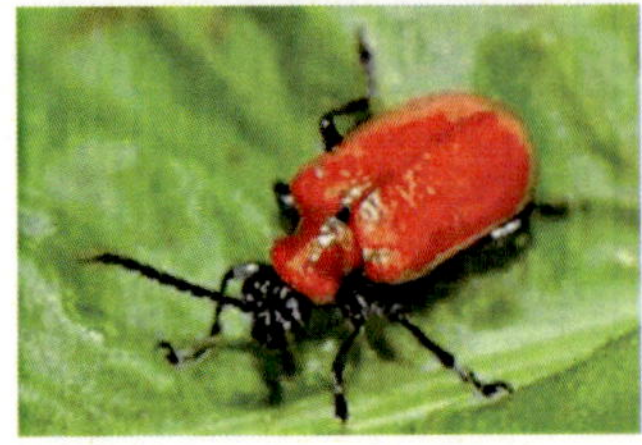
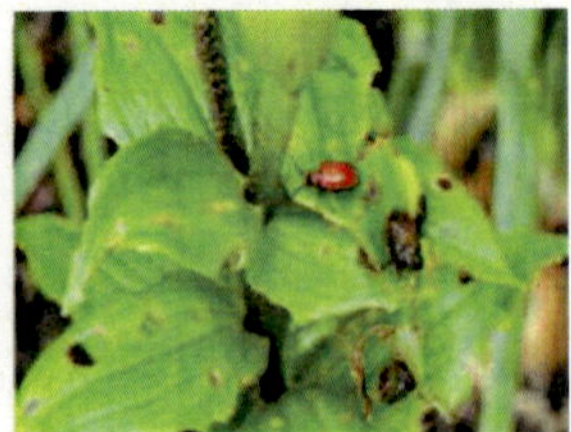

Adult beetle Grub with faecal shield Adult & grub feeding on leaves

Management

- Hand-picking adults, and grubs is effective in early infestations
- Dropping them into a soapy water solution reduces populations
- Removal of leaf litter and mulch helps eliminate overwintering adults
- Monitoring should be done during early spring as adults emerge
- The parasitoid wasp *Tetrastichus setifer* has shown promising results in Europe and North America (Haye & Kenis, 2004).
- Entomopathogenic fungi such as *Beauveria bassiana* is effective during initial period of infestation
- Neem-based insecticides and spinosad have shown moderate efficacy

Crescent-marked lily aphid : *Neomyzus circumflexus*

Purple-spotted lily aphid : *Macrosiphum lilii*

Family : Aphididae

Order : Hemiptera

Biology: Crescent-marked Lily Aphid

This aphid is known for a characteristic horseshoe-shaped marking on its abdomen. It's a relatively large aphid, reaching about 1/8 inch in length. Wingless forms are shiny, whitish, yellowish, or green.

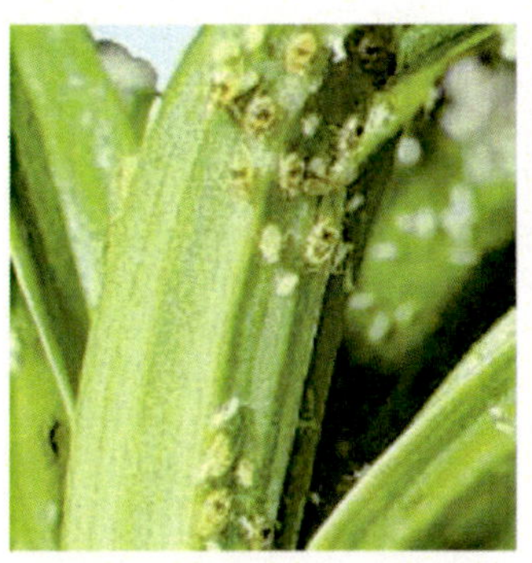

Crescent marks on the abdomen

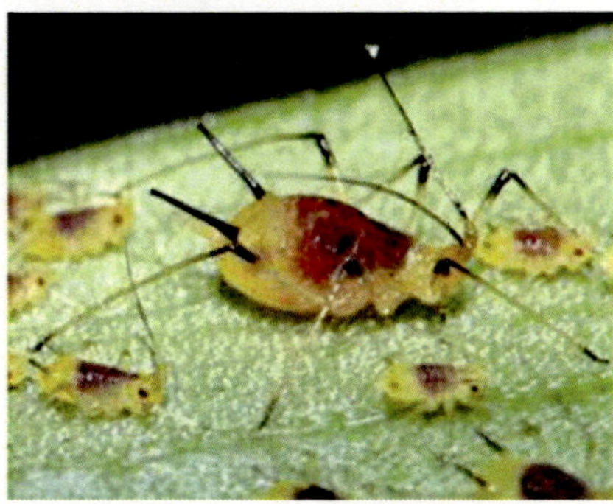

Purple marks on the abdomen

Purple-spotted Lily Aphid

This aphid is pale yellowish to yellowish-orange with long, black antennae and cornicles (structures that look like exhaust pipes). It has a conspicuous purple spot on its abdomen (Blackman & Eastop, 2000)

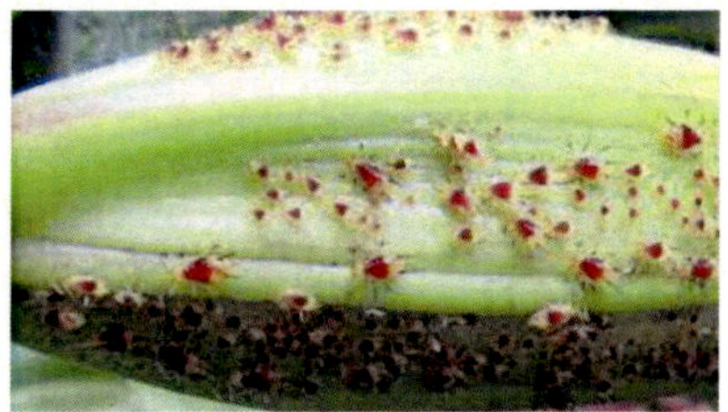

Purple-spotted aphid on lily bud

Nature and symptoms of damage

Feeding damage can result in twisting, cupping, or rolling of leaves, along with interveinal yellowing resulting in a classic sign of aphid sap extraction. Heavy infestations at growing points can cause stunted shoots, smaller flower buds, and deformation of flowers, as nutrient supply is compromised.

Management

- Inspect plants regularly, especially the undersides of leaves and buds.
- Remove and destroy heavily infested plant parts.
- Maintain good air circulation to reduce humidity favorable for aphid reproduction
- Botanical insecticides like neem (azadirachtin) are effective in early stages.
- Systemic insecticides like imidacloprid or acetamiprid may be used in severe infestations but should be restricted due to pollinator toxicity risks (Cloyd, 2009)

References

Blackman, R. L., & Eastop, V. F. (2000). Aphids on the World's Crops: An Identification and Information Guide (2nd ed.). John Wiley & Sons

Fox, R. M., & Collins, J. 2006. Lily Leaf Beetle Management in New England. University of Massachusetts Extension.

Haye, T., & Kenis, M. 2004. Biology of Tetrastichus setifer, a potential biological control agent of the lily leaf beetle in North America. Biocontrol, 49(3), 259–270. https://doi.org/10.1023/B:BICO.0000034604.36596.2e

LeSage, L. 1984. The lily leaf beetle, Lilioceris lilii (Scopoli), in Canada (Coleoptera: Chrysomelidae). The Canadian Entomologist, 116(3), 439–446. https://doi.org/10.4039/Ent116439-3

Sathe, T. V. 2015. Biology, intrinsic rate of increase and control of Indian lily moth Polytela gloriosae (Fab.) (Lepidoptera: Noctuidae). International Journal of Pharma and Bio Sciences. (6): 940 - 950.

Questions

1. What is the scientific name of the lily caterpillar?
   a) *Lilioceris lilii*
   b) *Polytela gloriosae*
   c) *Neomyzus circumflexus*
   d) *Macrosiphum lilii*
2. How do later instar larvae of *Polytela gloriosae* damage lily plants?
   a) By mining the bulbs
   b) By sucking sap from leaves
   c) By skeletonizing leaves and boring into stems
   d) By laying eggs in the soil
3. Which of the following statements about *Lilioceris lilii* larvae is TRUE?
   a) They feed singly and never in groups
   b) They are protected by a wax coating
   c) They cover themselves with their feces for defense
   d) They do not pupate in soil
4. What is a common symptom of *Macrosiphum lilii* infestation on lilies?
   a) Bulb rotting
   b) Purple discoloration of petals
   c) Sticky leaves with sooty mold
   d) Leaf miners in midrib
5. Which parasitoid has shown promise against the lily beetle in Europe and North America?
   a) *Trichogramma chilonis*
   b) *Tetrastichus setifer*
   c) *Encarsia formosa*
   d) *Aphidius colemani*
6. How many generations per year can *Lilioceris lilii* potentially have under ideal conditions?
   a) One
   b) Two
   c) Three
   d) Four
7. What is a characteristic marking of *Neomyzus circumflexus*?
   a) Purple spot on the thorax
   b) Yellow legs with black knees
   c) Horseshoe-shaped mark on abdomen
   d) Dark bands across the wings

8. Which of the following is NOT a recommended management practice for aphid infestation on lilies?
   a) Conservation of natural enemies
   b) Regular inspection of plants
   c) Use of systemic insecticides during flowering
   d) Spraying NSKE 5%
9. Where does pupation of the lily caterpillar *Polytela gloriosae* occur?
   a) Inside the stem
   b) Under leaf litter
   c) In a silken cocoon in soil
   d) On the leaf underside
10. Which group of chemicals should be used cautiously on aphids due to their impact on pollinators?
   a) Botanical insecticides
   b) Systemic neonicotinoids
   c) Fungicides
   d) Sulfur-based sprays

Answer Key

1	b	2	c	3	c	4	c	5	b	6	c	7	c
8	d	9	c	10	b								

23

Pests of Turfgrass

Turfgrass refers to a group of grass species cultivated to form a dense, uniform ground cover, primarily used in lawns, golf courses, sports fields, parks, and landscape areas. Turfgrass serves both aesthetic and functional purposes, including erosion control, temperature regulation, and dust suppression. Turfgrass ecosystems provide a favorable habitat for various insect pests and mites that affect roots, stems, and leaves, compromising turf quality, appearance, and playability.

Sl No.	Common name	Scientific name	Family and Order
Above-ground pests			
1	Common armyworm	*Mythimna unipuncta*	Noctuidae, Lepidoptera
2	Fall armyworm	*Spodoptera frugiperda*	Noctuidae, Lepidoptera
3	Yellowstriped armyworm	*Spodoptera ornithogalli*	Noctuidae, Lepidoptera
4	Black cutworm	*Agrotis ipsilon*	Noctuidae, Lepidoptera
5	Sod webworm	*Crambus spp*	Crambidae, Lepidoptera
6	Billbug	*Sphenophorus parvulus*, *S. venatus*	Curculionidae, Coleoptera
7	Chinch bug	*Blissus leucopterus*	Blissidae, Hemiptera
Below-ground pests			
8	White grubs	*Cyclocephala* spp	Scarabaeidae, Coleoptera
9	Termites	*Odontotermes* spp. *Microtermes spp.* *Coptotermes heimi*	Termitidae Rhinotermitidae Isoptera

Armyworms

Common armyworm : *Mythimna unipuncta*

Fall armyworm : *Spodoptera frugiperda*

Yellowstriped armyworm : *Spodoptera ornithogalli*

Family : Noctuidae

Order : Lepidoptera

Distribution: Andhra Pradesh, Tamil Nadu, Maharashtra, Gujarat, Punjab, Uttar Pradesh, Odisha, and other regions, *Mythimna separata* (oriental armyworm), is more prevalent in the northern and eastern states.

Common armyworm

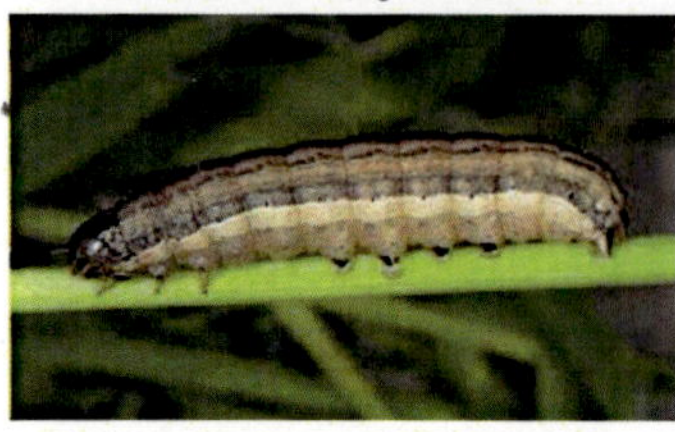

Larva of Common armyworm

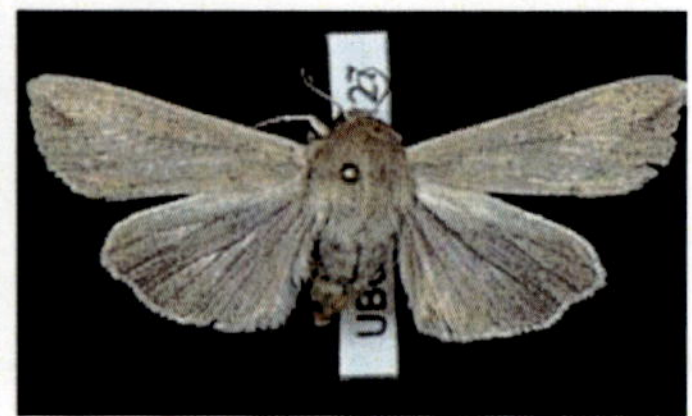

Adult of Common armyworm

Biology: Female moths lay eggs in clusters, often between leaf sheaths and blades, especially on dry grass. The eggs are initially pale yellow and darken before hatching. The larvae, also known as armyworms, go through several instars, feeding on grass blades. They are typically pale green initially, then turn yellow-brown to grey-green as they mature. They have a distinctive pattern of longitudinal lines on their bodies. Pupation occurs underground in a silken case. The pupa is typically 12-19 mm long and can be distinguished by the presence of hooks on the abdomen. The adult moths are nocturnal and have a distinctive white spot on each forewing. They are typically pale beige to reddish-brown

Fall armyworm

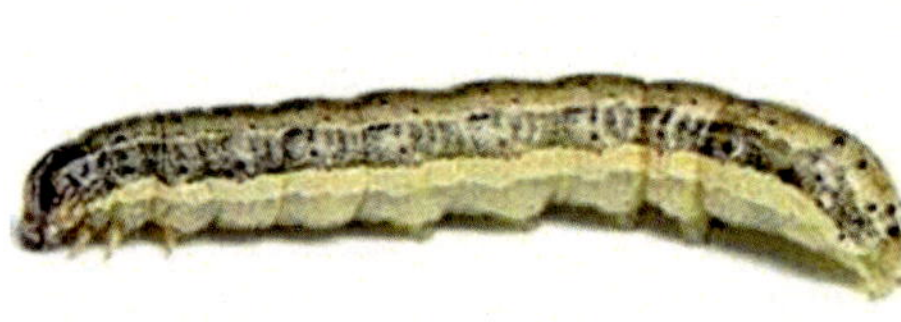

Spodoptera frugiperda-larva

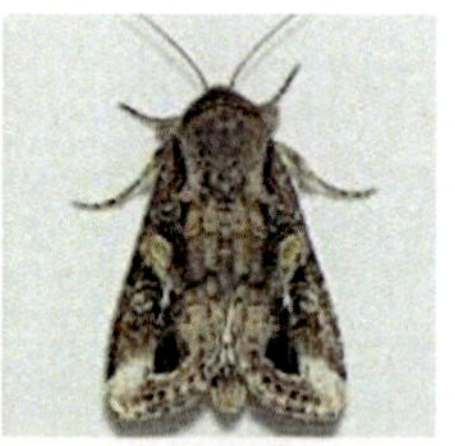

Adult of fall armyworm

Biology: Females lay eggs in masses, often on the underside of leaves, which hatch within a few days. Larvae, the feeding stage, go through six instars, with the larval stage lasting about 2-3 weeks. Larvae feed on grass blades, causing visible damage.

After the larval stage, the pupa develops in the soil or thatch. Adult moths emerge, mate, and the cycle repeats.

Yellowstriped armyworm

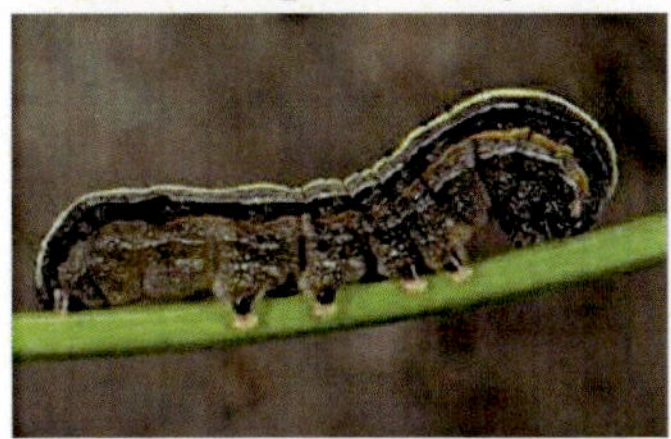
Yellowstriped armyworm

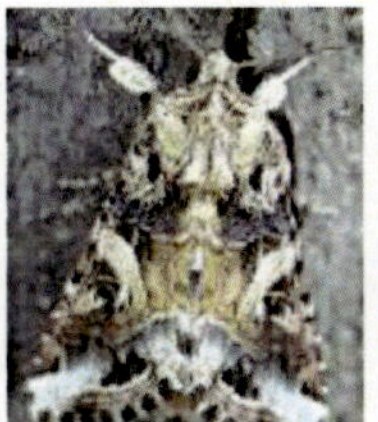
Adult

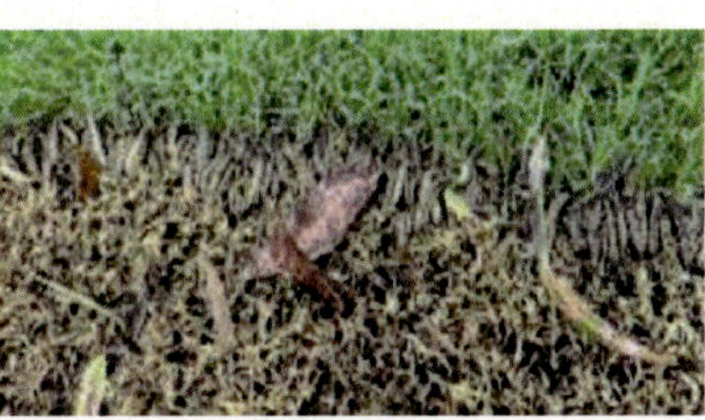
Damage caused by larvae

Female moths lay eggs in masses on foliage, trees, or buildings. The larvae hatch from the eggs and feed on green, tender foliage, initially in groups. They go through 6 instars, growing larger and more destructive with each stage. Mature larvae are typically 1.5-2 inches long, with a gray or yellow-green color and a tinge of pink, often exhibiting a distinctive pattern of white and yellow stripes. After about three weeks of feeding, the larvae burrow into the soil to pupate.

Nature of damage and symptoms

- Caterpillars are causing damage by feeding the leaves
- Sudden leaf skeletonization and turf stripped to the crown
- Grass blades that appear chewed, ragged, or have jagged tips
- Young armyworms may eat only the top layer of the grass blade, leaving a transparent, "windowpane" effect
- As armyworms feed, damaged areas may turn brown, and in severe cases, large patches of lawn can appear dead or dying
- In heavy infestations, the damage can appear to spread as armyworms move across the lawn in groups
- Green fecal pellets among the damaged areas can indicate armyworm activity

Management

- Apply bifenthrin at 45 g ai/acre, spinosad at 57 g ai/acre, or indoxacarb at 30 g ai/acre in late afternoon or evening.
- Use *Bt* var. kurstaki at 225–900 g/acre for early instars.
- Mow and remove clippings before treatment.
- Use soap flush (1 tbsp detergent in 4 L water/m^2) for monitoring.
- Encourage birds and predatory insects (Richmond, 2015).

Cutworm : *Agrotis ipsilon*, *Nephelodes minians*

Family : Noctuidae

Order : Lepidoptera

Distribution: Punjab, Haryana, Rajasthan, Uttar Pradesh, Tamil Nadu, and Andhra Pradesh. *N. minians* not found in India

Biology: Nocturnal feeders; *N. minians* active under snow cover (Redmond *et al.,* 2000).

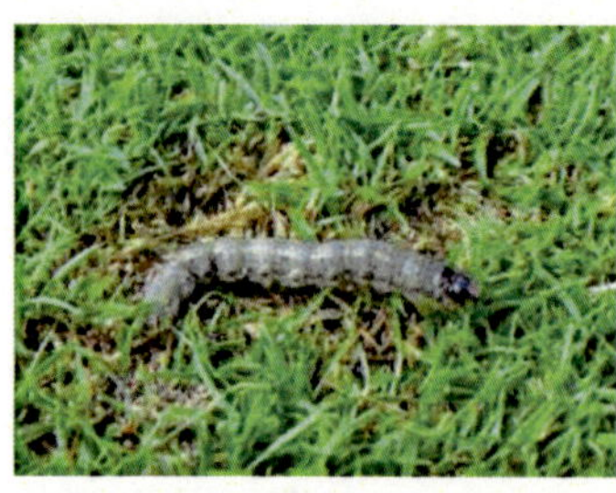

Larva of *Agrotis ipsilon*

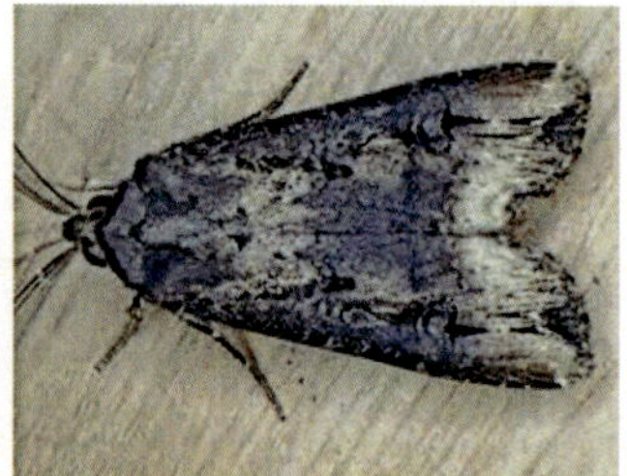

Adult of *Agrotis ipsilon*

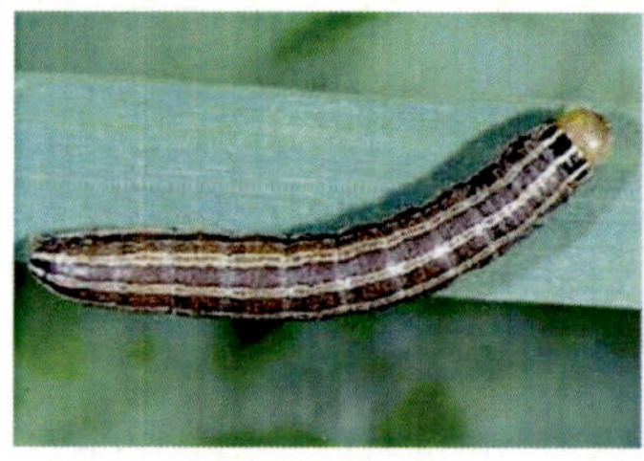

Larva of *N. minians*

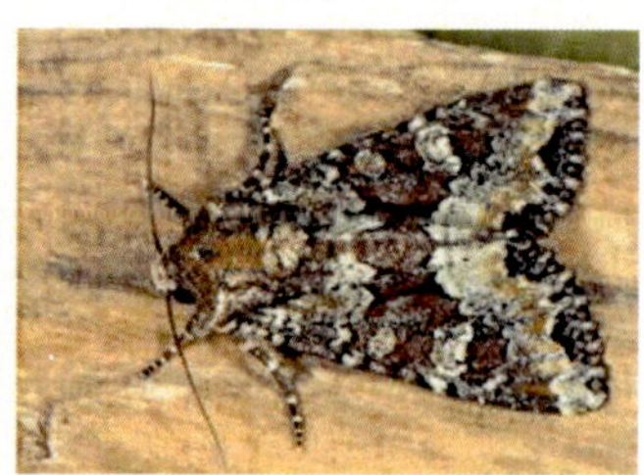

Adult of *N. minians*

Nature of damage and symptoms

Caterpillars feed on the leaf and stem. Small dead spots or depressions is seen on the stem and the caterpillars cut stem at soil level.

Management

- Apply deltamethrin at 23 g ai/acre or chlorantraniliprole at 90 g ai/acre in early evening hours
- During initial stages, apply *Bt kurstaki* at 225–450 g/acre for managing early-stage larvae
- Mow and dethatch to reduce habitat of the pest (Brandenburgh and Freeman, 2012).

Sod webworms : *Crambus spp.*

Family : Crambidae

Order : Lepidoptera

Distribution: Punjab, Maharashtra, Tamil Nadu, and parts of northeast India. Larvae tunnel in thatch and feed at night; 2–3 generations per year.

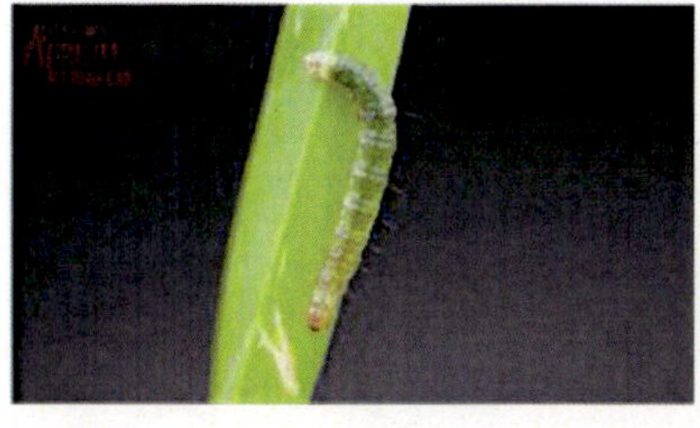

Larva

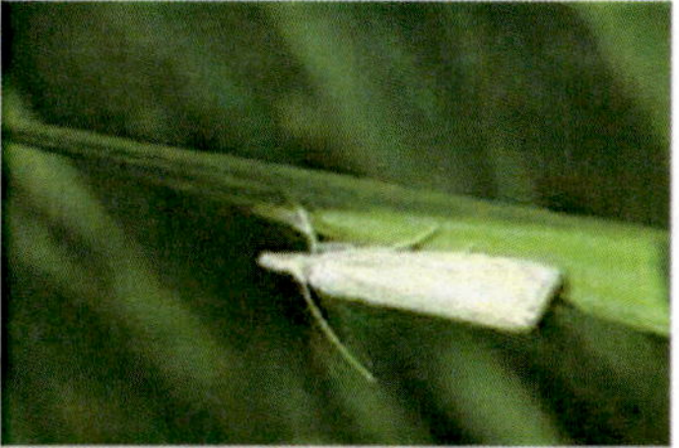

Adult

Nature of damage and symptoms

Brown patches, fecal pellets, and silk webbing in turf canopy.

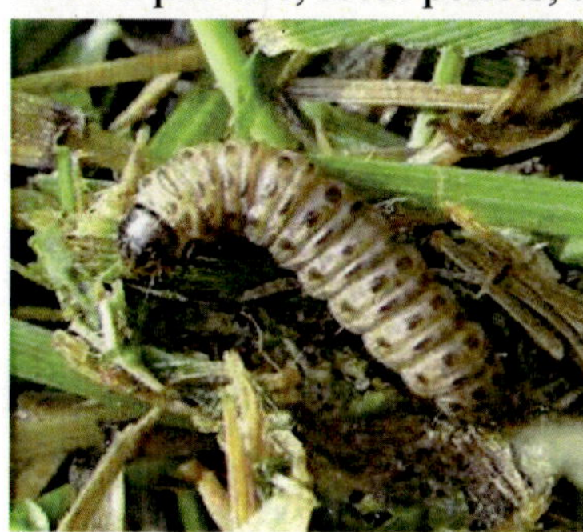

Larva feeding on turfgrass leaves

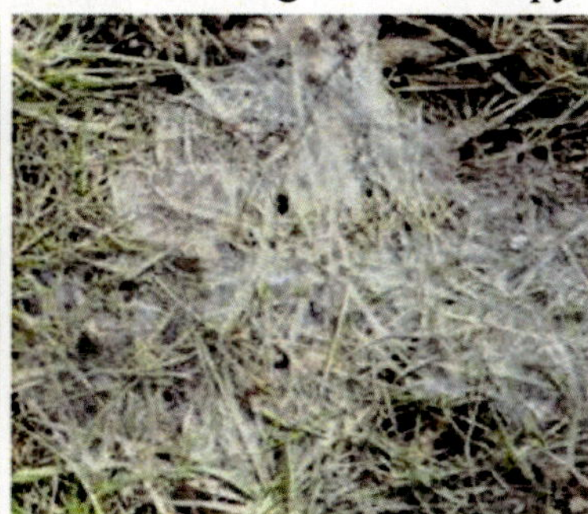

Webbing of sod webworm

Management

- Apply bifenthrin at 45 g ai/acre, spinosad at 57 g ai/acre, or chlorantraniliprole at 90 g ai/acre at early larval stages
- Apply Bt kurstaki at 225–900 g/acre during the initial period of infestation to managing young larvae
- Remove debris and mow before applying insecticide
- Encourage parasitic wasps and birds
- Irrigate lightly if label suggests post-treatment moisture (Richmond, 2015)

Billbugs : *Sphenophorus parvulus*, *Sphenophorus venatus*

Family : Curculionidae

Order : Coleoptera

Distribution: Native to southern U.S., Central America, and parts of South America.

Adults emerge in spring, lay eggs in stems. Grubs feed internally and are hidden.

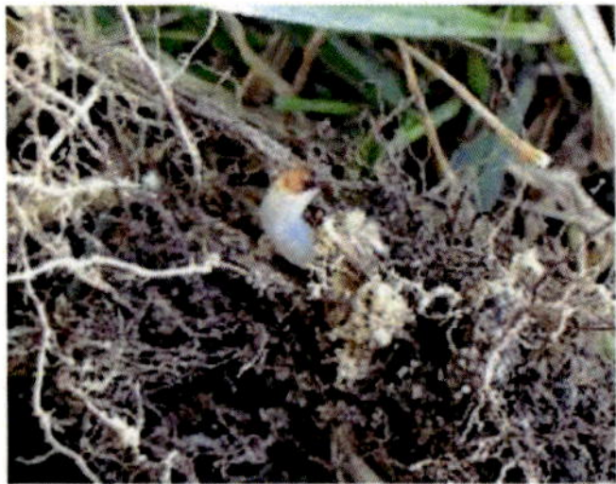

Grub of *Sphenophorus venatus*

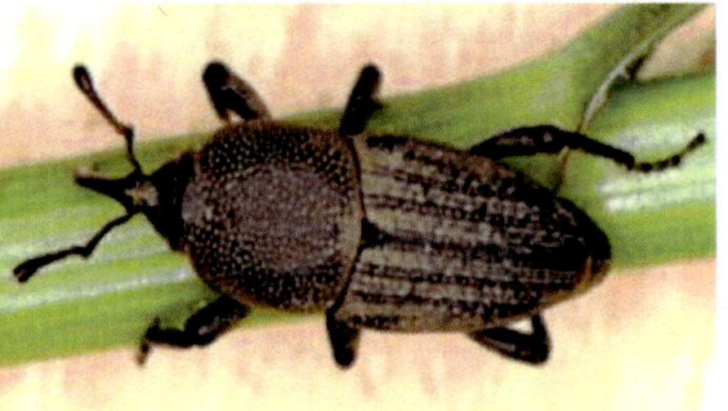

Adult of *Sphenophorus venatus*

Nature of damage and symptoms

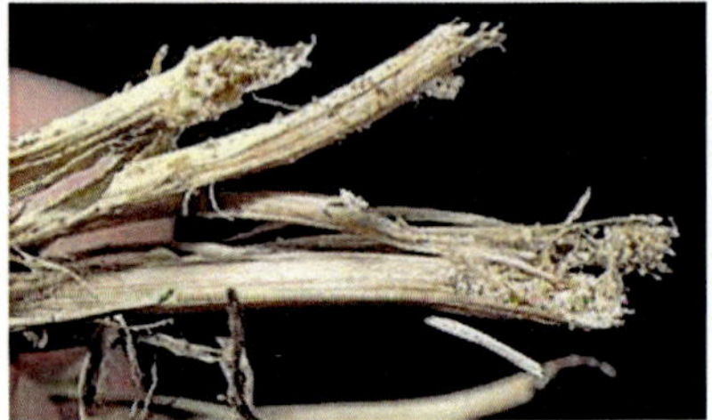

Tunneling made by the larvae

Adult weevils chew small, notched holes along the leaf margins of turfgrass. This damage is generally minor and cosmetic. Larvae are legless, creamy-white grubs with brown heads. They tunnel and feed inside stems, crowns, and roots of the grass. Turf breaks easily at crown with powdery frass; dead patches spread under dry stress.

Management

- Monitor adult emergence with pitfall traps
- Select resistant or endophyte-enhanced turfgrass
- Avoid drought and mow at 2.5–3.5 inches for plant resilience
- For adult suppression, apply bifenthrin at 45 g ai/acre in late April to early May
- Apply clothianidin at 113 g ai/acre or imidacloprid at 90 g ai/acre in mid-May to early June

Chinch bugs : *Blissus leucopterus hirtus*

Family : Blissidae

Order : Hemiptera

Distribution: Primarily found in North America, especially the U.S. and southern Canada

Biology: Eggs are laid in crevices near plant crowns, leaf sheaths, or in the thatch layer and are cylindrical, white to orange as they mature. Hatching in 7–10 days (warmer weather accelerates). Passes through 5 nymphal instars and the colour changes from reddish-orange to brownish and then turns black colour. Nymphal duration is about 3–4 weeks. Severe damage and highest population occur during hot, dry periods. Adults are about 3–4 mm long, black with white wings crossing over the back. Two forms viz., long-winged (macropterous) or short-winged (brachypterous) can be seen.

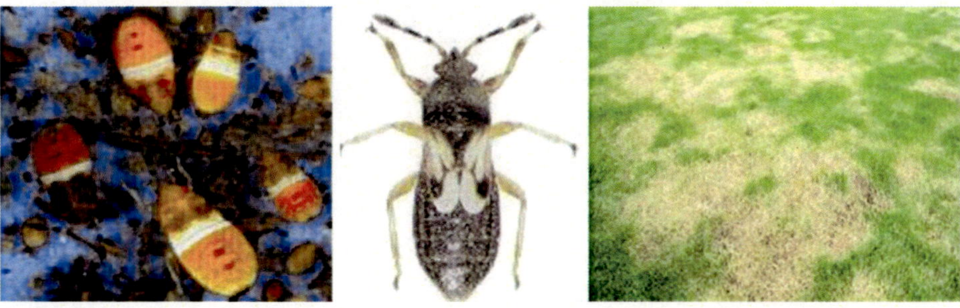

Nymphs Adult Damage symptom- dried patches

Nature of damage and symptoms

Both nymphs and adults feed by inserting their mouthparts into grass stems and leaf sheaths, usually at the base of the plant. Initial damage appears as small yellowish patches, often mistaken for drought. Yellow to brown wilting patches, with bugs visible at damage edges. Patches may coalesce into large dead areas, especially in hot, dry weather. Grass in damaged areas may pull up easily with little root resistance. On close inspection at the margin of the patch, numerous nymphs and adults can be seen.

Management

- Confirm infestation with flotation sampling (25+ bugs/ft^2)
- Irrigate during drought and reduce thatch to <1.25 cm
- Promote predators like *Geocoris spp.* (big-eyed bugs)
- Avoid broad-spectrum chemicals that suppress beneficial insects (Held and potter, 2004)
- Apply bifenthrin at 45 g ai/acre, zeta-cypermethrin at 23 g ai/acre, or thiamethoxam at 57 g ai/acre during peak nymph stage (June–July)

White grubs : *Cyclocephala* spp

Family : Scarabaeidae

Order : Coleoptera

Distribution: Sub-Himalayan region, central India, parts of the Deccan Plateau, northern, eastern, and northeastern states of India.

Biology: Larvae hatch mid-to-late summer and feed on roots. Most overwinter and resume feeding briefly in spring. Lifecycle duration varies by species.

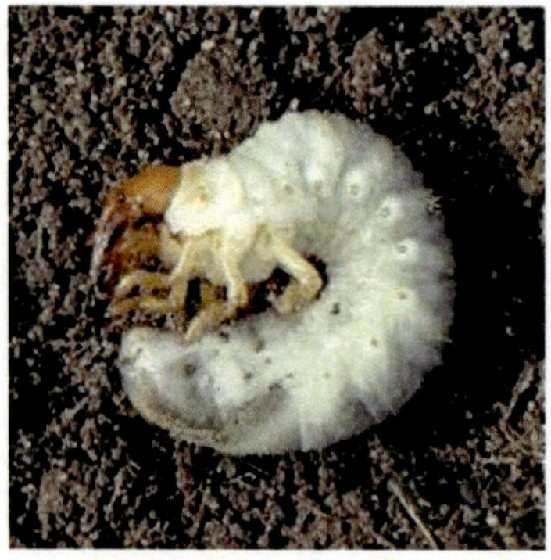

Grub of *Cyclocephala* spp

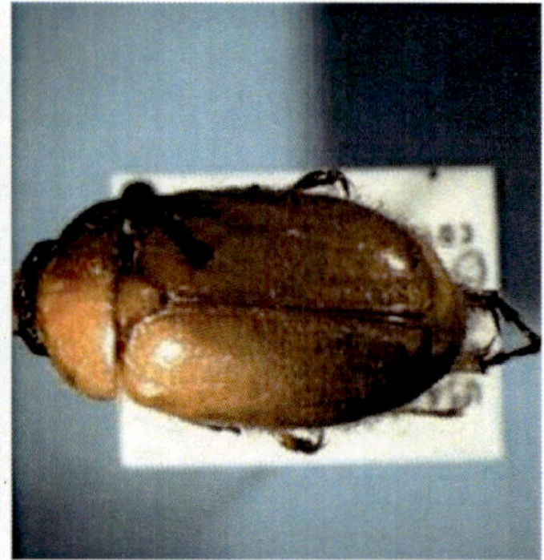

Adult of *Cyclocephala* spp

Nature of damage and symptoms

White grubs live below the soil surface and feed on turfgrass roots. Feeding severs roots and reduces the plant's ability to absorb water and nutrients. Wilting, root loss, and as a result affected turf lifts easily. Large brown patches and secondary damage from digging animals. Grass turns yellow or light green and wilts easily.

Management

- Maintain proper mowing and avoid irrigation during beetle egg-laying (Held and potter, 2004)
- Apply *Heterorhabditis bacteriophora* at 250 crore infective juveniles per acre during moist, shaded conditions (evening application best)
- Apply chlorantraniliprole at 90 g ai/acre in May–early June for long-lasting protection
- Irrigate with 6–12 mm water after granular application
- Apply imidacloprid at 90 g ai/acre or thiamethoxam at 57 g ai/acre preventively in late June to mid-July

Termites : *Odontotermes* spp. - Termitidae

Microtermes spp. - Termitidae

Coptotermes heimi - Rhinotermitidae

Termites, though typically known for damaging wood, can infest turfgrass and cause significant damage to lawns, golf courses, athletic fields, and nursery sod. These infestations are more common in warm, dry regions or during drought stress, when termites seek moisture from plant roots and organic matter in the soil.

Symptoms

- Patches of dead or dying grass (may resemble drought stress)
- Loosening of the turf — affected turf can be pulled up easily due to root pruning
- Presence of mud tubes or earthen runways on the surface or under thatch
- Soil mounds or small holes (used as ventilation)
- Hollowing of underground plant parts (roots, stolons, rhizomes)

Management

- Reduce thatch to <1.25 cm by dethatching or vertical mowing
- Irrigate deeply and regularly, especially during dry spells
- Remove wood debris, old tree roots, or stumps from the lawn area
- Use well-aerated, organic-matter-balanced soils
- Use of entomopathogenic fungi like *Metarhizium anisopliae* or *Beauveria bassiana*
- Application of nematodes like *Steinernema* spp.
- Chlorpyrifos 20 EC @ 2 ml/l (soil drench)
- Imidacloprid 17.8 SL @ 0.5 ml/l (soil application)
- Fipronil 5 SC @ 1–2 ml/l

References

Brandenburg, R. L., & Freeman, C. P. 2012. Turfgrass insect pests: biology, ecology, and management. In: Pests of Turfgrass (pp. 45-71), ACS Symposium Series.

Held, D. W., & Potter, D. A. 2004. Hazard assessment of insecticides to beneficial invertebrates in turfgrass: a review and synthesis. Environmental Entomology, 33(6), 1575–1583. https://doi.org/10.1603/0046-225X-33.6.1575

Redmond, C. T., Potter, D. A., & Spicer, P. G. 2000. Biology and management of the black cutworm Agrotis ipsilon in turfgrass. Crop Protection, 19(8–10), 509–515. https://doi.org/10.1016/S0261-2194(00)00073-2

Richmond, D. S. (2015). Turfgrass insect management (Publication No. E-61). Purdue University Cooperative Extension Service. https://extension.entm.purdue.edu/publications/E-61.pdf

Questions

1. Which of the following insecticides is recommended for *preventive* control of white grubs?

   a) Spinosad b) Imidacloprid

   c) Trichlorfon d) Carbaryl

2. The larval stage of *Spodoptera frugiperda* is commonly known as:

   a) Webworm b) Cutworm

   c) Armyworm d) Billbug

3. A suitable biological control agent for white grubs is:

   a) *Bacillus thuringiensis kurstaki*

   b) *Heterorhabditis bacteriophora*

   c) *Chrysoperla carnea*

   d) *Trichogramma chilonis*

4. What is the most appropriate timing to apply chlorantraniliprole against white grubs for long-lasting protection?

   a) September–October b) May–early June

   c) Late July–August d) January–February

5. Which turf pest creates silken tunnels in the thatch and is active mostly at night?

   a) Billbug b) Chinch bug

   c) Sod webworm d) Bronze cutworm

6. What is the preferred irrigation depth after applying granular insecticides for grubs?

   a) No irrigation required b) 1 mm

   c) 6–12 mm d) 25 mm

7. The recommended application rate of *Bt kurstaki* for early instar caterpillars is:

   a) 5–10 g/acre b) 225–900 g/acre

   c) 2.5 crore juveniles/acre d) 113 g/acre

8. Which insect pest injects toxic saliva into plant vascular tissues, leading to top-down browning?

   a) Armyworm b) Chinch bug

   c) Cutworm d) Webworm

9. Which pest is best monitored using pitfall traps during its adult emergence?
   a) Sod webworm
   b) White grub
   c) Billbug
   d) Armyworm

10. Endophyte-enhanced turfgrass varieties are particularly helpful against which of the following pests?
   a) White grubs
   b) Cutworms
   c) Chinch bugs
   d) Billbugs

Answer Key

1	b	2	c	3	b	4	b	5	c	6	c	7	b
8	b	9	c	10	d								

Index